Sociology as applied to medicine

Commissioning Editor: Timothy Horne
Development Editor: Clive Hewat
Project Manager: Andrew Palfreyman
Designer: George Ajayi
Illustrations Manager: Kirsteen Wright
Illustrator: Chartwell

Sociology as applied to medicine

Edited by

Graham Scambler BSc PhD

Professor of Medical Sociology,
Research Department of Infection and Population Health,
University College London,
London, UK

SIXTH EDITION

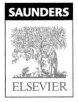

EDINBURGH LONDON NEW YORK OXFORD PHILADELPHIA ST LOUIS SYDNEY TORONTO 2008

SAUNDERS
ELSEVIER

© W.B. Saunders Company Limited 1997
© Harcourt Publishers Limited 2000
© 2003, Elsevier Limited. All rights reserved.

First edition 1982
Second edition 1986
Third edition 1991
Fourth edition 1997
Fifth edition 2003
Sixth edition 2008

ISBN: 978-0-7020-2901-1

British Library Cataloguing in Publication Data
A catalogue record for this book is available from the British Library

Library of Congress Cataloging in Publication Data
A catalog record for this book is available from the Library of Congress

---

Note

Neither the Publisher nor the Authors assume any responsibility for any loss or injury and/or damage to persons or property arising out of or related to any use of the material contained in this book. It is the responsibility of the treating practitioner, relying on independent expertise and knowledge of the patient, to determine the best treatment and method of application for the patient.

The Publisher

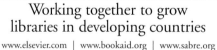

Working together to grow
libraries in developing countries

www.elsevier.com | www.bookaid.org | www.sabre.org

ELSEVIER   BOOK AID
            International   Sabre Foundation

  your source for books,
journals and multimedia
in the health sciences

www.elsevierhealth.com

The publisher's policy is to use paper manufactured from sustainable forests

Printed in China

Contents

CONTENTS

vi

Contributors

Mel Bartley, Professor of Medical Sociology, Department of Epidemiology and Public Health, UCL, London, UK

David Blane, Professor of Medical Sociology, Department of Primary Care and Social Medicine, Imperial College London, St. Dunstan's Road, London, UK

Iain Crinson, Lecturer in Medical Sociology, Division of Community Health Sciences, St George's, University of London, London UK

Ray Fitzpatrick, Professor of Public Health and Primary Care, Division of Public Health and Primary Care, University of Oxford, Oxford, UK

Judith Green, Reader in Sociology of Health, Health Services Research Unit, London School of Hygiene & Tropical Medicine, London, UK

Paul Higgs, Reader in Medical Sociology, Division of Research Strategy, UCL, London, UK

Moira Kelly, Lecturer in Medical Sociology, Centre for Health Sciences, Institute of Health Sciences Education, Barts and The London, Queen Mary's School of Medicine and Dentistry, London, UK

David Locker, Professor of Community Dentistry, Faculty of Dentistry, University of Toronto, Ontario, Canada

Nicholas Mays, Professor of Health Policy, Department of Public Health and Policy, London School of Hygiene and Tropical Medicine, London, UK

Myfanwy Morgan, Reader in Sociology of Health, Department of Public Health Sciences, King's College London, London, UK

James Nazroo, Professor of Sociology, School of Social Sciences, University of Manchester, Manchester, UK

Annette Scambler, Visiting Lecturer in Medical Sociology, Department of Dental Public Health, King's College London, London, UK

Graham Scambler, Professor of Medical Sociology, Research Department of Infection and Population Health, UCL, London, UK

Fiona Stevenson, Lecturer in Medical Sociology, Department of Primary Care and Population Sciences, UCL, London, UK

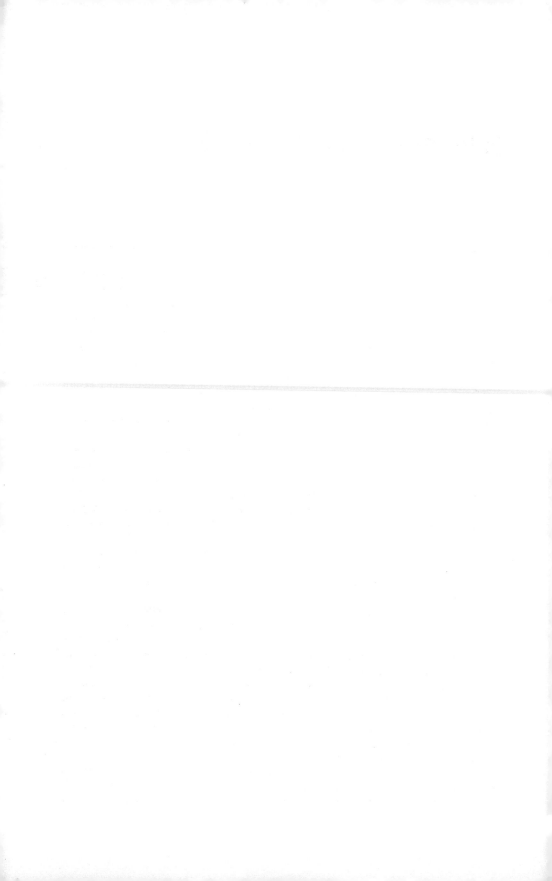

Foreword to the first edition

Students of medicine and of other related disciplines may be forgiven for feeling that their schools and colleges insist that they learn more and more about an increasing number of aspects of the human condition in health and illness. There was a halcyon time, not so long ago, when the pre-clinical curriculum consisted of one course in human anatomy and another in physiology; the clinical phase involved merely learning the skills needed to recognize the signs and symptoms of a wide but ultimately limited range of diseases. Moreover, there was little institutional pressure on students to study since they were free to repeat examinations until they passed them.

The picture is very different today. Knowledge of the molecular structure of living beings and the factors which determine natural and pathological growth and decay has expanded exponentially in the last fifty years and continues to do so. Students are expected to know a good deal about the theories and research methods of the scientific disciplines, the 'ologies', which have led to this increased knowledge, as well as about the implications of their findings for medical practice. More and more disciplines claiming relevance to medical knowledge and practice jostle each other for a place in the pre-clinical curriculum; new clinical specialities want medical students to be exposed at some time during their clinical studies to what they have to offer. All make claims to the indispensable nature of their own contribution to the curriculum. Meanwhile, medical students are no longer free to work at their own pace. Examinations weed out those who cannot satisfy their teachers after a maximum of two failures. The pressures are those of the institution. Students of other health professions, such as nursing, dentistry, pharmacy and optometry, are exposed to broadly comparable pressures in the process of qualifying as practitioners.

Sociology is one of the disciplines which has recently claimed the attention of the medical and other related health professions and their students. Its formal introduction into the curriculum as a basic medical science, which by the 1980s had taken place in most of the medical schools of the United Kingdom, was a radical innovation. Compared with most of the other new subjects it involves a break away from the traditional preparation for medicine based exclusively on the detailed study of parts of the biological organism which we call the human body. Its focus is not on the human individual per se: it is on the two-way relationships between the individual and society. Sociology as applied to medicine is concerned specifically with those aspects of the relationship which influence the experiences of health and illness in individuals and the response to them of others – relatives, doctors, nurses, administrators and governments.

Not surprisingly, not all those already involved in medical education welcomed the advent of sociological teaching. Some of the staff involved in teaching the traditional laboratory based or clinical subjects saw in it an intrusion of a largely unknown and untested quantity competing for the students' limited span of attention time. They were unfamiliar with its methods or potential and sceptical about its contribution to the making of a good practitioner. Some students, expecting the medical curriculum to resemble in essence the pre-medical natural science courses they had taken prior to entry, also needed to be persuaded that sociology was relevant to their preparation as future doctors, especially when they felt themselves to be under pressure to absorb all that the teachers of subjects which were more thoroughly examined put before them.

Such early doubts have not entirely disappeared, but they have substantially diminished. Indeed, the General Medical Council's recommendations for medical education in the 1980s are even more insistent than earlier recommendations on the necessity for broadening the students' basic understanding of the social context of health and illness and of social determinants of medical practice and health service provision. This then is the major task and challenge for those responsible for the teaching of sociology as applied to medicine, and the contributors to this book are to be congratulated for providing a concise introduction to the subject.

In this book, which will form an admirable basic text upon which teachers and students can build, the contributors have shown how some of the theories, concepts and methods developed by sociologists can illuminate aspects of human experience in health and illness. They look at how such socially determined factors as marital status, social class and family composition influence the pattern of morbidity and mortality. They show that medical perceptions of what constitutes mental or physical illness are not necessarily shared by the populations served and that the absence of shared perceptions may frustrate much medical effort. They look at the variety of ways in which old age, death and ethnicity are regarded and treated and the dilemmas which such variety can pose for practitioners. They explore the social origins of contemporary systems of health care in order to obtain greater understanding of their present problems. They examine too the various interpretations which can be placed upon the collective and individual behaviour of members of the medical profession, and on the expansion of medical concern and metaphors into many aspects of social life. This list does not exhaust their concerns and there are many other developments in the sociology of health and illness which cannot be covered in a volume of this size.

It seems to me impossible to argue that acquaintance with such findings and with the methods and conceptual frames of the discipline on which they are based is not an essential ingredient in the preparation of the doctor for medical practice whether it be in general practice, an age-band or body-system speciality, or community medicine. He or she needs it at the very least for protection against the very real hazard of frustration and unhappiness when it proves difficult to implement medical measures; but above all it is needed if the medical and other health-related professions are to make their greatest potential contribution to the welfare of the populations they are privileged to serve.

Margot Jefferys
August 1981

Preface

It is perhaps surprising that after a quarter of a century Margot Jefferys' wise and encouraging words of introduction to the first edition of *Sociology as Applied to Medicine* still resonate. The case for asking, even requiring, medical and other students of the health professions to engage with the multiple ways in which health-related phenomena, from individual behaviours through classifications of and strategies for coping with medically defined disease to the funding of healthcare systems, are embedded in the social world remains undeniable. Not only is this social world patterned in various identifiable ways – by class, gender, ethnicity and age for example – but these patterns themselves demand explanation. It is rare for explanations in social sciences like sociology, or indeed the theories of which they are part, to be decisive and to command the assent of the entire community of sociologists let alone that of the wider public. This does not mean that sociology is an unscientific discipline, but that its subject matter – the ways in which an individual's thoughts and behaviours are grounded and evolve in the social world, against the background of cultural norms and expectations and the structures of states and market places – is obdurately complex and resistant to easy answers to 'why' questions. There are no laws in sociology, and if the natural and life sciences too are, or ought to be, characterized by a readiness to rethink and re-theorize, sociologists are only too aware of the fallibility of their latest explanations.

The social world of the late 1970s and early 1980s when this textbook first saw the light of day differs from the social world of 2008. The Soviet bloc has gone, the Cold War is history, and many people have a sense of inhabiting a more uni-dimensional if not necessarily safer planet. Global considerations now impose themselves on individuals and on national governments alike. It is not a matter of chance that the British National Health Service is under constant reform. Medical and other health students and workers cannot be expected to become experts in the 'how' and 'why' of such momentous social change. It is incumbent on those charged with introducing them to sociological perspectives not to recruit them to the discipline but to equip them to 'think sociologically': this is a defence against the naivety that too often passes for common sense. Sociology may not be well placed to deliver laws but it remains a vital resource for discerning, even explaining, modes of interpretation presented as neutral but in fact emanating from points of view that reflect particular interests. These 'interests' may be associated with the state, with private entrepreneurs, with religious bodies, with the medical or other health care professions, even with those of sociologists.

If thinking sociologically is one aim of courses in sociology as applied to medicine, sociologists have a responsibility also to inform their students of the nuts and bolts of health-related change. Theories in sociology must always be responses to the available evidence, for or against. This is as true of theories of individual help-seeking behaviour and the subtle dynamics of doctor-patient encounters as it is of those of national and global health care reform. *Sociology as Applied to Medicine* began as a collective project rooted in the experience of medical school based teachers within the University of London who felt medical students needed a text written *for them*. If the aim was to encourage them to see with a 'sociological eye', one of the crucial objectives was to parade before them an array of *issues*, and the pertinent *research findings*, that they, *as practitioners*, should be aware of and for which a considered response was required. The brief has since extended to embrace health students and workers beyond the compass of the medical profession.

We have endeavoured collectively – and this remains very much a collective enterprise – to summarize in a concise and accessible way an enormous and complex body of literature. In this edition we have stuck to our evolving brief: we have borne in mind the requirements not just of medical students but of *all* students oriented to health and health care. Contributors have changed, as is in some ways fitting. For this sixth edition we are joined by Mel Bartley, Iain Crinson, Judy Green, Moira Kelly and James Nazroo, but have lost Ian Rees Jones. We acknowledge in particular the role of Margot Jefferys, whose pioneering career, influence and prescience helped launch this initiative, and Donald Patrick, senior co-editor of the early editions. We acknowledge too the past input of Ellie Scrivens and, especially, Sheila Hillier. We offer special thanks to our students, from whom all teachers learn, or fail to learn at their peril, some of whom have taken the trouble to offer their own feedback. All chapters have been reviewed and many substantially revised or re-written. As editor, my thanks go to my fellow contributors and colleagues and to all those students who have taken the trouble over the years to provide feedback.

Graham Scambler 2008

Social aspects
of disease

CHAPTER

1

Society and changing patterns of disease

Ray Fitzpatrick

One of the most important recent developments in ideas about health care and illness has been the widespread recognition that social and economic conditions have a major effect on patterns of disease and death rates. A wide range of sources – historical, medical and sociological – have provided the evidence for such influences. This chapter considers how lines of influence from society and the economy can be traced to patterns of disease.

The starting-point of this analysis is the dramatic variation to be found in death rates both in the past and at present. For example, the death rate per annum has virtually halved in England and Wales over the past 150 years: in 1851 it was 22.7 per 1000 population and by 1999 it had fallen to 10.6. Another way to express the difference over this period is in terms of the average number of years an individual could expect to live at birth, i.e. life expectancy. A man or woman born in 1840 could, on average, expect to live to 40 and 43 years, respectively, whereas by 1999 life expectancy had risen to 75 and 80 years, respectively. However, such differences in overall mortality rates disguise a more complex picture if we look at particular age groups. The higher death rates of the mid-nineteenth century were much more severe in particular age groups, especially in infancy and childhood. Thus, future life expectancy for those who have reached the age of 45 years has improved only slightly over the last 100 years, and not nearly as dramatically as has the life expectancy of a child at birth.

The higher death rates and lower life expectancies are not of course simply an historical phenomenon. At present, many under-developed countries have much lower life expectancies than England; for example, in 1999, life expectancies for men and women in Ethiopia were 41 and 43 years, and for Sierra Leone 33 and 35 years, respectively. Under-developed countries with higher death rates resemble nineteenth-century England and Wales in that infant and child mortality are one of the main reasons for lower life expectancy.

VARIATION IN DISEASE PATTERNS IN HUMAN SOCIETY

The diseases encountered by humans have not remained the same over time. The history of humans might be viewed as a progressive victory over disease, but this is an over-simplification. Although some diseases are less important than in the past, others have become more important. Complex social and biological processes have altered the balance between humans and disease. A number of authorities (McKeown 1979, Powles 1973) now agree on three characteristic disease patterns in historical sequence.

Preagricultural disease patterns

Before about 10 000 BC, indeed for most of the evolution of humans as a distinct species, humans lived as hunter–gatherers, that is, without any form of settled agriculture for subsistence. Although conclusions based on such early evidence are somewhat speculative, anthropologists and epidemiologists have argued that the infectious diseases that were later to become major causes of illness and death were relatively uncommon at this stage of social evolution. Furthermore, diseases that are sometimes described as diseases of civilization, such as heart disease and cancer, were less common than at the present time (Powles 1973). It is likely that mortality in adults arose from environmental and safety hazards, for example hunting accidents and exposure.

Diseases in agricultural society

Knowledge of the diseases that plagued agricultural societies is more certain. These were predominantly the infectious diseases, which for purposes of discussion can be divided into the following:

1. air-borne diseases, such as tuberculosis

2. water-borne diseases, such as cholera

3. food-borne diseases, such as dysentery

4. vector-borne (i.e. carried by rats or mosquitoes) diseases, such as plague and malaria.

In England and Wales, and in Europe generally, the plague was a particularly important cause of death and at its most virulent, in the Black Death of 1348, it killed one-quarter of the English population. It last occurred on any large scale in England and Wales in 1665, and disappeared from Europe shortly after. The plague was spread by the fleas carried by black rats. Its disappearance was due to the replacement of the black rat by the brown rat, which was much less prone to infest human habitations.

Malaria was never as great a health problem in England and Wales as it has been in the tropics, where conditions are ideal for the natural life cycle of both vector and parasite. By the mid-nineteenth century, when reliable vital statistics were available in

England and Wales and the country's economy was changing from agricultural to industrial, the major causes of death were tuberculosis, bronchitis, pneumonia, influenza and cholera.

The modern industrial era of disease

By the mid-twentieth century, infectious diseases had become relatively unimportant causes of death in England and Wales and in the western world in general, although some infectious diseases, such as influenza, remained common causes of death, particularly in the elderly. The infectious diseases have been replaced as major causes of death by the so-called degenerative diseases, cancer and cardiovascular disease.

Because of these changes in patterns of death, the major medical problems of today are chronic illnesses such as atherosclerosis, diabetes and osteoarthritis. These are all problems involving multiple risk factors, rather than a single cause. Their onset is quite early in life; they tend to be progressive; and they appear in all modern societies. Fries (1983) argues that there appear to be quite definite limits to the extension of the human lifespan, so that life expectancy at age 100 years has barely changed in the past 80 years. However, if one looks at such indices as age at first heart attack or age-specific lung cancer rates in the USA, there have been quite definite improvements in recent years. Fries concludes that health policy should make the compression of morbidity a major objective. Combining medical and social approaches to reducing the risk factors for chronic illnesses such as atherosclerosis would result in a life in which serious illness and decline in functioning were increasingly confined to later ages and the years of vigorous life extended.

This dramatic increase in importance of the chronic degenerative diseases is characteristic of almost all countries that have undergone industrialization, although the exceptions and the variations in rates from one country to another provide important and intriguing problems for the medical and social scientist. Japan, for example, has a much lower incidence of heart disease than comparable industrialized societies. On the other hand, the level of stomach cancer is considerably higher in Japan than, for example, the USA.

Explaining changes in disease prevalence

It would be all too easy to regard changes in disease patterns as the inevitable consequences of medical and technical progress without further explanation. Close examination of the major influences on disease patterns, however, uncovers a complex picture that is increasingly recognized as important for the understanding of disease in the contemporary world. The study of how disease patterns have changed indicates the pervasive influence of social and economic factors on disease prevalence.

Three main factors seem important in the changes in disease patterns that followed the transition from nomadic hunting and gathering to agricultural life. First, the development of cereals such as wheat allowed agricultural societies to feed more mouths and hence support higher population densities. Evidence from epidemiological studies, however, shows that many infectious organisms thrive when human populations grow above certain densities. Second, agricultural work necessitated permanent settlement, whereas hunter–gatherers moved settlement periodically in search of fresh food sources. However, in the absence of sanitation and awareness of its importance, permanent settlement often led to the contamination of water supplies by waste products, which increased the risks of infection from a number of organisms. Third, the development of cereals as the major source of food, although supporting greater numbers of people, paradoxically narrowed the range and quality of diet, a factor that crucially reduced resistance to infection.

More careful examination is needed to explain the remarkable changes in death rates and the decline in significance of mortality from infectious disease that occurred with the transition from agricultural to industrial economies. The victory over death and diseases in the nineteenth and twentieth centuries still represents the most dramatic improvement in health in the history of human kind. Death rates for the various infectious diseases did not decline simultaneously. Tuberculosis, the most common cause of death in the nineteenth century, began to decline in the first half of that century, as indicated in Fig. 1.1.

There are a limited number of possible explanations for such a marked decline in mortality from an infectious organism. Box 1.1 shows the competing explanations that have been offered, not only for the decline of tuberculosis but for the wide range of infectious diseases for which mortality rates declined dramatically in the course of the nineteenth century in Britain and other parts of western Europe. It is possible that a change occurred in the virulence of the organism itself or that the genetic immunity of the population improved. Both these possibilities are generally discounted. There is no theoretical reason why the organisms responsible for tuberculosis and a number of other infectious diseases should fortuitously change in their virulence at approximately the same period. It is very unlikely that genetic immunity could improve in such a short time as the selection processes implied would require dramatic increases in mortality rates across a range of diseases. For these reasons, the first and third explanations in Box 1.1 are normally rejected as unlikely. The most convincing explanation for the decline in mortality from tuberculosis and, later in the century, from air-borne diseases such as pneumonia, is that of greater acquired resistance. An increased resistance to infection resulted from improvement in nutritional intake as agricultural techniques improved and transportation of produce became faster and more efficient. Much of the nineteenth century also saw unprecedented increases in real wages and the standard of living in Britain. It is also possible to argue for the significance of nutrition with contemporary evidence. In many third world countries today, diseases such as measles or tuberculosis have a much higher fatality, especially among the very young in populations whose resistance is reduced by malnutrition. McKeown cites the conclusion of the World Health Organization report that one-half to three-quarters of all statistically recorded deaths of infants and young children

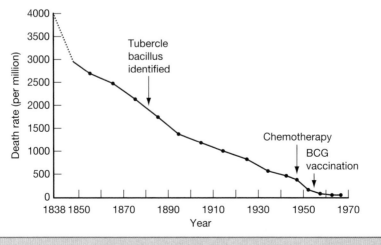

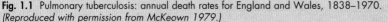

Fig. 1.1 Pulmonary tuberculosis: annual death rates for England and Wales, 1838–1970. (Reproduced with permission from McKeown 1979.)

BOX 1.1 Possible explanations for the decline of mortality from infectious disease in Britain in the nineteenth century

- Decline in virulence of organisms: organisms responsible for diseases, for example tuberculosis and bronchitis, became less lethal as a result of changes in their biological properties
- Reduction in exposure of humans to infectious organisms: for example, through changes in domestic housing and urban planning or through reduced contamination of food and water supplies
- Genetically induced increase in resistance of humans to infection: human genes associated with resistance to infection might be favoured by Darwinian selection processes and thus individual and population resistance increased over time
- Acquired resistance of humans to infection: general fitness brought about by improved nutrition resulted in greater resistance in terms of probability of: (1) being infected; and/or (2) recovering from infection
- Specific medical interventions: rates of recovery from infectious diseases were improved by developments in medical treatment and therefore mortality rates were reduced

are attributed to a combination of malnutrition and infection (McKeown 1979). However, the role of the second possible explanation in Box 1.1 – reduced exposure to infectious organisms – is also of importance. The incidence of illness and mortality from water-borne diseases such as cholera declined somewhat later in the nineteenth century, largely as the result of concerted efforts by the public health movement to prevent the contamination of drinking water supplies by sewage; gastroenteric infectious diseases came under control by the beginning of the twentieth century, resulting in a dramatic impact on infant mortality. The sterilization and more hygienic transportation of milk in particular, and improved food hygiene in general, constitute another form of environmental change that produced the decline in infectious disease mortality.

Thus, most of the decline in death rates achieved in Britain and in the western world generally by the Second World War can be attributed to environmental factors such as improvements in food and hygiene, which were the products of economic development. Other social changes, such as the decline in the birth rate, reduced the demand for food and housing resources. Improved housing and better personal hygiene also played their role in reducing mortality rates.

Historians still dispute the precise nature of the changes that brought about the decline in mortality rates just described. The nature of that debate can, with some simplification, be termed one between the 'public health' form of explanation and the 'invisible hand' version of events (Box 1.2). The debate is of more than purely historical interest because it mirrors and has implications for current debates. Even now, some would argue that improvements in the economy and wealth are the most effective ways of producing improvements in the health of modern populations ('the invisible hand' (Guha 1994)). Others would argue that more direct and political intervention is required by a modern public health movement to address the ills described later in this chapter (Szreter 1988). Box 1.2 shows how difficult it is to disentangle claims, even with historical hindsight!

The global burden of disease

There is a danger of focusing excessively on changing patterns of disease in developed countries. A ranking of the top ten causes of death and disability combined for the world as a whole in 1999 shows that five of the top ten causes primarily affect younger children: lower respiratory tract infections, conditions arising during the perinatal period,

BOX 1.2	The debate between 'public health' and 'the invisible hand' to explain improved life expectancy in nineteenth century Britain

The 'public health' explanation emphasizes deliberate government interventions:

- The public health movement improved water supplies, housing standards, regulation of food sold to public
- Increased income of working classes sometimes coincided with deteriorating death rates because of migration into more unhygienic industrial towns
- The 'invisible hand' explanation emphasizes benefits of rising incomes:
- Some areas of London enjoyed improved death rates in the nineteenth century before reforms to water supplies
- Studies of claims to insurance societies show that while working class sickness rates due to infectious disease were stable, deaths from the same causes declined
- In some nineteenth century towns, such as Mansfield, deaths from infectious disease remained high despite excellent water supplies
- The greatest benefit of improved diet is upon the capacity of infants and children to survive infectious disease

diarrhoeal diseases, childhood vaccine-preventable diseases and nutritional deficiencies (Michaud et al 2001). Two further causes are infectious diseases largely associated with poverty in developing countries: malaria and HIV. There is an unfinished agenda of child-hood and infectious diseases responsible for the majority of ill health in the modern world.

THE HISTORICAL ROLE OF MEDICINE

To this point nothing has been said about the role that medical intervention (the last possible explanation listed in Box 1.1) has played in the relationship between man and disease. At first glance, this might seem an important omission, given that medical knowledge was accumulating throughout the period and that hospitals had grown in number since the latter part of the eighteenth century. The evidence that McKeown and others have gathered, however, suggests that very little of the decline in mortality rates can be attributed to improvements in medical care. They list a range of evidence against the role of specific medical interventions having a substantial effect on mortality:

- Hospitals and surgical procedures were actually harmful. When Florence Nightingale began to reform the hygienic conditions in hospitals, it was widely thought that hospitals constituted a risk to health; in other words, one stood a high risk of cross-infection – contracting a disease from other patients – because wards were unsegregated as well as unhygienic. Similarly, despite the advances in surgery made possible by the development of anaesthetics, there is little evidence that surgical procedures made any impact on life expectancy in the nineteenth century (McKeown & Brown 1969).

- Drugs were largely ineffective. Before the twentieth century a large armoury of medicines appears to have been available to the Victorian doctor. However, only a few, such as digitalis, mercury and cinchona, used in the treatment of heart disease, syphilis and malaria, respectively, would be recognized by modern standards as having specific efficacy and, in any case, dosages were unlikely to have been appropriate.

The first drugs that can be shown to have influenced mortality rates did not appear until the end of the 1930s. Antibiotics, which are used in the treatment of a wide range of bacterial infections, were developed in the 1930s and 1940s. Prophylactic immunization

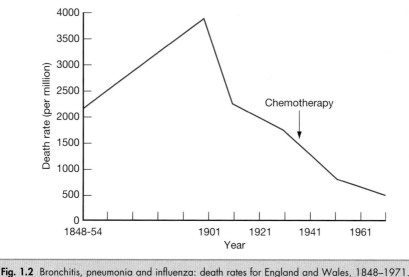

Fig. 1.2 Bronchitis, pneumonia and influenza: death rates for England and Wales, 1848–1971. *(Reproduced with permission from McKeown 1979.)*

against such diseases as whooping cough and polio dates from the 1950s. In the case of these medical breakthroughs, however, it is easy to overstate the contribution that they made to mortality rates. The decline in mortality for most infectious diseases took place before the introduction of antibiotics. The period of decline for tuberculosis can be seen in Fig. 1.1, and the mortality rates for bronchitis, pneumonia and influenza are shown in Fig. 1.2. Moreover, it is difficult to distinguish between the improvements in disease mortality that can be attributed to the introduction of treatment or immunization and those due to the continuing influence of improving social and economic conditions. The immunization programmes for diphtheria and polio probably brought about the greatest improvements that can be attributed to specific medical intervention.

DISEASE RATES AND SOCIAL FACTORS IN MODERN SOCIETY

The association between diseases and social and economic circumstances is not a purely historical phenomenon. In many parts of the third world life expectancy at birth is much lower than in Europe or North America. Many aspects of the environment in the third world provide much more favourable conditions for the spread of infectious diseases than those that prevailed in historical Europe. For example, tropical ecology is particularly favourable for the vectors of diseases such as malaria (the mosquito) and sleeping sickness (tsetse fly). Nevertheless, it is the extremely low standard of living above all else that produces high mortality rates in countries such as Bangladesh and Ethiopia.

In countries like Britain, the social and environmental factors that are responsible for many kinds of commonly occurring disease are somewhat different and will require different explanation. The association between standard of living and the risk of disease, however, is still apparent in the social-class differences in illness and mortality rates discussed in Chapter 8. It is evident that environmental factors, whether in the home or at work, continue to play an important role in influencing the risks of illness and mortality.

The report of the Research Working Group on Inequalities in Health (DHSS 1981) makes clear in many of its recommendations which aspects of the social and economic environment it considers responsible for inequalities in health in Britain. Its proposed strategy largely targets poverty and low income:

● Benefits such as the maternity grant and child benefits need to be increased to reduce child poverty.

● Major programmes are needed in housing improvement, the prevention of accidents to children and the provision of school meals.

● More action is needed to prevent accidents in the work place, largely in manual occupations.

These recommendations are a clear reminder that, for large sections of society, health is harmed by material deprivation in terms of income, diet and housing, rather than because of the 'diseases of affluence'.

Although environmental conditions associated with poverty increase the risk of disease, many kinds of disease are now associated with behaviour that might have little or nothing to do with poverty. Increasingly, the mass media focuses attention on the role that over-eating or inappropriate diet, smoking and excessive alcohol consumption have in a wide variety of disorders such as heart disease, diabetes, lung cancer and cirrhosis of the liver.

The association between smoking and lung cancer has been established beyond all reasonable doubt. It is important to recognize, however, that contemporary health risks associated with behaviour are just as certainly a function of current social conditions as were the infectious health risks associated with the social conditions of the nineteenth century. This is an essential point to grasp, because it is all too easy to view behaviour such as smoking as simply reflecting an individual's decisions and preferences. To focus on an individual smoker would not only lead to erroneous and oversimplified explana-tions of the causes of his or her behaviour but, more importantly, it might lead to misguided or naive attempts to change that behaviour (Box 1.3).

The example of smoking illustrates that disease is as much a reflection of the economy today as it has been in the past. Diet is another example. It has been estimated (Lock & Smith 1976) that 56% of women and 52% of men in Britain over the age of 40 years are at least 15% overweight. The mortality risks of men who are 10% overweight are one-fifth higher than average, especially in mortality associated with diabetes and vascular disease. Clearly, over-eating is a major health risk. Burkitt (1973) and others have argued that inappropriate diet is also a problem. He argues that diverticular disease, cancer of the bowel, diabetes and indeed various venous diseases such as varicose veins and deep vein thrombosis, can all be linked to lack of fibre. Populations that have diets with a high fibre content seem relatively free of many such diseases. In Britain, the daily fibre intake from bread has been reduced to about one-tenth of its level in 1850, and the consumption of sugar and other refined carbohydrates has almost doubled. Again, the statistics of change do not reveal the causal links. Changes in diet have reflected changes in the food-producing industries, which are now concentrated in a small number of multinational companies whose main concern is to produce standardized, well-accepted and easily transported commodities: nutritional values have taken second place to the expansion of profits.

Another essentially modern form of health hazard can be identified in the 6000 deaths and 80 000 serious injuries that occur annually as a result of road traffic accidents. Doll (1983) makes the point that the rate per million of deaths on the roads is actually lower now than it was in the 1930s and is in this sense a testament to the beneficial effects of legislation with regard to prevention. Nevertheless, some 2000 hospital beds are occupied

BOX 1.3 Smoking: A product of the economy as much as of individual behaviour?

Who smokes is socially patterned:

- 13% of men and 14% of women in social class 1 are smokers (see Chapter 8 for the definition of the five social classes)
- 44% of men and 33% of women in social class V are smokers
- Attitudes and behaviour are influenced by:
  - advertising and marketing strategies
  - governmental health warnings
  - taxation
- Effective health policies require evidence of social factors; there is no point in increasing spending on health education to alter the behaviour of groups who do not respond to such influences

Economic significance of cigarettes:

- An analysis of smoking should include political, economic and health issues
- An increase in taxation would make cigarettes cost-prohibitive to some, but this would result in a decline in revenue
- A reduction in smoking would lead to a decrease in National Health Service costs but an increase in pensions, as greater numbers would live to old age
- A reduction in the tobacco industry would reduce the amount of sickness absence but lead to unemployment in areas dependent on the industry

every day by the victims of road traffic accidents (Butler & Vaile 1984), which places a considerable demand on healthcare resources. The risk of having an accident as a motor-cyclist is 18 times higher than the risk to car drivers, and much more still could be achieved to prevent accidents to this group by, for example, legislation on training and testing riding ability.

It might seem that an analysis of the relationship of social and economic factors to health is unhelpful because it points to features of our economic system that are central, firmly established and difficult to change. If this is the case, then another parallel is suggested with the nineteenth-century problems of environmental disease. The changes in sanitation, urban planning and building that were required to transform the pattern of infectious diseases in Victorian times were similarly regarded as unrealistic and resisted for long periods by politicians and business interests; but the reforms were adopted slowly and growing awareness of the relationship between commercially promoted behaviours such as smoking and unhealthy eating in our own time should help to speed the process of securing reforms.

A multidisciplinary committee has produced a major report to assess the effectiveness of existing public health policies and to stimulate new national strategies (Smith & Jacobson 1988). Six areas of current lifestyles that influence health were identified, for which research evidence of harmful effects is strong and support for the feasibility of action is clear cut:

1. tobacco

2. diet

3. physical activity

4. alcohol

5. sexuality

6. road safety.

Similarly, five areas of preventive services were identified where evidence is very strong that public health interventions could now produce dramatic improvements:

1. maternity services

2. dental health

3. immunization

4. early cancer detection (breast and cervix)

5. detection of high blood pressure.

The approach in each of these 11 priority areas is to identify precise quantitative targets and make specific recommendations to public bodies and institutions. Thus, one of a number of specific nutritional targets is to increase the total dietary fibre intake from 20 g per person per day to 30 g. The list of agencies to which nutritional targets and specific actions are recommended includes the food industry, local authorities, health authorities and government. The committee's view is that agencies need specific targets to stimulate action and to provide a ready means of monitoring results.

THE ECONOMY AND HEALTH POLICY IN MODERN SOCIETY

Some of the most recent research on the relationship between the economy and health suggests that, even in modern societies, economic factors play the predominant role in determining patterns of illness, and that the role of health services is negligible by comparison. Four different views of how the economy generally, and patterns of employment and income in particular, can affect health are evaluated here (Box 1.4).

Unemployment and health

Brenner (1977) has argued that most of the variation in annual overall mortality rates for the USA can be explained statistically in terms of changes in the annual level of employment, provided that a time lag of 5 years is allowed for unemployment to have its effect on health. This impact is produced in two ways: first, unemployment reduces family income and, therefore, the material standard of living; second, the individual loses a sense of meaning and purpose found at work and experiences increased fears about the future and tension at home. This results in greater vulnerability to ill health. From USA data, Brenner concluded that a 1% increase in unemployment, if sustained for 5 years, was statistically responsible for nearly 37 000 extra deaths. Similar results have been found from analyses of data collected in England and Wales and in Sweden (Brenner 1979).

BOX 1.4   Alternative models of the economy and health

- Unemployment is a major cause of ill health
- Rapid economic growth is a major cause of ill health
- Particular forms of employment are causes of ill health:
  - 'job-strain' model
  - 'effort–reward imbalance' model
- Income distribution is a major cause of ill health

Rapid economic growth and health

This work has been challenged by Eyer (1977), who argues that the influence on health of experience such as unemployment generally occurs within a much shorter time than the 5-year lag that Brenner allows. If this is the case, the association between unemployment and mortality is considerably reduced. Instead, Eyer argues that death rates increase at the time of business booms, when employment rates are high. He explains the association between employment and mortality in terms of four connected social factors that attend business cycles.

1. Economic booms increase workers' migration, which weakens the social networks that normally protect individuals against disease.

2. 'Stress' through overwork in times of business peaks increases ill health.

3. The unhealthy consumption of alcohol and tobacco increases.

4. Conversely, during low periods of the economy, social networks are strong and act to protect individuals.

Similar deleterious effects upon health of rapid economic growth have been detected in history. To return to the evidence of nineteenth century Britain, it can be argued that it was the disruption caused by rapid economic growth that resulted in little or no overall increase in life expectancy in the middle of that century. Mortality rates were particularly poor in the rapidly growing industrial cities such as Manchester, Glasgow and Liverpool. Rapid economic growth was associated with large-scale immigration of the rural poor into cities, growing social divisions between rich and poor within cities and a decline in willingness of those in power to fund environmental and public health protection (Szreter 1999). Szreter argues that the 'invisible hand' of rapid economic growth alone proved harmful to health and that only a deliberate public health movement in the second half of the nineteenth century restored the improving trends in life expectancy associated with economic growth.

Forms of employment and health

It is increasingly argued that the nature of work processes need to be examined for possible health effects. One very influential theory is associated with the work of Karasek & Theorell (1990). According to the 'job–strain' model, individuals who have very demanding jobs but who see themselves as having very little control over their work, experience not only higher levels of stress than others but also elevated cardiovascular disease. A number of studies have been carried out in Sweden and the USA to support this approach. A related model – the effort–reward imbalance model – argues rather similarly that those whose work is demanding and stressful, but who perceive themselves as insufficiently rewarded for their efforts, are also more prone to distress as well as to cardiovascular disease (Siegrist et al 1990). Rewards are not primarily monetary but prospects of status enhancement or promotion. Both models, when tested on work forces, have been found to demonstrate the highest levels of risk in semi- and unskilled manual workers.

Income distribution and health

One final model of the effects of the economy on health argues that it is the relative degree of inequality in incomes within a country that influences health (Wilkinson 1994). The evidence to support this model comes from international comparisons of countries where it is claimed that countries with the smallest spread and least inequality of incomes from top to bottom (e.g. Japan and Sweden) have higher life expectancies than those with large income differentials (such as the USA and the UK). The emphasis of the model is, therefore, not on how absolute income influences health but how people attach meaning to disadvantage in ways that actually harm them.

Of the four models outlined, only the role of unemployment has been researched to any great extent. The other three need further investigation. Bunn (1979) examined national statistics for the incidence of ischaemic heart disease in Australia. He found that economic recessions and their associated problems of high unemployment were associated not only with subsequently higher levels of heart disease mortality, but also with increased rates of drug prescribing. The latter he interpreted as a potential indicator of the stress of the recession, which resulted in increased general practitioner (GP) prescribing. One of the most convincing pieces of statistical evidence to support this research is the Office of Population Censuses and Surveys (OPCS) Longitudinal Study (OPCS 1984). This found that men who were unemployed in 1971, and their wives, experienced a 20% higher mortality rate than those men employed in the following 10 years (Moser et al 1987).

Other studies, instead of looking at correlations in national statistics, have examined at close hand the experiences of unemployed families. Fagin (1981) examined in detail a small sample of families in which the male breadwinner had been without work for at least 16 weeks. In many families the breadwinners developed clinical depression, loss of self-esteem, insomnia and suicidal thoughts, much of which necessitated psychotropic drug treatment by their GP. Physical symptoms included asthmatic attacks, backache and skin lesions. The health of younger children in some families also seemed to be affected.

MODERN MEDICINE AND HEALTH

The issues raised by these contrasting approaches are far from being resolved. All four models at least agree in placing the main responsibility for health and illness on economic policy rather than on the health services. This controversial position is partly shared by more radical writers who are more concerned with analysing directly the contribution of modern medicine to health. Perhaps the best known is Illich (1977), who argues that medicine has played a very small role in improving health and that its contribution has actually been negative, insofar as it has:

● raised public expectations of 'wonder cures', which in reality are ineffective

● extended too far the kinds of problem that are thought to be medical

● been responsible for large amounts of iatrogenic (medically induced) illness

● decreased the ability of individuals to cope with their own illness by fostering a debilitating dependency on the expert (see Chapter 12).

Illich's own solution is first to break down the monopoly of medicine in health care, so that there is a 'free market' in which anyone can practise healing, and second to reverse the social trend towards dependency by restoring the value of personal responsibility.

This approach, which is attractive to many advocates of 'alternative medicine' and self-help groups, is rejected as mistaken and utopian by writers such as Navarro (1975) because it wrongly blames the medical profession and a 'gullible' public for aspects of ill health that are best understood as products of a capitalist economy. It is this that directly creates much illness, maintains an unequal distribution of illness and encourages a very inappropriate healthcare system for treating illness once it has occurred. Hence, Navarro advocates radical political changes in society as the only solution to the kinds of problems that have been identified in this chapter.

Other writers, such as McKeown and Powles, place more emphasis on the need to reform health care rather than concerning themselves with wider issues of social change. First, they argue that, because much disease is caused environmentally, preventive medicine in teaching, research and practice should concentrate on the prevention of disease rather than treatment after it has occurred. Not only has prevention had a significant impact in the past, it appears to be a simple, more humane and sound means of reducing disease for the present.

Second, these analysts also maintain that healthcare resources and energy have become too concentrated on high technology and hospital-based acute medicine at the expense of preventive and community resources. In the light of the evidence reviewed above, it seems that there is an unwarranted faith in technological medicine. With the possible exception of antibiotics and immunization, few improvements in health can be attributed to breakthroughs in laboratory medicine. Cochrane (1972) argues that all too few medical procedures have been submitted to rigorous evaluation of their effectiveness (see Chapter 18).

Third, it is argued that another shift in the emphasis of medicine is needed, that from cure to care. Because medicine can claim few cures to be effective, it must confront the task of caring for the sick with greater zeal and effectiveness. Caring necessitates concern with the quality of life of the ill and reduction in any handicap or disadvantage consequent to disease. However, financial and other resources, reflecting medical values, are at present spent more in efforts in acute medicine than in the psychiatric or geriatric units. Medical education perpetuates such values because it is conducted predominantly in acute hospitals where consultants maintain traditional values in their teaching.

Clearly, these arguments are controversial and have not gone unchallenged. Lever (1977) has argued that inferences about current health planning based on historical patterns are hazardous. To prove that environmental factors were the most important determinants of mortality in the past does not necessarily prove that environmental measures will produce such beneficial effects in the present. Given limited funds for health services, a major shift towards environmental and preventive health care would be a major gamble. Whatever the merits of such points, it has to be acknowledged that at present insufficient resources have been committed to such preventive services as health education and occupational medicine, compared with expenditure on hospital technology, to allow any serious examination of their potential role.

It might also be argued that analysts like McKeown are too pessimistic in their interpretation of the impact of medical treatments, which have been shown to have led to markedly improved survival rates for many forms of childhood cancers and Hodgkin's disease and cancer of the testis amongst adult cancers (Doll 1990). Moreover, the debate has tended to focus on death rates, thereby ignoring substantial benefits that could have been derived from medical treatments in improving individuals' quality of life, for example by mitigating symptoms of pain, discomfort or disability (see Chapter 18). There is now very firm evidence that rates of physical disability among the elderly are declining in the USA (Cutler 2001). This is very striking evidence of movement towards the 'compression of morbidity' discussed earlier in this chapter, given the popular assumption (supported by some evidence) that longer life expectancy will be associated with increased levels of disability. The 25% reduction in disability in the elderly observed since 1982 cannot easily be explained but is almost certainly due to a combination of:

- improved medical treatments such as drugs and joint replacement surgery for arthritis and cataract surgery for visual impairment

- behavioural changes such as reduced smoking and improved diet that, as well as improving mortality, also reduce disability from respiratory disease, stroke and heart disease

- greater availability of adaptive devices such as devices to aid walking and walk-in showers that reduce the disabling consequences of chronic disease.

Such analyses challenge the excessively negative critiques of modern medicine. However, they do so by showing the limitations of opposing medical with social interventions (both are involved) and by demonstrating the need to move beyond mortality as the sole outcome of interest.

At present, much work remains to be done regarding the influence that social and economic factors exert on health. At the same time, controversial debates continue unresolved about the priorities in efforts and expenditure that are most appropriate to modern patterns of illness.

References

Brenner M 1977 Health costs and benefits of economic policy. International Journal Health Services 7:581–623

Brenner M 1979 Mortality and the national economy. Lancet ii:568–573

Bunn A 1979 Ischaemic heart disease mortality and the business cycle in Australia. American Journal of Public Health 69:772–781

Burkitt D 1973 Some diseases characteristic of modern Western civilization. British Medical Journal 1:274–278

Butler J, Vaile M 1984 Health and health services. Routledge & Kegan Paul, London

Cochrane A 1972 Effectiveness and efficiency: random reflections on the health service. Nuffield Provincial Hospitals Trust, London

Cutler D 2001 The reduction in disability among the elderly. Proceedings of the National Academy of Sciences USA 98:6546–6547

Department of Health and Social Security (DHSS) 1981 Inequalities in health. HMSO, London

Doll R 1983 Prospects for prevention. British Medical Journal 286:81–88

Doll R 1990 Are we winning the fight against cancer? An epidemiological assessment. European Journal of Cancer 26:500–508

Eyer J 1977 Does unemployment cause the death rate peak in each business cycle? International Journal of Health Services 7:625–662

Fagin L 1981 Unemployment and health in families. Department of Health and Social Security (DHSS), London

Fries J 1983 The compression of morbidity. Milbank Memorial Fund Quarterly 61:397–419

Guha S 1994 The importance of social intervention in England's mortality decline: the evidence reviewed. Social History of Medicine 7:89–114

Illich I 1977 Limits to medicine. Medical nemesis: the expropriation of health. Penguin, Harmondsworth

Karasek R, Theorell T 1990 Healthy work. Basic Books, New York

Lever A 1977 Medicine under challenge. Lancet i:353–355

Lock S, Smith T 1976 The medical risks of life. Penguin, Harmondsworth

McKeown T 1979 The role of medicine: dream, mirage or nemesis, 2nd edn. Blackwell Scientific, Oxford

McKeown T, Brown R 1969 Medical evidence related to English population changes in the eighteenth century. In: Drake M (ed) Population in industrialisation. Methuen, London

Michaud CM, Murray CJ, Bloom BR 2001 Burden of disease – implications for future research. Journal of the American Medical Association 285:535–539

Moser K et al 1987 Unemployment and mortality: comparison of the 1971 and 1981 longitudinal study census samples. British Medical Journal 294:86–90

Navarro V 1975 The industrialization of fetishism or the fetishism of industrialization: a critique of Ivan Illich. International Journal of Health Services 5:351–371

Office of Population Censuses and Surveys (OPCS) 1984 Mortality statistics. HMSO, London

Powles J 1973 On the limitations of modern medicine. Science, Medicine and Man 1:1–30

Siegrist J et al 1990 Low status control, high effort at work and ischaemic heart disease: prospective evidence from blue-collar men. Social Science and Medicine 31:1127–1139

Smith A, Jacobson B (eds) 1988 The nation's health: A strategy for the 1990s. Kings Fund, London

Szreter S 1988 The importance of social intervention in Britain's mortality decline c. 1850–1914: a reinterpretation of the role of public health. Social History of Medicine 1:1–38

Szreter S 1999 Rapid economic growth and 'the four Ds' of disruption, deprivation, disease and death: public health lessons from nineteenth-century Britain for twenty-first century China. Tropical Medicine and International Health 4:146–152

Wilkinson R 1994 The epidemiological transition: from material scarcity to social disadvantage? Daedalus 123:61–78

17

CHAPTER 2

Social determinants of health and disease

David Locker

In Chapter 1, evidence was presented to indicate that the improvements in health observed during the eighteenth and nineteenth centuries were the product of rising standards of living and sanitary reform. This illustrates the general principle that the health of a population is closely tied to the physical, social and economic environment. This chapter expands on this point of view by examining some of the social factors that have been linked to health and disease. Over the past 40 years research in this field has grown significantly, with relatively new disciplines such as social epidemiology and psychophysiology devoted to the investigation of the links between the social environment, psychological and emotional states, physiological change and disease. The broad implication of this work, and the view of health it embodies, is that health and illness are social, as well as medical, issues.

THEORIES OF DISEASE CAUSATION

Before the rise of modern medicine, disease was attributed to a variety of spiritual or mechanical forces. It was interpreted as a punishment by God for sinful behaviour or the result of an imbalance in body elements or 'humours'. Many infectious diseases were ascribed to a life of vice or a weak moral character or believed to be due to 'miasma', that is, bad air arising out of dirt and decaying organic matter. The ancient Greeks rejected the notion that disease was a punishment for sin or the consequence of witchcraft and saw disease as being related to the natural environment or the way in which human populations lived and worked. However, they failed to recognize that many diseases were contagious. The idea that disease could be passed from person to person arose in the Middle Ages and coexisted with the belief that disease was linked to evil behaviour. For example, by the mid-nineteenth century there was good evidence that cholera could be transmitted by close personal contact with a cholera victim. The observation that outbreaks occurred at great distances from existing cases led to the idea that the disease could also be transmitted in the water supply. John Snow, a physician who investigated the London cholera epidemics of 1848–9 and 1853–4, provided convincing evidence that the disease was spread by water contaminated by the excretions of cholera victims. While this provided a means to control epidemics of the disease it was not for another 40 years that the organism causing cholera was identified. However, Snow's work did illustrate the important principle that epidemics of disease could be controlled without knowing the biological mechanisms involved.

Ideas about disease that emerged during the late nineteenth century were influenced by two developments that provided a philosophical and empirical basis for the biomechanical approach characteristic of modern medical practice. These developments were the 'Cartesian revolution', which gave rise to the idea that the mind and body were independent, and the doctrine of specific aetiology, which flowed from the discovery of the microbiological origins of infectious disease. These effectively denied the influence of social and psychological factors in disease onset. Rather, the body was viewed as a machine to be corrected when things go wrong, by procedures designed to neutralize specific agents or modify the physical processes causing disease. These ideas have been progressively challenged as the monocausal view of disease has been modified by multicausal models of disease onset. The key features of these theories of health and disease are summarized in Box 2.1.

The germ theory of disease

During the second half of the nineteenth century, the work of Ehrlich, Koch and Pasteur revealed that the prevailing health problems of the time were the product of living organisms which entered the body through food, water, air or the bites of insects or animals. In 1882, Koch identified and isolated the bacillus causing tuberculosis, and between 1897 and 1900 the organisms responsible for 22 infectious diseases were identified. This work gave rise to the idea that each disease had a single and specific cause. This was embodied in Koch's postulates, a set of rules for establishing causal relationships between a micro-organism and a disease. These state that, to be ascribed a causal role, the agent must always be found with the disease in question and not with any other disease. This doctrine and its monocausal approach came to dominate medical research and practice. As a result, research effort moved from the community to the laboratory and concentrated on the identification of the noxious agents responsible for a given disease, while medical practice became devoted to the destruction or eradication of that agent from individuals already affected (Najman 1980).

Multicausal models of disease

Although the infectious organism theory of disease made a significant contribution to explaining and solving the major health problems of its time, it has serious limitations

BOX 2.1	Theories of disease causation: Key ideas

Germ theory
- Disease is caused by transmissable agents
- A specific agent is responsible for one disease only
- Medical practice consists of identifying and neutralizing these agents

Epidemiological triangle
- Exposure to an agent does not necessarily lead to disease
- Disease is the result of an interaction between agent, host and environment
- Disease can be prevented by modifying factors which influence exposure and susceptibility

Web of causation
- Disease results from the complex interaction of many risk factors
- Any risk factor can be implicated in more than one disease
- Disease can be prevented by modifying these risk factors

General susceptibility
- Some social groups have higher mortality and morbidity rates from all causes
- This reflects an imperfectly understood general susceptibility to health problems
- This probably results from the complex interaction of the environment, behaviours and life-styles

Socioenvironmental approach
- Health is powerfully influenced by the social and physical environments in which we live
- Risk conditions integral to those environments damage health directly and through the physiological, behavioural and psychosocial risk factors they engender
- Improving health requires political action to modify these environments

in terms of our understanding of disease processes. The most important of these is that not all those exposed to pathogens become ill: an organism or other noxious agent is a necessary, but not a sufficient, cause of disease. The *epidemiological triangle* approach sees disease as the product of an interaction between an agent, a host and the environment. Agents are biological, chemical or physical factors whose presence is necessary for a disease to occur. Host factors include personal characteristics and behaviours, genetic endowment and predisposition, immunological status and other factors which influence susceptibility, while environmental factors are external conditions other than the agent that influence the onset of disease. These can be physical, biological or social in nature. For example, the extent of HIV transmission in a population is the result of multiple agent, host and environmental factors (Box 2.2). In this respect, all diseases, including infections, are multifactorial and have multiple causes. One of the benefits of this broader view is that the health of a population may be promoted by procedures which modify susceptibility and exposure as well as by procedures which attack the agent involved in the disease. That is, disease can be prevented as well as cured.

The epidemiological triangle is useful in understanding infectious disorders, but is less useful with respect to chronic, degenerative disorders such as heart disease, stroke and arthritis, for here no specific agent can be identified against which individuals and populations may be protected. Many contemporary medical problems are better understood in terms of a *web of causation*. According to this concept, disorders such as heart disease develop through complex interactions of many factors which form a hierarchical causal web of events. These factors may be biophysical, social or psychological and may promote or inhibit the disease at more than one point in the causal process. Ultimately, they determine the level of disease in a community. This is illustrated with respect to heart disease in Fig. 2.1. Since many of these factors can be modified, prevention offers better prospects

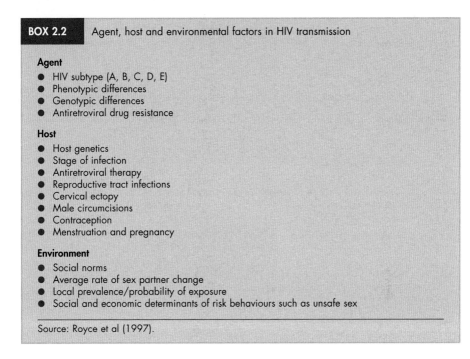

BOX 2.2   Agent, host and environmental factors in HIV transmission

Agent
- HIV subtype (A, B, C, D, E)
- Phenotypic differences
- Genotypic differences
- Antiretroviral drug resistance

Host
- Host genetics
- Stage of infection
- Antiretroviral therapy
- Reproductive tract infections
- Cervical ectopy
- Male circumcisions
- Contraception
- Menstruation and pregnancy

Environment
- Social norms
- Average rate of sex partner change
- Local prevalence/probability of exposure
- Social and economic determinants of risk behaviours such as unsafe sex

Source: Royce et al (1997).

for health than cure. It is also important to note that many of the factors implicated in heart disease have been identified as increasing the risk of other disorders, such as stroke and cancer.

The theory of general susceptibility

The theory of general susceptibility has emerged over the past 20 years and departs in important ways from monocausal and multicausal models of disease. It is not concerned with identifying single or multiple risk factors associated with specific disorders, but seeks to understand why some social groups seem to be more susceptible to disease and death in general. For example, numerous studies have shown that social class, measured by occupation, education, income or area of residence, is closely related to health, even in countries with nationalized and egalitarian healthcare systems such as the National Health Service (NHS) in the UK (see Chapter 8).

The socioenvironmental approach

During the late 1980s, the theory of general susceptibility became more explicitly formulated as the socioenvironmental approach. This approach is not so much concerned with the causes of disease, rather it seeks to identify the broad factors that make and keep people healthy. In its concern with populations rather than individuals, it forms the basis for the health promotion strategies described in Chapter 17. One framework concerning the determinants of health identifies five broad factors that can be targeted in order to improve population health: the social and economic environment; the physical environment; personal health practices; individual capacity and coping skills; and health services. An expanded list along with a rationale for each broad factor is presented in Box 2.3.

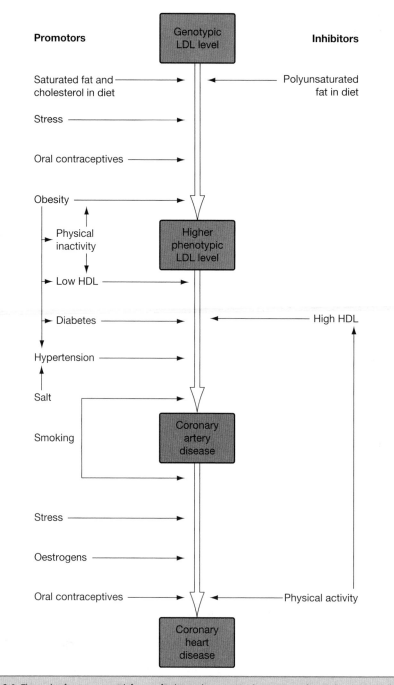

Fig. 2.1 The web of causation: risk factors for heart disease. LDL/HDL = Low density lipoproteins/high density lipoproteins.
(Reproduced with permission from Mausner & Kramer 1985.)

BOX 2.3   Social and environmental determinants of health

Income and social status
There is a close association between income and health so that health improves at each step up the income and social hierarchy. In addition, societies with a high standard of living in which wealth is more equally distributed are healthier, irrespective of the amount spent on health services.

Social support networks
Support from family, friends and social organizations is associated with better health. Moreover, people living in communities with higher levels of social cohesion tend to be healthier.

Education
Higher levels of education are associated with better health. Education increases opportunities for income and job security and equips people with the means to exert control over their life circumstances.

Employment and working conditions
Hazardous physical working environments and the injuries they induce are important causes of health problems. Moreover, those with more control over their work and jobs which involve fewer stress-inducing demands are healthier. However, unemployment, particularly if long term, is associated with poorer health.

Physical environments
The quality of air, water influence the health of populations. So do features of the constructed physical environment, such as housing, roads and community design.

Personal health practices and coping skills
Social environments which encourage healthy choices and healthy lifestyles are key influences on health as are the knowledge, behaviours and skills which influence how people cope with challenging life issues and circumstances.

Healthy child development
Prenatal and early childhood experiences can have a powerful effect on development and health throughout the life span.

Health services
Although not a major determinant of population health, health services can, if appropriately organized and delivered, prevent disease and help promote and maintain health.

Source: Federal, Provincial and Territorial Committee Advisory Committee on Population Health (1994).

23

Other factors which have been cited as determinants of health include social exclusion in the form of racism and discrimination, food and transportation (Wilkinson & Marmot 1998).

According to Labonte (1993), social and environmental factors constitute risk conditions which have a direct effect on health and well-being and also affect health through the numerous psychosocial, behavioural and physiological risk factors which they engender (Fig. 2.2). One implication of the model presented in Fig. 2.2 is that material deprivation and a lack of control over important dimensions of one's life are the main issues that need to be addressed in promoting the health of the population. It is no accident that those countries where the income gap between the rich and the poor is narrowest have the lowest overall mortality rates. As a consequence, social and political change, including income redistribution, may be necessary to modify the health experience of lower socioeconomic groups.

24

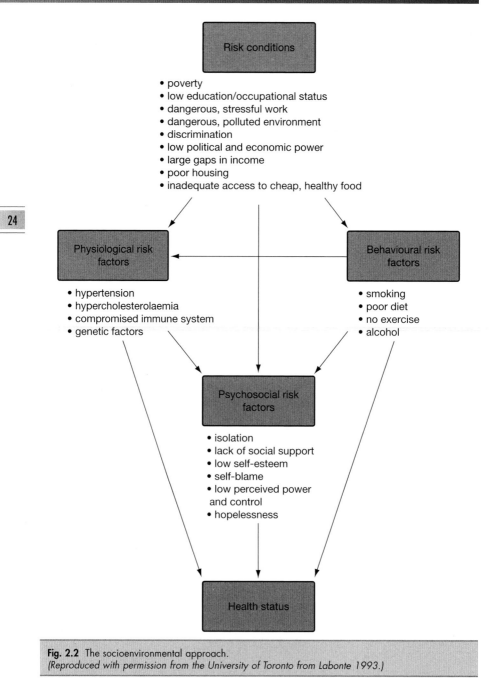

Fig. 2.2 The socioenvironmental approach.
(Reproduced with permission from the University of Toronto from Labonte 1993.)

These theories of the causes of disease have been presented in a more or less historical sequence. From the brief descriptions offered it is clear that the role ascribed to the physical, social and psychological environment increases as we have progressed from the germ theory of disease to socioenvironmental models of health. The latter completely overturns the doctrine of specific aetiology central to the former, for broad non-specific social and psychological factors are seen to be associated with a variety of disease outcomes and ultimately the health and well-being of the population.

It would, however, be a mistake to assume that the role of social and psychological factors as causes of disease has been realized only in modern times. Many of the so-called 'pre-scientific' explanations of disease gave recognition to the part played by such factors. In many cultures, disease is still seen in social terms, as the outcome of a lack of harmony in social relationships. In the context of modern medical history the idea that disease can be brought about by psychological influences was integral to the work of Freud, who explained disorders such as asthma and gastric ulcers as the product of unresolved psychological conflict. Freud's work gave rise to the notion that some diseases were 'psychosomatic' whereas others were not. The contemporary view is that social and psychological factors are implicated in all diseases, although the mechanisms by which they influence health are complex and variable.

25

SOCIAL AND PSYCHOLOGICAL FACTORS AND HEALTH

The research effort invested in studies of social and psychological factors and health is substantial and the body of work that has been produced is difficult to summarize. One reason for this is that a wide variety of factors having a potential influence on health and disease have been studied. As the discussion of theories of disease indicated, these factors fall into three broad types: socioenvironmental, behavioural and psychological.

Clearly, there are close links between many of these factors, and contemporary models of illness attempt to specify how and when they are involved in the mechanisms leading to disease. Even though behaviours such as smoking are individual acts, a number of social and cultural factors influence whether someone will become a smoker and continue to smoke. These factors include 'cultural themes associated with smoking such as relaxation, adulthood, sexual attractiveness and emancipation; the socioeconomic structure of tobacco production, processing, distribution and legislation; explicit and continual advertising by the tobacco companies and the influence of peers, siblings and significant others' (Syme 1986).

Some of the social and psychological factors having an influence on health and explanations of their role as causes of disease are reviewed below.

Social and cultural change

Most of the early studies of social factors and disease onset were concerned with the effects of social and cultural change. They included studies of industrialization and urbanization, migration and social, occupational and geographical mobility. The major disease outcome studied was coronary heart disease since this is predominantly a disease of industrialized, urbanized nations. Some populations isolated from western culture have low blood pressure which does not rise with age. However, blood-pressure levels and coronary heart disease rates increase when these populations move to urban settings.

A number of studies conducted during the 1960s and early 1970s found higher rates of disease among people who changed jobs, place of residence or life circumstances. For example, one study found that men reared on farms who moved to urban centres to take middle-class jobs had higher rates of coronary heart disease than men who continued to work on the farm or who took up labouring jobs in cities (Syme et al 1964). Similar observations have been made with respect to cancer.

A number of mechanisms might be responsible for the negative effects of social and cultural change on health. The adverse effects may be the direct result of change itself, a product of the circumstances to which individuals move or the product of personal characteristics which predispose individuals to both mobility and poor health. One study which attempted to evaluate these explanations compared rates of heart disease among Japanese immigrants to California and Hawaii with those of Japanese men still living in Japan (Marmot et al 1975). Coronary heart disease and mortality rates were highest among those living in California and lowest in Japan. Among those living in California, some had become 'acculturated' and had adopted western lifestyles, whereas others retained traditional Japanese ways. The former had disease rates up to five times as high as the latter. This suggests that being mobile is not, in itself, the important factor, rather it is the change in the environment in which these people lived that explained the increase in disease risk.

Social support

One of the earliest studies of the relationship between social environment and health was undertaken by the French sociologist Durkheim and published in 1897. In this work Durkheim pioneered the use of statistical methods for exploring and explaining differences in suicide rates across different social groups. Although suicide is an individual act, these differences in rates have persisted over time and across cultures. Durkheim explained suicide in terms of the social organization of these groups, particularly the extent to which individuals were integrated into the group, and the way in which this encouraged or deterred individuals from suicide. High rates of suicide were associated with groups that had very high and very low levels of integration.

More recent studies of social ties and health have focused on the relationship between social support and well-being. Some of this early work looked at differences in health according to marital status. The single, widowed and divorced have higher mortality rates than the married, the differences being much larger for men than for women (Table 2.1). These differences, which were first observed and reported in the mid-nineteenth century, have been remarkably consistent over time, and are consistent across cultures and healthcare systems. Only a small part of the differences in mortality rates can be explained by the selective effects of marriage (Morgan 1980).

One possible explanation of these differences is that marital status has an influence on psychological states and life-styles (Gove 1979). Studies have shown that the married

TABLE 2.1	Mortality, all causes: ratio of mortality rate of the unmarried to the mortality rate of the married; whites aged 25–64 years, USA 1960		
Marital status		**Sex**	**Ratio**
Single		Male	1.96
		Female	1.68
Widowed		Male	2.64
		Female	1.77
Divorced		Male	3.39
		Female	1.95

Reproduced with permission from the University of Chicago Press from Gove (1979).

tend to be happier and more satisfied with life than the unmarried, they are less likely to be socially isolated and have more social ties. In a society in which marriage and family life are a central value, being married gives meaning and significance to daily life, promotes a sense of well-being and is a source of social and emotional support. This explanation tends to be supported by data on marital status and specific causes of death. Variations in mortality rates are large where psychological states or aspects of life-style play a direct role in death, as in suicide or death from accidents, or are associated with acts such as smoking or alcohol consumption. Large differences are also observed with respect to diseases such as tuberculosis, where family factors may influence entry into medical care, willingness to undergo treatment or the availability of help and support.

An influential study which clearly demonstrated that integration into the community has a direct effect on health was undertaken by Berkman & Syme (1979). They followed a random sample of adults over a 9-year period. At the start of the study a social network score was calculated for each subject based on marital status, contacts with friends and relatives and membership of religious and other social groups. Over the 9-year period of the study those with low network scores were more likely to die than those with high network scores. After controlling for other factors such as weight, cigarette smoking, alcohol consumption, physical activity, health practices and health status at baseline, mortality rates for the socially isolated were two to three times higher than those with extensive social networks. These early findings have been confirmed in a number of other longitudinal studies. For example, a 6-year study of men in Finland found that risk of death was highest among those who reported having few persons to whom they gave or from whom they received support. Lack of participation in social organizations, having few friends and not being married were associated with mortality after taking into account baseline health and other risk factors including income (Kaplan et al 1994).

Other evidence suggests that social integration and social support have a broad influence on health. Early studies found that they were linked to heart disease, complications of pregnancy and emotional illness. More recent studies have found that social integration exerts a protective effect on the incidence of non-fatal myocardial infarction in men aged 50 and over (Vogt et al 1992) while social isolation increased the risk of stroke in a study of male health professionals in the USA (Kawachi et al 1996). There is also strong and consistent evidence to show that lack of social support, social isolation and not being married have an influence on long-term survival among men following an initial myocardial infarction (Williams et al 1992). More recent studies have found that social support predicts survival in dialysis patients (Thong et al 2007), patients with acute myeloid leukaemia (Pinquart et al 2007) and among women following diagnosis of breast cancer (Kroenke et al 2006). In the last study women who were socially isolated before diagnosis had a 66% increased risk of all cause mortality and a two-fold increase in breast cancer mortality over women who were socially integrated. Other studies have found that social support was related to levels of residual disability following a stroke and was related to the onset of depression and degree of disability among rheumatoid arthritis patients (Fitzpatrick et al 1991). A 2-year follow-up study of people with disabilities living alone found that people with few social contacts were more likely to deteriorate in physical and psychosocial functioning than people with high levels of contact with others (Patrick et al 1986). However, the greatest and most significant difference between those with and without social support occurred among those reporting an adverse life event during the period of the study.

Social support refers to a fairly broad category of events and includes practical assistance, financial help, the provision of information and advice and psychological support.

A 10–year study of elderly women in Finland examined the effect of practical support and emotional support on mortality and found that the risk of death was 2.5 times higher in those lacking emotional support (Lyyra & Heikkinen 2006). However, a large scale Swedish study found that having diverse sources of support was associated with better health outcomes, with economic support, social contacts and the opportunity to discuss personal problems being the most important (Ostberg & Lennartson 2007).

The mechanisms by which social and emotional support enhances or protects health are not known. One hypothesis concerning this mechanism has emerged in the context of studies of the negative health impact of stressful life circumstances. This research suggests that such support acts as a buffer against adverse events that would otherwise have health-damaging effects. In their research on the social origins of depression, Brown & Harris (1978) found that social support was protective only in the context of a severe life event. Certainly, social support has been shown to be associated with reduced psychological distress and enhanced coping when the life event in question is the onset of a medical condition such as cancer (Baider et al 2003). Although studies suggest that social support enhances coping and the ability to tolerate stressful life circumstances, it is also possible that it exerts an influence via psychological, hormonal and neurophysiological pathways.

Life events

A more comprehensive attempt to assess the influence of life experiences such as bereavement and unemployment is to be found in studies of life events and health. This approach emerged at the end of the 1960s with the development of instruments such as the Social Readjustment Rating Scale (SRRS). This scale consists of a list of 42 events, each of which involves personal loss or some degree of change in roles or personal relationships. Each event is given a score depending on how much life change it involves. Scores for an individual are totalled to give a numerical estimate of the amount of life change experienced in a defined period, usually the past year. A number of studies have shown that there is some relationship between scores on this scale and future changes in health.

There have been a number of criticisms of this method of measuring the frequency and severity of life events. Perhaps the most important is that scales such as the SRRS fail to take account of variations in the meaning and significance of life events. The birth of a child, for example, may be a positive event for some women but a negative event for others, depending on the social context in which it occurs. More sophisticated measures of life events have been developed which take account of variations in the meaning of life events based on contextual factors (Brown & Harris 1978).

A second criticism of the SRRS is that it focuses on major life events and ignores less severe but more common life difficulties. A measure which attempts to assess such difficulties is the Hassles Scale (Kanner et al 1981). Its proponents claim that measures of life stress based on daily 'hassles' are better predictors of changes in physical and psychological health than measures based on major life events.

Clearly, the measurement of life stress is a complex issue and establishing a relationship between such stress and negative health outcomes is challenging. Many studies showing such a relationship have design weaknesses making interpretation of their results difficult.

One particularly noteworthy study is that conducted by Brown & Harris (1978) which was mentioned above in connection with social support. This was an investigation of the social and economic circumstances causally implicated in the onset of depression in women. Using measures that were context sensitive, they were able to show a clear relationship between life events with long-term threatening implications and the onset of depression in women. Events with short-term implications, no matter how stressful, were not associated with depression. However, whether or not a woman became depressed after an event involving long-term threat depended on the presence of four 'vulnerability factors'. These were: the absence of a close, confiding relationship with a spouse or other person, loss of mother before age 11 years, lack of employment outside the home, and having three or more children under the age of 15 living at home. The greater the number of these factors present, the greater was the likelihood of depression following an event with long-term threatening implications. Brown & Harris (1978) believe that these vulnerability factors produce ongoing low self-esteem and an inability to cope with the world. These interact with life events to produce generalized feelings of hopelessness and, subsequently, depression.

Life events have also been implicated in the mechanisms leading to physical disorders. They have been linked to disturbances in the control of diabetes, to diseases such as duodenal ulcer, and to abdominal pain leading to appendectomy (Creed 1981).

29

Occupational hierarchies and the organization of work

The physical environments in which people work are often hazardous and damaging to health. Air pollution at work, exposure to carcinogens, working with machinery and industrial accidents take a large toll on the health of manual workers. However, the psychosocial environments in which we work can also have a negative impact on health. Two models that identify important aspects of the psychosocial work environment are the demand-control model and the effort-reward imbalance model (Marmot et al 1999). The former suggests that jobs that combine a high level of psychological demands with low levels of control and skill utilization lead to stress and increase the risk of illness such as coronary heart disease. The latter suggests that jobs which combine a high degree of effort but low levels of gain in the form of financial or emotional rewards, employment security or career advancement lead to emotional distress, job strain and illness.

Evidence in support of the demand-control model comes from a study of British civil servants conducted in the mid-1980s which explored the links between the organization of their work and health outcomes (Marmot & Theorell 1988). None of the subjects in the British study were living in poverty; nevertheless, there were differences in health status according to occupational grade. Those in the lowest grade had mortality rates three times that of those in the highest grade, higher rates of onset of heart disease and higher rates of sickness absence. These differences were directly related to the degree of control in the workplace. Another noteworthy finding was that although blood pressure levels were similar for low and high-grade civil servants when at work, they declined much more for the latter than the former when they were at home. This study concluded that a lack of freedom to make decisions at work, particularly when jobs are stressful or psychologically demanding, is linked both to at-risk behaviours such as smoking, physiological risk factors such as high blood pressure and health outcomes such as heart disease. A follow-up of study participants a decade later confirmed these findings. Those with job strain, a combination of low decision latitude and high demands, were at the greatest risk for the onset of coronary heart disease (Kuper & Marmot 2003) with the effects being greatest among younger individuals. One factor which may explain this link is psychological distress; data from the same study indicated that the risk of onset of angina was predicted by anxiety and sleep disturbance (Nicholson et al 2005). Studies from Sweden have also found a higher risk of myocardial infarction among men in high demand/low control jobs, with this association being particularly evident among manual workers (Hallqvist 1998).

To date, few studies have explored the effort-reward imbalance model. However, these studies indicated that chronic stress associated with effort-reward imbalance results in a two to six-fold increase in the risk of onset of heart disease (Bosma et al 1998, Siegrist et al 1990). This increased risk could not be explained by other biomedical or behavioural risk factors. More recent evidence concerning effort-reward imbalance comes from the longitudinal study of British civil servants cited above. This indicated that an increase in effort-reward imbalance over time was associated with the onset of angina in men and these increases were more common in lower grade civil servants (Chandola et al 2005). However, this relationship was not observed in women. Other studies have documented the adverse effects of effort–reward imbalance on mental health, musculoskeletal and gastrointestinal disorders, sleep disturbance and sickness absence.

Unemployment

Although the physical and social environments in which we work can have a negative effect on health, so can unemployment. There are two main reasons why unemployment could conceivably affect health (Marmot & Madge 1987). First, it is related to standards of living and the material conditions of life, and second it is a stressful event which may become chronic and deprive an individual of a social role, meaningful daily existence and contact with others.

Two approaches are evident in studies of unemployment and health and both are subject to problems in interpretation, largely because it is difficult to separate the effects of unemployment from the effects of other social and economic conditions (Marmot & Madge 1987). The first of these approaches attempts to demonstrate an association between unemployment rates and mortality rates and the way these co-vary with the ups and downs of the economic cycle. The most recent of this work was conducted by Brenner (1979) and is reviewed in Chapter 1. The second approach attempts to assess the health of people who are, or have recently become, unemployed. Since ill health can lead to unemployment as well as vice versa, such studies need to be conducted carefully before it can be concluded that unemployment is a cause of poor health. Nevertheless, evidence from well-designed research does suggest that the unemployed experience more illness, have higher blood pressure, poorer psychological health and increased mortality (Jin et al 1996, Montgomery et al 1999, Turner 1995). Poverty, stress and insecurity, particularly housing insecurity, have all been implicated in the onset of the health problems following unemployment (Nettleton & Burrows 1998).

Although a recent review of 104 studies confirmed that the unemployed have worse physical and psychological health than their employed counterparts, it indicated that the magnitude of the effects varied according to the length of unemployment, and according to individual characteristics such as age, gender and coping resources. (McKee-Ryan et al 2005). The most marked effects tended to be observed among younger persons and males (Artazcoz et al 2004, Reine et al 2004). Contextual factors such as the local unemployment rate did not influence the health effects of being unemployed. It is also the case that other employment transitions, such as starting maternity leave or staying home to look after family members, can lead to compromised psychological well-being among women (Thomas et al 2005).

Health behaviours

There are many behaviours which can have a positive or negative impact on health. Diet, exercise, drinking, smoking, use of illegal drugs are examples which have been the subject of numerous investigations. These behaviours are often characterized as being the result of individual choice and personal responsibility even though it is more useful to see them as the product of social circumstances (Jarvis & Wardle 1999). Evidence that they are linked to social contexts is to be found in data showing that behaviours likely to promote health are less common in groups subject to poverty and social deprivation while behaviours likely to damage health are more common. For example, the percent of smoking among both men and women is inversely related to occupational class and education. However, a broad range of circumstances are related to smoking (Jarvis & Wardle 1999). Rates are higher among the unemployed, those living in rented accommodation, those without access to a car and those who are divorced, separated or single parents. Clearly, material deprivation and factors which indicate stressful social and personal circumstances all predict whether or not an individual will smoke. The highest rates of all are found among groups characterised by combinations of these factors. There is also evidence to suggest that rates of smoking cessation are substantially lower in deprived compared to non-deprived groups even though there appears to be little difference between these groups in terms of wanting to quit smoking. One reason for this may be that nicotine dependence is strongly related to deprivation. Another reason is that the social environments in which deprived groups live and work are less conducive to quitting. One implication of this research is that smoking rates among the deprived are unlikely to decline unless the social circumstances which foster smoking and nicotine dependence are addressed.

■ Sense of coherence

Much of the work on psychosocial factors and health attempts to identify those that increase the risk of specific diseases or poor health overall. By contrast Antonovsky's salutogenic theory attempts to identify individual characteristics that promote health (Antonovsky 1987). The central concept of this theory is sense of coherence (SOC). Individuals with a high SOC tend to be resilient in the face of stress; they perceive events as less stressful, are able to mobilize resources to deal with stressors and possess the commitment, motivations and desire to cope. SOC has been linked to the adjustment to the onset of chronic illness such as cancer and rheumatoid arthritis (Buchi et al 1998) and has been found to be strongly associated with health behaviours such as alcohol use and smoking (Glanz et al 2005). A study of premenopausal women found that those with a strong SOC had lower systolic blood pressure and total cholesterol than those with a weak SOC (Lindfors et al 2005), while longitudinal studies of men suggested that a strong SOC is associated with the delayed onset of cancer (Poppius et al 2006) and cancer mortality (Surtees et al 2006). Studies have also indicated that the role of SOC may be as moderator of the effects of stressful life events (Richardson & Ratner 2005).

PEOPLE, PLACES AND HEALTH

Although a great deal has been made of the links between social and physical environments and health, it is rare for these environments themselves to be the focus of research. The overwhelming tendency has been to look at the characteristics of individuals rather than the characteristics of the places in which they live. However, as evidence begins to accumulate, it is clear that the immediate neighbourhood in which one lives can have an impact on health. Simply put, poor people living in wealthier neighbourhoods have better health than similarly poor people living in poor neighbourhoods (Blaxter 1990). For example, data from the Whitehall II study (Stafford & Marmot 2003) found that 12.3%

of High Grade civil servants living in the most deprived areas had poor health compared with 35.9% of Low Grade employees. Among those living in the least deprived areas the percent with poor health was 8.8% for High Grade and 19.7% for Low Grade employees. Such neighbourhood effects have been found for a variety of health outcomes including mortality and coronary heart disease.

MacIntyre et al (1993) have argued that findings such as these indicate a need for research to discover precisely which features of local areas either damage or promote health. Although some research is available which tries to link aspects of the physical environment, such as air pollution or water hardness, to diseases such as bronchitis and cancer, there is very little work that tries to identify the social, cultural or economic characteristics of areas that affect health. The importance of such work is clear; we may be able to improve health by changing places rather than people.

As an example of this kind of research, MacIntyre et al (1993) compared two areas of Glasgow to identify differences in the living environments they provided. One was in the north west of the city and had relatively low mortality rates; the other was in the south west of the city and had high mortality rates. They found differences between the areas such that living in the north west would be more conducive to good health than living in the south west. Healthy foodstuffs were more available and cheaper in the north west, there were more sporting and recreational facilities, better transport services, better health services, less crime and a less hostile environment. Even though two people might have the same personal characteristics (the same income, family size and composition, and housing tenure, for example) the one living in the north west would be advantaged compared to the one in the south west in ways likely to be related to physical and mental health. A more recent study conducted in Scotland and England identified additional features of neighbourhood social and physical environments that were predictive of poor health (Cummins et al 2005). These were: poor quality physical environment, a more left wing political climate, lower political engagement, high unemployment, low access to private transport or low transport wealth. Interventions to change these features of the environment offer one way of improving the health of local populations.

■ Social cohesion and social capital

Another community-level factor which is associated with health is that of social cohesion. This is a difficult idea to grasp but essentially refers to 'the extent of connectedness and solidarity among groups in society' (Kawachi & Berkman 2000). At the individual level it is indicated by a personal sense of connectedness to a community which can be aggregated to provide an area level indicator of social cohesion (Patterson et al 2004). Cohesive communities are ones in which there is a high level of participation in communal activities and high levels of membership of community groups (Stansfield 1999). Important components of social cohesion seem to be the friendliness and support of neighbours, opportunities for interaction with other members of the community and lack of fear of violence and crime. Recent evidence has indicated that both individual and area level social cohesion is associated with at-risk behaviours such as smoking (Patterson et al 2004).

Social cohesion is one component of what has come to be called social capital. This is measured at an area level by the percentage who feel that people can be trusted and by the 'density of associational life'; that is, the per capita membership of groups such as church groups, fraternal organizations, sports clubs and labour unions (Kawachi & Kennedy 1997). Emerging evidence suggests that social capital is associated with an area's overall mortality rate, as well as rates of death from cancers and heart disease (Kawachi & Kennedy 1997, Kawachi et al 1997, Wilkinson 1996). It has also been shown to be associated with self-rated health and violent crime (Kawachi et al 1999). Consequently, interventions which improve the physical characteristics of a community so as to promote feelings of safety and perceptions of the friendliness of an area have resulted in improvements in the mental health and self-esteem of residents (Halpern 1995).

The main conclusion to be drawn from this and the other research summarized above is that patterns of health and disease are largely the product of social and environmental influences. Although health and illness may involve biological agents and processes, they are inseparable from the social settings in which people live. Ultimately, it is these which influence the challenges people encounter in daily life and their capacity to manage them. Changing these environments is one way in which the health of a community can be improved. However, the nature of communities and the social determinants of health they embody are shaped by public policies and these are influenced by the social, economic and political forces that influence governments. Gaps in our knowledge of how these forces operate and the lack of professional and public understandings of the social determinants of health are barriers to improvements of the environments in which people live (Raphael 2006).

THE SOCIAL CAUSES OF DISEASE: BIOLOGICAL PATHWAYS

Although the evidence linking socioenvironmental factors and health is compelling, the question remains as to how social factors operate to influence health and disease. Psychoneuroimmunology, an emerging and sometimes controversial field of knowledge, is beginning to provide evidence of the biological pathways linking social factors and disease and filling in the gaps in the social stress–illness model. Although there are a number of formulations of this model, most assume that stressors (threatening environmental circumstances) give rise to strains (psychological and physiological changes) which increase an individual's susceptibility to disease. There is evidence to suggest that stress, or its outcome in the form of depression, leads to a number of changes in the human body. It interferes with the normal functioning of neuroendocrine, autonomic metabolic and immune systems, leads to increased heart rate and respiration, dilatation of blood vessels to the muscles and alterations in gastrointestinal function. These changes are believed to cause disease directly or render an individual more prone to disease (Brunner & Marmot 1999).

The most recent evidence of the biological correlates of stress-inducing social environments comes from the study of British civil servants cited in many of the sections above. Some of their extensive findings are as follows:

- Stress at work is associated with metabolic syndrome, a group of metabolic risk factors in the same person that increase the risk of heart disease and stroke. These include, abdominal obesity, blood fat disorders, high blood pressure, insulin resistance and elevated C-reactive protein. Those with chronic work stress were more than twice as likely to have the syndrome than those without work stress (Chandola et al 2006).

- Men whose work was characterized by effort-reward imbalance and over-commitment had higher cortisol and systolic blood pressure levels with the effect on systolic blood pressure being marked in low status over-committed men (Steptoe et al 2004).

- There is a strong inverse relationship between employment grade and plasma viscosity. In turn, plasma viscosity was associated with a number of other biological factors such as fibrinogen, triglycerides and fasting insulin (Kumari et al 2005). In a related study, men with low job control showed greater fibrinogen responses to acute stress than did those with high job control (Steptoe et al 2003a).

These and other analyses of data from the study suggest that the influence of employment status on cardiovascular disease may be the outcome of differences in stress related activation of autonomic and neuroendocrine processes (Hemingway et al 2005, Steptoe et al 2003b).

However, this essentially simple model is more complex than it seems. The link between stressors and illness is mediated by a number of factors that may increase or decrease an individual's vulnerability when faced with a stressor. Social factors such as social support and psychological variables such as personality characteristics, perceptual processes and coping styles, interact in complex ways to affect health outcomes. Moreover, as the socioenvironmental approach suggests, behavioural responses to environmental stressors in the form of health-damaging activities such as smoking also play an important role (Najman 1980). However, while the specification of these biological and behavioural pathways strengthens the credibility of the research evidence, the implications of that evidence are clear. Changing the social circumstances of low status or economically deprived groups is necessary to improve population health.

References

Antonovsky A 1987 Unravelling the mystery of health – how people manage stress and stay well. Jossey-Bass, London

Artazcoz L, Benach J, Borrel C, Cortes I 2004 Unemployment and mental health: understanding the interactions among gender, family roles and social class. American Journal of Public Health 94:82–88

Baider L, Ever-Hadani P, Goldzweig G 2003 Is perceived family support a relevant variable in psychological distress? A sample of prostate and breast cancer couples. Journal of Psychosomatic Research 55:453–460

Berkman L, Syme S 1979 Social networks, host resistance and mortality: a nine-year follow-up of Alameda County residents. American Journal of Epidemiology 109:186–204

Blaxter M 1990 Health and lifestyles. Tavistock-Routledge, London

Bosma H, Peter R, Siegrist J, Marmot M 1998 Alternative job stress models and the risk of heart disease. American Journal of Public Health 88:68–74

Brenner M 1979 Mortality and the national economy. Lancet ii:568–573

Brown G, Harris T 1978 The social origins of depression. Tavistock, London

Brunner E, Marmot M 1999 Social organization, stress and health. In: Marmot M, Wilkinson R (eds) Social determinants of health. Oxford University Press, Oxford

Buchi S, Sensky T, Allard S et al 1998 Sense of coherence: a protective factor for depression in rheumatoid arthritis. Journal of Rheumatology 25:869–875

Chandola T, Sigerist J, Marmot M 2005 Do changes in effort-reward imbalance at work contribute to an explanation of the social gradient in angina? Occupational and Environmental Medicine 62:223–230

Chandola T, Brunner E, Marmot M 2006 Chronic stress at work and the metabolic symdrome: prospective study. British Medical Journal 332:521–525

Creed F 1981 Life events and appendicitis. Lancet i:1381–385

Cummins S, Stafford M, Macintyre S et al 2005 Neighbourhood environment and its association with self-rated health: evidence from Scotland and England. Journal of Epidemiology and Community Health 59:207–213

Federal, Provincial and Territorial Advisory Committee on Population Health. Strategies for Population Health: Investing in the Health of Canadians. Ottawa: Minister of Supply and Services Canada, 1994

Fitzpatrick R, Newman S, Archer R, Shipley M 1991 Social support, disability and depression: a longitudinal study of arthritis and depression. Social Science and Medicine 33: 605–611

Glanz K, Maskarinec G, Carlin L 2005 Ethnicity, sense of coherence and tobacco use among adolescents. Annals of Behavioral Medicine 29:192–199

Gove W 1979 Sex, marital status and mortality. American Journal of Sociology 79:45–67

Hallqvist J, Diderichsen F, Theorell Y et al and the SHEEP study 1998 Is the effect of job strain on myocardial infarction due to interaction between high psychological demands and low decision latitude. Results from the Sweden Heart Epidemiology Program. Social Science and Medicine 46:1405–1415

Halpern D 1995 Mental health and the built environment. More than bricks and mortar? Taylor and Francis, London

Hemingway H, Shipley M, Brunner E et al 2005 Does autonomic function link social position to coronary risk? The Whitehall II Study. Circulation 111:3071–3077

Jarvis M, Wardle J 1999 Social patterning of health behaviours: the case of cigarette smoking. In: Marmot M, Wilkinson R (eds) Social determinants of health. Oxford University Press, Oxford

Jin RL, Shah CP, Sroboda TJ 1996 The impact of unemployment on health: a review of the evidence. Canadian Medical Association Journal 153:529–540

Kanner A, Coyne J, Schaefer C, Lazarus R 1981 Comparison of two modes of stress measurement: daily hassles and uplifts versus major life events. Journal of Behavioural Medicine 4:1–39

Kaplan G, Wilson T, Cohen R et al 1994 Social functioning and overall mortality: prospective evidence from the Kuopio ischemic heart disease risk factor study. Epidemiology 5:495–500

Kawachi I, Kennedy P 1997 Health and social cohesion: why care about income inequality? British Medical Journal 314:1037–1041

Kawachi I, Berkman L 2000 Social cohesion, social capital and health. In: Berkman L, Kawachi I (eds) Social epidemiology. Oxford University Press, New York

Kawachi I, Colditz G, Ascherio A 1996 A prospective study of social networks in relation to toal mortality and cardiovascular disease in men in the USA. Journal of Epidemiology and Community Health 50:245–251

Kawachi I, Kennedy P, Lochner K 1997 Social capital, income inequality and mortality. American Journal of Public Health 87:1491–1499

Kawachi I, Kennedy P, Glass R 1999 Social capital and self-rated health: a contextual analysis. American Journal of Public Health 89:1187–1194

Kroenke C, Kubzansky L, Schernhammer E et al 2006 Social networks, social supprt and survival after breast cancer diagnosis. Journal of Clinical Oncology 24:1105–1111

Kumari M, Marmot M, Rumley A, Lowe G 2005 Social, behavioural and metabolic determinants of plasma viscosity in the Whitehall II Study. Annals of Epidemiology 15:398–404

Kuper H, Marmot M 2003 Job strain, job demands, decision latitude and risk of coronary heart disease within the Whitehall II study. Journal of Epidemiology and Community Medicine 57:147–153

Labonte R 1993 Health Promotion and Empowerment: Practice Frameworks. Centre for Health Promotion, University of Toronto. Issues in Health Promotion no. 3

Lindfors P, Lundberg O, Lundberg U 2005 Sense of coherence and biomarkers of health in 43-year-old women. International Journal of Behavioural Medicine 12:98–102

Lyyra TM, Heikkinen RL 2006 Perceived social support and mortality in older people. Journal of Gerontology 61:S147–S152

MacIntyre S, MacIver S, Soomans A 1993 Area, class and health: should we be focusing on places or people? Journal of Social Policy 22:213–234

Marmot M, Madge N 1987 An epidemiological perspective on stress and health. In: Kasl S, Cooper C (eds) Stress and health: issues in research methodology. Wiley, Winchester

Marmot M, Theorell T 1988 Social class and cardiovascular disease: the contribution of work. International Journal of Health Services 18:37–45

Marmot M, Syme L, Kagan A 1975 Epidemiological studies of heart disease and stroke in Japanese men living in Japan, Hawaii and California. Prevalence of coronary and hypertensive disease and associated risk factors. Americal Journal of Epidemiology 102:514–525

Marmot M, Siegrist J, Theorell T, Feeny A 1999 Health and the psychosocial environment at work. In: Marmot R, Wilkinson R (eds) Social determinants of health. Oxford University Press, Oxford

Mausner J, Kramer S 1985 Epidemiology: an introductory text. W.B. Saunders, Philadelphia

McKee-Ryan F, Song Z, Wanberg C, Kinicki A 2005 Psychological and physical well-being during unemployment: A meta-analytic study. Journal of Applied Psychology 90:53–76

35

Montgomery S, Cook D, Bartley M, Wadsworth M 1999 Unemployment in young men predates symptoms of depression and anxiety resulting in medical consultation. International Journal of Epidemiology 28:95–100

Morgan M 1980 Marital status, health, illness and service use. Social Science and Medicine 14A:633–643

Najman J 1980 Theories of disease causation and the concept of general susceptibility: a review. Social Science and Medicine 14A:231–237

Nettleton S, Burrows B 1998 Mortgage debt, insecure home ownership and health: an exploratory analysis. Social Science & Illness 20:731–753

Nicholson A, Fuhrer R, Marmot M 2005 Psychological distress as a predictor of CHD events in men: the effect of persistence and components of risk. Psychosomatic Medicine 67:522–530

Ostberg V, Lennartson C 2007 Getting by with a little help: the importance of various types of social support for health problems. Scandinavian Journal of Public Health 35:197–204

Parkes C, Benjamin B, Fitzgerald R 1969 Broken heart: a statistical survey of increased mortality among widowers. British Medical Journal 1:740–744

Patrick D, Morgan M, Charlton J 1986 Psychosocial support and change in the health status of physically disabled people. Social Science and Medicine 22:1347–1354

Patterson J, Eberly L, Ding Y, Hargreaves M 2004 Associations of smoking prevalence with individual and area level social cohesion. Journal of Epidemiology and Community Health 58:692–697

Pinquart M, Hoffken K, Silbereisen R, Wedding U 2007 Social support and survival in patients with acute myeloid leukaemia. Care in Cancer 15:81–87

Poppius E, Virkkunen H, Hakama M, Tenkanen L 2006 The sense of coherence and the incidence of cancer – role of follow-up time and age at baseline. Journal of Psychosomatic Research 61:205–211

Raphael D 2006 Social determinants of health: present status, unanswered questions and future directions. International Journal of Health Services 36:651–677

Reine I, Novo M, Mammarstrom A 2004 Does the association between health and unemployment differ between young people and adults? Results from a 14 year follow-up study with a focus on psychological health and smoking. Public Health 118:337–345

Richardson C, Ratner P 2005 Sense of coherence as a moderator of the effects of stressful life events on health. Journal of Epidemiology and Community Health 59:979–984

Royce R, Sena A, Cates W, Cohen M 1997 Sexual transmission of HIV. New England Journal of Medicine 336:1072–1078

Siegrist J, Peter R, Junge A et al 1990 Low status control, high effort at work and ischemic heart disease: prospective evidence from blue collar men. Social Science and Medicine 31:1127–1134

Stafford M, Marmot M 2003 Neighbourhood deprivation and health: does it affect us all equally? International Journal of Epidemiology 32:357–366

Stansfield S 1999 Social support and social cohesion. In: Marmot M, Wilkinson R (eds) Social determinants of health. Oxford University Press, Oxford

Steptoe A, Kunz-Ebrecht S, Owen N et al 2003a Influence of socioeconomic status and job control on plasma fibrinogen responses to acute mental stress. Psychosomatic Medicine 65:137–144

Steptoe A, Kunz-Ebrecht S, Owen N et al 2003b Socioeconomic status and stress-related biological responses over the working day. Psychosomatic Medicine 65:461–470

Steptoe A, Sigerist J, Kirschbaum C, Marmot M 2004 Effort-reward imbalance, overcommitment and measures of cortisol and blood pressure over the working day. Psychosomatic Medicine 66:323–329

Surtees P, Wainwright N, Luben R et al 2006 Mastery, sense of coherence and mortality: evidence of independent associations from the EPIC-Norfolk Prospective Cohort Study. Health Psychology 25:102–110

Syme S 1986 Social determinants of health and disease. In: Last J (ed) Public health and preventative medicine. Appleton-Century-Crofts, Norwalk CT

Syme S, Hyman M, Enterline P 1964 Some social and cultural factors associated with the occurrence of coronary heart disease. Journal of Chronic Diseases 17:277–289

Thomas C, Benzeval M, Stansfeld S 2005 Employment transitions and mental health: an analysis from the British household panel survey. Journal of Epidemiology and Community Health 59:243–249

Thong M, Kaptein A, Krediet R et al 2007 Social support predicts survival in dialysis patients. Nephrology Dialysis Transplantation 22:845–850

Turner JB 1995 Economic context and the impact of unemployment. Journal of Health and Social Behaviour 35:213–219

Vogt T, Mullooly J, Ernst D et al 1992 Social networks as predictors of ischemic heart disease, cancer, stroke and hypertension: incidence, survival and mortality. Journal of Clinical Epidemiology 45:659–666

Wilkinson R 1996 Unhealthy societies: from inequality to well-being. Routledge, London

Wilkinson R, Marmot M (eds) 1998 Social determinants of health: the solid facts. WHO Regional Office for Europe

Williams R, Barefoot J, Califf R 1992 Prognostic importance of social and economic resources among medically treated patients with angiographically documented coronary heart disease. JAMA 267:520–524

Social factors in medical practice

CHAPTER

3

Health and illness behaviour

Graham Scambler

Definitions of 'health' and 'illness' vary within cultures, subcultures and communities, and even within households – between generations for example. There can also be gaps between lay and medical concepts. The primary focus of this chapter is on lay beliefs about, and attitudes towards, health and illness, and on the various ways in which these, together with a host of other social factors, can influence people's behaviour when faced with what they perceive to be threats to their well-being.

Consideration is given first to differences in people's perspectives on health and illness. A brief review is then given of studies of the prevalence of illness and disease in the community. Special attention is paid to those factors known to influence help-seeking behaviour, and especially to those known to affect whether or not people who define themselves as ill consult a physician, usually a general practitioner. Finally, self-help and sources of help other than allopathic medicine are considered, ranging from informal lay networks to alternative therapies.

PERCEPTIONS OF HEALTH AND ILLNESS

The modern study of how lay people define health and illness was pioneered by Herzlich (1973) with her research with 80, largely middle-class, adults in France. She identified three different metaphors to describe the way people talked about health and illness:

● *Illness as destroyer*, involving loss, isolation and incapacity;

● *Illness as liberator*, referring to a lessening of burdens;

● *Illness as occupation*, meaning freedom from responsibility, excepting the need to combat the disease.

Analysing their accounts of health and illness, she found that illness was generally perceived as external and as a product of a way of life, notably urban life. This covered not merely pathological agents such as germs, but also accidents and diseases like cancer and various mental disorders. Health, on the other hand, was perceived as internal to the individual, with three different and discernible dimensions: (1) an absence of illness ('health in a vacuum'); (2) a 'reserve of health', determined by constitution and temperament; and (3) a positive state of well-being or 'equilibrium'.

Several studies in Britain have since led to similar distinctions. Pill & Scott (1982) interviewed mothers from working-class backgrounds with young children. They encountered definitions of health in terms of the absence of illness. A functional definition of health was also common, that is, in terms of the capacity to perform or cope with normal roles. As in Herzlich's study, a positive definition of health was apparent as well, although among Pill & Scott's sample it was associated with being cheerful and enthusiastic rather than with a state of equilibrium.

Such a positive dimension was missing, however, from the accounts of mothers and daughters in socially disadvantaged families questioned by Blaxter & Paterson (1982). References were made to health as the absence of illness, but the majority seemed to have a functional definition of health. They also had a functional definition of illness, many of them distinguishing between normal illness, which they accommodated, and serious illness, like cancer, heart disease and tuberculosis, which called for radical adjustment and change. These conceptions of health and illness, especially the lack of a positive definition of health, clearly reflected the high prevalence of health problems among the sample.

Reviewing these and other studies, Blaxter (1990) writes: 'Health can be defined negatively as the absence of illness, functionally, as the ability to cope with everyday activities, or positively, as fitness and well-being'. She adds that health also has moral connotations, which are as salient in modern urban communities as they were among pre-modern or primitive societies. There is a sense in which people feel a duty to be healthy and experience illness as failure. Health can be seen in terms of will-power, self-discipline and self-control.

Increasingly relevant too, it might be added, is an emphasis on what has been called 'body maintenance'. This is linked to innovative forms of entrepreneurial activity and to 'consumerism' (see Chapter 12). The body becomes a site of pleasure and a representation of happiness and success. As Nettleton (1995) puts it, 'to look good is to feel good'. Health education echoes the commercialization of body maintenance. Thus, Featherstone (1991) argues that common to the media treatment of body maintenance and to health education is the 'encouragement of self-surveillance of bodily health and appearance as well as the incentive of lifestyle benefits'. He goes on to refer to the 'transvaluation' of activities like jogging and slimming, which have been re-evaluated in light of their putative health benefits. The most conspicuous example of the commercialization of healthy life-styles is probably the 'fitness industry', its products ranging from exercise machines and videos to special stylish clothing.

Monaghan (2001) takes this line further to consider what he calls the 'vibrant pleasures'. He too argues that only recently has the body been linked to health as opposed to illness. In his ethnographic study of bodybuilding, he emphasizes the importance to participants of 'looking good' and 'feeling good'. As one interviewee put it: 'It's all to do with looks, and I would rather look good on the outside. That's what bodybuilding is. It's not for fitness reasons, it's all visual'. Monaghan maintains that 'a crucial point of overlap between 'risk-inducing' bodybuilders and 'health conscious' fitness enthusiasts more generally (e.g. weight-trainers, joggers, participants in step aerobics) is a shared attempt to embody and display a sense of empowerment and self-mastery'. It is simplistic to stereotype bodybuilding as injurious to health and as intimately associated with drug use. Rather, 'embodied pleasures', epitomized in the gym by 'the rush', and the perceived psychosocial benefits of anaerobic exercise, together with the imagery of muscle, are more directly relevant in sustaining people's consumption of (risky) bodybuilding technologies.

Finally, an interesting and important general distinction is drawn by Bury (2005) between 'health as an attribute' and 'health as a relation'. The notion of health as an attribute is associated with the medical profession. Doctors tend to make the assumption that illness or disease is a property or attribute of the individual, an 'it' which a person has or harbours. The idea of health as a relation, on the other hand, is typically associated with lay thinking. The focus here is not on the biological determinants at work in the individual's body, but on the social or psychosocial forces that influence the pattern and expression of illness. This can be understood in two ways, either in terms of the 'social creation' of patterns of illness through inequalities or environmental factors; or in terms of the 'social production' of illness in individuals through the 'contingencies and negotiations that surround its identification, naming and treatment'.

Bury is careful to point out that it is not in fact always accurate to associate an attributional perspective with doctors and a relational perspective with lay people. He considers the case of osteoarthritis, a common disorder in later life, involving progressive deteriorioation in the joints of the body, especially the hips. As this disorder is linked with age, people often discount the aches and pains which accompany it as features of the ageing process itself, treating them as 'normal', or at least trying to do so (Sanders et al 2002). One result is that the reporting of such symptoms is highly variable. At the same time the fit between symptoms and degree of disease progression is often difficult for doctors to judge. Patients with low levels of pain may have severely affected joints, and people in considerable pain may not show signs of physical changes. When and how to intervene thus becomes a matter for negotiation. So the medical model cannot easily operate within an entirely attributional perspective. Similarly, a relational view of health is not always characteristic of lay thinking. An attributional perspective has become attractive over recent years to some lay people, especially in the context of contentious disorders. Disorders like Myalgic Encephalomyelitis (ME) or Chronic Fatigue Syndrome (CFS) and Gulf War Syndrome are examples. In such cases it is people as would-be patients who are claiming that illness results from an underlying biological attribute and doctors who are warning against the 'medicalization' of 'non-diseases'. Bury suggests that ways of seeing and dealing with health and illness should be recognized as dynamic.

ILLNESS AND DISEASE IN THE COMMUNITY

The national 'Health and lifestyles' survey (Blaxter 1990) found that 71% of participants defined their health as at least 'good'. This did not mean that none of these people had symptoms of illness or, indeed, medically defined disease. For example, many disabled and/or elderly people defined their health as 'excellent', clearly meaning 'my health is excellent despite my disability/considering my advanced years'. Comparisons were made between participants' own assessments of their health and a series of objective measures. Although there was a general correspondence between the two, most obviously at the extremes, 10% of men and 7% of women in the top category of health, objectively measured, described their health as only 'fair' or 'poor'; and as many as 40% of those with undoubted health problems, objectively measured, described their health as 'good' or 'excellent'.

More recent data from the 2001 Census indicate that 91% of people in private households in England and Wales reported 'good/fairly good' health (Office for National

Statistics 2006). The age-standardized rates (all ages) of 'good/fairly good' health were similar for men and women. Children aged under 16 were reported as having the best health, with 99% having 'good/fairly good' health. For those aged 16 and over, the age-specific rates of 'good/fairly good' health declined with age. The least healthy section of the population comprised people aged 75 and over, 72% of whom said they were in 'good/fairly good' health. Predictably, there were substantial variations in reported health status by socio-economic group (see Chapter 8).

The overall proportion of people reporting a long-term illness or disability that restricted their activities was 18% (Office for National Statistics 2006). The age-standardized rates were again similar for men (16%) and women (15%). In general, the rates increased with age, first slowly and then sharply from the age of 45, further accelerating in later life. The level was lowest in children aged under 5 (3%), and highest for people aged 90 and over (75%). There was once more an association with socio-economic group.

Interestingly, the findings of a recent Swedish study of self-rated health suggested a strong relation between poor self-rated health and mortality in all the subgroups investigated, greater at younger ages, and similar among men and women and among people with and without chronic illness. The authors put forward the idea that self-rated health might be a useful outcome measure (Burstrom & Fredlund 2001).

The rate of reporting of individual symptoms of illness is high. The findings by Wadsworth et al (1971) remain typical of retrospective studies in this area. Of their sample of 1000 adults, 95% had experienced symptoms in the 14 days prior to interview and only one in five had consulted a doctor. In a prospective study (Scambler et al 1981) a sample of women aged 16–44 years kept 6-week health diaries in which they recorded any disturbances in their health. Symptoms were recorded on an average of one day in three. Table 3.1 shows the 10 most frequently recorded symptoms and also how often these precipitated medical consultations and the ratio of medical consultations to symptom episodes. Overall, there was one medical consultation for every 18 symptom episodes.

It might be thought that most symptoms not precipitating consultations are mild and not indicative of disease requiring medical intervention. Ingham & Miller (1979) found that symptom severity for seven selected symptoms was indeed greater in consulters than in non-consulters. There is convincing evidence, however, that general practitioners are often not consulted for disease that would undoubtedly respond to treatment. Epsom (1978) carried out a seminal investigation of the health status of a sample of adults using a mobile health clinic. Of the 3160 people investigated, 57% were referred to their general practitioners for further tests and possible treatment. Major diseases detected included seven instances of preinvasive cervical cancer, one confirmed case of carcinoma of the breast and one active case of pulmonary tuberculosis. A follow-up study of those referred to their general practitioners indicated that 38% of the findings had not previously been known to the general practitioners and that 22% of the findings made known to the general practitioners for the first time were judged serious enough to warrant hospital referrals. Thus a significant clinical iceberg exists: the professional health services treat only the tip of the sum total of ill health.

The existence of a clinical iceberg has important implications. Most obviously there is the problem of unmet need: many people of all ages are enduring avoidable pain, discomfort and handicap. There is a gap in other words between the need for and the demand for health care. It must be remembered, however, that any substantial increase in the existing level of demand would swamp the primary care services. Many general practitioners also argue that there is currently a widespread tendency for people to consult for trivial, unnecessary or inappropriate reasons: in one national study, one-quarter of the general practitioners questioned felt that half or more of their surgery consultations fell into this

| TABLE 3.1 | Symptom episodes and medical consultations recorded in health diaries |||||

Main types of symptom recorded	No. of symptom episodes	Percentage of total number of symptom episodes	Mean length of symptom episodes (days)	No. of occasions on which symptom episode precipitated medical consultation	Ratio of consultations to symptom episodes
Headache	180	20.9	1.3	3	1:60
Changes in energy, tiredness	109	12.6	1.4	0	–
Nerves, depression or irritability	74	8.6	1.7	1	1:74
Aches or pains in joints, muscles, legs or arms	71	8.2	1.6	4	1:18
Women's complaints like period pain[a]	69	8.0	1.7	7	1:10
Stomach aches or pains	45	5.2	1.5	4	1:11
Backache	38	4.4	1.6	1	1:38
Cold, flu, or running nose	37	4.3	4.1	3	1:12
Sore throat	36	4.2	2.4	4	1:9
Sleeplessness	31	3.6	1.5	1	1:31
Others	173	20.0	1.9	21	1:8
Total	863	100.0	1.7	49	1:18

Reproduced with permission from Scambler et al (1981).
[a] Stomach aches and pains and backache were classified as period pains if so defined by the women themselves.

45

category (Cartwright & Anderson 1981). Basic to these issues, of course, is the question of how to define 'need'.

UNDERSTANDING ILLNESS BEHAVIOUR

A number of studies have documented the sociodemographic characteristics of users and non-users of medical services. It is known, for example, that women consult more than men, children and the elderly more than young adults and the middle-aged. Social class, ethnic origin, marital status and family size are other factors that have been shown to be related to utilization. These studies tell us who does and does not make use of the services, rather than why. To begin to answer the more complex question of why people seek or decline to seek professional help is to begin to theorize about what is conventionally referred to as illness behaviour. According to Quah (2002), however, the term illness behaviour is outmoded. She distinguishes between three aspects or dimensions:

- *preventive behaviour*, referring to activity undertaken for the purpose of preventing illness;

- *illness behaviour*, denoting the activity of a person who is ill in order to define the illness and seek a solution;

- *sick role behaviour*, or the formal response to symptoms, including the seeking of formal help and subsequent action of a person as a patient.

Blaxter (2004) adds that preventive behaviour and health-promoting behaviour are also sometimes distinguished. Preventive acts may include the use of specific services such as immunization, dental care or breast self-examination (health viewed 'within a model of not-diseased'). Health-promoting acts, on the other hand, refer to lifestyle habits like exercising, eating healthily (health viewed positively or holistically).

It is crucial to recognize that whether or not people consult their doctors does not depend only on the presence of disease, but also on how they, or others, respond to its symptoms. Mechanic (1978) has listed 10 variables known to influence consulting behaviour (Box 3.1). Mechanic acknowledges that this list is far from exhaustive and that, in reality, different variables tend to interact together. He also introduces a basic underlying distinction between 'self-defined' and 'other-defined' illness: the major difference is that, in the latter, individuals tend to resist the definitions that others attempt to impose upon them, and it might be necessary to bring them into treatment under great pressure, even involuntarily. As it is not possible to explore all the multifarious and interrelated influences on illness and consulting behaviour here, six broad categories have been selected for emphasis.

Cultural variation

The significance of cultural factors in determining how symptoms are interpreted has been well documented, perhaps most convincingly in studies of ethnicity and the experience and reporting of pain. In a pioneering study conducted in New York, Zborowski (1952) found that patients of Old-American or Irish origin displayed a stoical, matter-of-fact attitude towards pain and, if it was intense, a tendency to withdraw from the company of

---

BOX 3.1   Mechanic's variables known to influence illness behaviour

1. Visibility, recognizability or perceptual salience of signs and symptoms
2. The extent to which the symptoms are perceived as serious (that is, the person's estimate of the present and future probabilities of danger)
3. The extent to which symptoms disrupt family, work and other social activities
4. The frequency of the appearance of the signs or symptoms, their persistence, or their frequency or recurrence
5. The tolerance threshold of those who are exposed to and evaluate the signs and symptoms
6. Available information, knowledge and cultural assumptions and understandings of the evaluator
7. Basic needs that lead to denial
8. Needs competing with illness responses
9. Competing possible interpretations that can be assigned to the symptoms once they are recognized
10. Availability of treatment resources, physical proximity, and psychological and monetary costs of taking action (not only physical distance and costs of time, money and effort, but also such costs as stigma, social distance and feelings of humiliation)

Reproduced with permission of The Free Press from Mechanic (1978).

others. In contrast, patients of Italian or Jewish background were more demanding and dependent and tended to seek, rather than shun, public sympathy. Subsequent research has both corroborated Zborowski's findings and afforded support for the more general view that there is a marked cultural difference in the interpretation of and response to symptoms between so-called Anglo-Saxon and Mediterranean groups. It is tempting to assume that such cultural variation is explicable in terms of socialization alone, namely that differences in illness behaviour merely reflect different culturally learned styles of coping with the world at large. The authors of a study of Anglo-Saxon, Anglo-Greek and Greek groups in Australia, however, have suggested that other factors might also be important. They found, for example, that immigrant status and, relatedly, the stress of adapting to a majority culture, played a significant part in accounting for the different patterns of illness behaviour among the Anglo-Saxon and Mediterranean groups (Pilowski & Spence 1977). In short, cultural patterns might vary, depending on the social context.

■ Symptoms and knowledge of disease

Studies have indicated that symptoms that present in a 'striking' way, for example, a sharp abdominal pain or a high fever, are more likely to be interpreted as illness and to receive prompt medical attention than those that present less dramatically. Consultation in such circumstances might simply be a function of the pain or discomfort; alternatively, it might be a function of the degree of incapacitation or disruption engendered by the pain or discomfort (see 'Triggers' below). Many distressing symptoms are not indicative of serious disease; but, equally, some serious diseases, for example some cancers, rarely appear in a striking fashion: their onset can be slow and insidious. The actions of potential patients are thus also dependent on their knowledge of disease and on their capacity to differentiate between diseases that are threatening/non-threatening and that can/cannot be effectively treated.

A study by Corner and colleagues (2006) of the experiencee of health changes and reasons for delay in seeking care prior to a diagnosis of lung cancer is pertinent here. They found that individuals, regardless of the disease stage or their social background, failed to recognize symptoms they experienceed over many months prior to their eventual diagnosis as serious or warranting attention. Even when severe, symptoms were often attributed to everyday causes and not as indicative of ill health. There was a discernible reluctance to seek help for symptoms among some because they were unsure whether what they were experiencing was normal or not.

■ Triggers

Although many of the symptoms people experience are recognized as indicating disease processes, it is not necessarily the case that treatment is sought. What, when and if action to resolve any problems is undertaken often depends on a number of other factors. Zola (1973) has looked at the timing of decisions to seek medical care. He found that most people tolerated their symptoms for quite a time before they went to a doctor, and that the symptoms themselves were often not sufficient to precipitate a consultation: something else had to happen to bring this about. He identified five types of trigger:

1. the occurrence of an interpersonal crisis (e.g. a death in the family)

2. perceived interference with social or personal relations

3. 'sanctioning' (pressure from others to consult)

4. perceived interference with vocational or physical activity

5. a kind of 'temporalizing of symptomatology' (the setting of a deadline, e.g. 'If I feel the same way on Monday...', or 'If I have another turn...').

The decision to seek professional help is, then, very much bound up with an individual's personal and social circumstances. Zola also found that, when doctors paid insufficient attention to the specific trigger that prompted an individual or that an individual used as an excuse to seek help, there was a greater chance that the patient would eventually break off treatment.

■ Perceptions of costs and benefits

Doctors and other healthcare personnel tend to assume that a rational individual will report any symptoms that are causing him or her distress or anxiety; in other words, they take it for granted that the restoration of 'good health' is a natural first priority. Good health, however, is one goal among others; it is not always supreme. At any given time a person might deem obtaining treatment, which might involve hospitalization, to be less important or urgent than, for example, looking after young children or a dependent mother at home, preparing for an examination, being at work or going on holiday. Thus the value an individual attaches to good health varies in accordance with his or her perception of the benefits versus the costs of its accomplishment. The 'health belief model' represents one sustained attempt to bring together all those factors – from the demographic to the psychological – that influence an individual's assessment of the costs and benefits involved in seeking help.

■ Lay referral and intervention

It is comparatively rare for someone to decide in favour of a visit to the surgery without first discussing his or her symptoms with others. Scambler et al (1981) found that three-quarters of those participating in their study discussed their symptoms with some other person, usually a relative, before seeking professional help. Freidson (1970) has claimed that, just as doctors have a professional referral system, so potential patients have lay referral systems: 'the whole process of seeking help involves a network of potential consultants from the intimate confines of the nuclear family through successively more select, distant and authoritative laymen until the 'professional' is reached'. Freidson has himself produced a model in terms of: (1) the degree of congruence between the subculture of the potential patient and that of doctors; and (2) the relative number of lay consultants interposed between the initial perception of symptoms and the decision whether or not to go to the doctor. Thus, for example, a situation in which the potential patient participates in a subculture that differs from that of doctors and in which there is an extended lay referral system would lead to the 'lowest' rate of utilization of medical services. In line with this example, one Scottish study reported that a high degree of interaction with interlocking kinship and friendship networks might well have 'inhibited' women in social class V from using antenatal care services (McKinlay 1973).

Occasionally, lay persons might take it upon themselves to intervene and to initiate medical consultations (see Mechanic's other-defined illness, above). This is most common when symptoms are perceived to be serious or life-threatening or when the sufferer is temporarily incapable of self-help: parents might take action on behalf of a child, a wife on behalf of a husband who is psychotic or who has experienced a tonic–clonic seizure.

Scambler (1989) found that four out of five first consultations for epilepsy were other-initiated, many of them involving the calling of an ambulance. It has been suggested, however, that lay persons who are not members of the sufferer's family might be less likely than those who are to tolerate delays in help-seeking resulting from the normalization or denial of symptoms. Finlayson & McEwen (1977), for example, have described how the wives of some men tried in vain to persuade their husbands to see a doctor in the hour preceding myocardial infarction.

Access to healthcare facilities

Ease of access to healthcare facilities has obvious implications for usage. Tudor-Hart (1971) has argued that what he terms an 'inverse care law' applies in Britain; that is, the provision of health care is inversely related to the need for it (i.e. poor facilities in depressed areas characterized by high morbidity and good, or better, facilities in affluent areas characterized by low morbidity). He relates this to the market economy: the more prosperous areas attract the most resources, including skilled health workers, in both primary and secondary care. The degree of equity of access to healthcare services is in fact not easy to determine (Goddard & Smith 2001). In one recent study of the coverage of minor surgery, child health surveillance and chronic disease management for asthma and diabetes in relation to both population need and to key organizational features of general practice in the 481 primary care groups (PCGs) in England, the authors found little evidence of poorer service availability for PCGs with higher population need; but they did find evidence that the inverse care law might be geographically specific, and particularly pronounced for London PCGs (Baker & Hann 2001). It has often been shown that, as the distance between home and general practice increases, the likelihood of consultation diminishes; this is particularly true for elderly or disabled people, who are relatively immobile (Whitehead 1992).

SELF-CARE, SELF-HELP AND ALTERNATIVE THERAPY

The fact that only a small minority of all symptoms are presented to a doctor suggests that self-care, and especially self-medication, could be of considerable importance. Wadsworth et al (1971) found that self-treatment with non-prescribed medicines and home remedies is indeed extremely common. Dunnell & Cartwright (1972) found lower consultation rates among people who reported self-medication. They also found that in a 2-week period the ratio of non-prescribed to prescribed medicines taken by adults was approximately two to one; 67% of their sample had taken one or more non-prescribed medicines during this period. Moreover, only one in 10 of the non-prescribed medicines consumed had been first suggested by a doctor; most were recommended by members of lay referral systems. The data suggested that adults tended to use self-medication as an alternative to medical consultation. Anderson et al (1977) provide support for this interpretation, but add that whereas self-medication seems to be more popular among non-users than among users of the primary-care services, non-users are also less inclined than users to obtain medical help for potentially serious symptoms. Dunnell & Cartwright (1972) found that, for children, self- or parent-medication seemed to be used more as a supplement to medical consultation.

A more recent survey in the UK found that in response to minor ailments in the previous two weeks, over a quarter of adults had used an over-the-counter medicine, while 14% had used a prescription medicine already in the house (British Market Research Bureau 1997). The types of problems treated in this way included headaches, athlete's

49

foot, dandruff, heartburn, migraine, vaginal candidiasis and period pains. According to Stevenson and her colleagues (2003), doctors do not ask patients about the use of over-the-counter medicine, and patients do not tell them.

Of particular interest too is the rapid growth of self-help groups. Some, like Alcoholics Anonymous, have been established for a long time and are well known, but there are many newer and less well-known groups – for people with schizophrenia, skin diseases, depression, hypertension, cancer, the parents of handicapped children, victims of disasters, and so on. Some of these were the brainchildren of health workers who are still active within them, but many operate quite independently of the formal health services; in fact, the impetus for the formation of a number of groups has been the lack of adequate understanding, care, treatment or support from the various health professions. Some commentators regard self-help groups as a poor substitute for people who are starved of 'real' services. Others, like Robinson (1980), argue that 'it is the professional health services which should be seen as specific technical, organizational or expert assistance'; they contend that self-help should be regarded as one of the basic components of primary health care.

Kelleher (1994) notes that although many of the activities of self-help groups can be seen as complementary to the work of health professionals, some also reflect 'a subversive readiness to question the knowledge of doctors and to assert that experiential knowledge has value'. Developing this theme, he suggests that self-help groups might constitute a new social movement. His argument is that modern medicine, like other 'expert systems', has become increasingly limited in its capacity to comprehend human suffering and to engage with patients; it pays far too little attention, for example, to how people with chronic illnesses define their own situations experientially and 'cope' on an everyday basis. Self-help groups, whether or not they comprise a social movement, allow people to diverge from the medical perspective and, if necessary, to challenge and interrogate it. Kelleher (2001) has also argued that some self-help groups at least afford participants a genuine opportunity to construct their own personal and/or joint narratives, thereby 're-socializing people to see themselves as normal people with diabetes/epilepsy/schizophrenia'.

Apart from simply ignoring symptoms, another alternative to consulting a doctor or pursuing some form of self-care or self-help is to rely on complementary and alternative medicine (CAM). Fulder (2005) identifies the following common features of CAM:

- the notion that self-healing is paramount;

- working with, not against, symptoms;

- individuality;

- integration of human facets ('holism');

- no fixed beginning or ending;

- conformity to universal principles, such as Ch'i in Chinese medicine.

In her comprehensive study of medicines in society, Britten (in press) maintains that self-care and self-help and CAM make up what sociologists call the lifeworld. Thomas et al (1991) estimated that in 1987 there were 1909 registered, non-medical practitioners of non-orthodox health care, that is, of acupuncture, chiropractic, homoeopathy, medical herbalism, naturopathy and osteopathy, working in Britain (Table 3.2). The same authors report that of the 70 600 patients seen by this group of practitioners in an average week, 78% were attending for musculoskeletal problems. About 36% of the patients had not received previous medical care for their main problem; 18% were receiving concurrent non-orthodox and medical care.

TABLE 3.2	Main treatments and multiple treatments offered by registered non-orthodox practitioners (estimated numbers (%))			
Main treatment	Registered practitioners (%)		Practitioners in each group offering multiple treatments and having membership of only one association	
Acupuncture	507	27	100	20
Chiropractic	290	15	6	2
Homoeopathy	93	5	12	13
Medical herbalism	115	6	45	39
Naturopathy with osteopathy	128	7	41	32[a]
Osteopathy	680	36	34	5
Member of more than one association	96	5	–	
Total	1909	100	238	12

Reproduced with permission from Thomas et al (1991).
[a] Practitioners offering at least one treatment in addition to naturopathy and osteopathy.

CAM are growing much more rapidly than orthodox allopathic medicine. If non-registered practitioners offering therapies beyond those considered by Thomas and his colleagues are included, then it has been estimated that there are approximately 50 000 practitioners at work in the UK (that is, 60% more than the number of GPs) (Fulder 1996). A series of *Which?* surveys in Britain found that one in seven of the magazine's readers had used some form of alternative or complementary practice in 1986, one in four in 1992, and one in three in 1995; findings supported by regional studies funded by health authorities (Emslie et al 1996). Studies in other European countries and the USA reveal these British figures as fairly typical. Users are, it seems, more likely to be women, middle-aged, middle class and conscious of their health and of healthy living (Cant & Sharma 1999).

The increasing popularity of non-orthodox therapy might in part be a function of people's disillusionment with biomedicine. Practitioners themselves stress their longer consultations and a holistic orientation that concerns itself 'with complete wellness, not just symptomatology' (Bakx 1991). However, Saks (1994) cautions that although alternative therapists, like self-help groups, are now offering a real challenge to the mode of practice of orthodox medicine, there is little evidence as yet that the legitimacy of medical authority is being seriously undermined.

To summarize, it has been shown that very often the decision whether to consult a doctor is not simply a function of the degree of pain or disability associated with symptoms, or of their perceived seriousness. What Hannay (1980) has termed 'incongruous referral behaviour' is commonplace. The heterogeneous assembly of factors that are known to influence decisions about medical consultation has been indicated. It has been stressed too, however, that the study of illness behaviour is not concerned exclusively with whether or not people visit doctors. On the basis of anthropological work, Kleinman (1985) suggested that there are typically three major arenas of care in what he calls 'local health care systems': popular, folk and professional (Fig. 3.1).

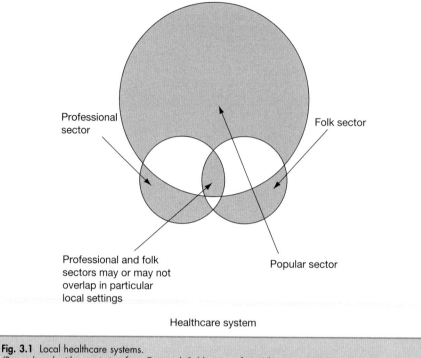

Fig. 3.1 Local healthcare systems.
(Reproduced with permission from Tavistock Publications from Kleinman 1985.)

Most health care takes place in the popular sector, which embraces self-care, including self-medication, and those self-help groups that function independently of professional health workers. The folk sector comprises non-professional 'specialists' who offer some form of alternative or non-orthodox therapy. Professionalization, Kleinman contends, has a tendency to distance practitioners from patients and to lead to a focus on (medically defined) disease as opposed to (patient defined) illness. Of the professional sector in western societies he writes: 'Western-oriented biomedicine seems to be the more extreme example of this trend, perhaps because biomedical ideology and norms are more remote from (one almost wants to say estranged from) the life world of most patients' (Kleinman 1985).

Scambler (2002) associates Kleinman's popular, folk and professional sectors of local healthcare systems with different and distinctive 'relations of healing' (Table 3.3). The popular sector, he suggests, is characterized by relations of caring. He makes the point that it remains largely women who assume day-to-day responsibility for looking after

TABLE 3.3	Sectors of local healthcare systems and their relations of healing (adapted from Scambler 2002)	
Sector		**Relations of healing**
Popular		Caring
Folk		Restoring
Professional		Fixing

those who are ill in this sector, not only those who are chronically or permanently ill but also children and partners who have mundane illnesses like flu. Arguably, the 'unpaid health work' done here underwrites the more specialist 'paid health work' on offer in the other sectors (see Chapters 9 and 16). The folk sector is characterized by relations of restoring, reflecting the holist philosophies that often underpin the endeavours of alternative or complementary practitioners. Finally, the professional sector gives rise to relations of fixing. The emphasis here is on the onus placed on doctors to treat disease within the confines of the 'sick role' (Chapter 4) so that people can resume their normal responsibilities as expeditiously as possible. Needless to say, this differentiation of relations of healing does not imply, for example, that doctors cannot or do not either care or restore, merely that Kleinman's sectors of local healthcare systems are distinguished in part by their own specific paradigms, modes or relations of healing.

Kleinman (1985) considers that the major challenge is to 're-work medicine's paradigm of clinical practice to make it more responsive to indigenous patient values, beliefs and expectations'. Agree or disagree, there is no question that the study of illness behaviour must address itself to the popular and folk as well as to the professional sectors of local healthcare systems.

References

Anderson J, Buck C, Danaher K, Fry J 1977 Users and non-users of doctors – implications for care. Journal of the Royal College of General Practitioners 27:155–159

Baker D, Hann M 2001 General practitioner services in primary care groups in England: is there equity between service availability and population need? Health and Place 7:67–74

Bakx K 1991 The 'eclipse' of folk medicine in Western society. Sociology, Health and Illness 13:20–57

Blaxter M 1990 Health and lifestyles. Tavistock/Routledge, London

Blaxter M 2004 Health. Polity, Cambridge

Blaxter M, Paterson E 1982 Mothers and daughters. Heinemann Educational, London

British Market Research Bureau 1997 Everyday Health Care: A Consumer Study of Self-Medication in Britain. British Market Research Bureau, London

Britten N Medicines and society: prescribing and medicine taking in their social context. Palgrave, London (in press)

Bury M 2005 Health and illness. Polity, Cambridge

Burstrom B, Fredland P 2001 Self rated health: is it as good a predictor of subsequent mortality among adults in lower as well as higher social classes? Journal of Epidemiology and Community Health 55:836–840

Cant S, Sharma U 1999 A new medical pluralism? Alternative medicine, doctors, patients and the state. UCL Press, London

Cartwright A, Anderson R 1981 General practice revisited: a second study of patients and their doctors. Tavistock, London

Corner J, Hopkinson J, Roffe L 2006 Experience of health changes and reasons for delay in seeking care: a UK study of the months prior to the diagnosis of lung cancer. Social Science and Medicine 62:1381–1391

Dunnell K, Cartwright A 1972 Medicine-takers. Prescribers and hoarders. Routledge & Kegan Paul, London

Emslie M, Campbell M, Walker K 1996 Complementary therapies in a local health care setting. Part 1: is there a public demand? Complementary Therapies in Medicine 4:39–42

Epsom J 1978 The mobile health clinic: a report on the first year's work. In: Tuckett D, Kauffert J (eds) Basic readings in medical sociology. Tavistock, London

Featherstone M 1991 The body in consumer culture. In: Featherstone M, Hepworth M. Turner B (eds) The body: social processes and cultural theory. Sage, London

Finlayson A, McEwen J 1977 Coronary heart disease and patterns of living. Croom Helm, London

Freidson E, 1970 Profession of medicine. Dodds Mead, New York

Fulder S 1996 The handbook of alternative and complementary medicine, 3rd edn. Oxford University Press, Oxford

Fulder S 2005 The basic concepts of alternative medicine and their impact on our views of health. In: Lee-Treweek G, Heller T, Spurr S et al (eds) Perspectives on complementary and alternative medicine: a reader. Routledge, London

Goddard M, Smith P 2001 Equity of access to health care services: theory and evidence from the UK. Social Science and Medicine 53:1149–1162

Hannay D 1980 The iceberg of illness and trivial consultations. Journal of the Royal College of General Practitioners 30:551–554

Herzlich C 1973 Health and illness. Academic Press, London

Ingham J, Miller P 1979 Symptom prevalence and severity in a general practice. Epidemiology and Community Health 33:191–198

Kelleher D 1994 Self-help groups and their relationship to medicine. In: Gabe J, Kelleher D, Williams G (eds) Challenging medicine. Routledge, London

Kelleher D 2001 New social movements in the health domain. In Scambler G (ed) Habermas, critical theory and health. Routledge, London

Kleinman A 1985 Indigenous systems of healing: questions for professional, popular and folk care. In: Salmon J (ed) Alternative medicines: popular and policy perspectives. Tavistock, London

McKinlay J 1973 Social networks, lay consultation and help-seeking behaviour. Social Forces 53:255–292

Mechanic D 1978 Medical sociology, 2nd edn. Free Press, New York

Monaghan L 2001 Looking good, feeling good: the embodied pleasures of vibrant physicality. Sociology of Health and Illness 23:330–356

Nettleton S 1995 The sociology of health and illness. Polity Press, Cambridge

Office for National Statistics (ONS) 2006 Health status – higher groups report best health. HMSO, London www.statistics.gov.uk (archived Jan 2006)

Pill R, Scott N 1982 Concepts of illness causation and responsibility: some preliminary data from a sample of working-class mothers. Social Science and Medicine 16:43–52

Pilowski I, Spence N 1977 Ethnicity and illness behaviour. Psychological Medicine 7:447–452

Robinson D 1980 The self-help component of primary care. Social Science and Medicine 14A:415–421

Saks M 1994 The alternatives to medicine. In: Gabe J, Kelleher D, Williams G (eds) Challenging medicine. Routledge, London

Sanders C, Donovan J, Dieppe P 2002 The significance and consequences of having painful and disabling joints in older age: co-existing accounts of normal and disrupted biographies. Sociology of Health and Illness 24:227–253

Scambler G 1989 Epilepsy. Routledge, London

Scambler G 2002 Health and social change: a critical theory. Open University Press, Buckingham

Scambler A, Scambler G, Craig D 1981 Kinship and friendship networks and women's demand for primary care. Journal of the Royal College of General Practitioners 26:746–750

Stevenson F, Britten N, Barry C et al 2003 Self-treatment and its discussion in medical consultations: how pluralism is managed in practice. Social Science and Medicine 57:513–527

Thomas K, Carr J, Westlake L, Williams B 1991 Use of non-orthodox and conventional health care in Great Britain. British Medical Journal 302:207–210

Tudor-Hart J 1971 The inverse care law. Lancet i:405–412

Wadsworth M, Butterfield W, Blaney R 1971 Health and sickness: the choice of treatment. Tavistock, London

Whitehead M 1992 The health divide, 2nd edn. Penguin, London

Zborowski M 1952 Cultural components in response to pain. Journal of Social Issues 8:16–30

Zola I 1973 Pathways to the doctor: from person to patient. Social Science and Medicine 7:677–889

54

CHAPTER

4

The doctor–patient relationship

Myfanwy Morgan

The essential unit of medical practice is the consultation between doctor and patient. Such meetings are a frequent and regular occurrence, with over half a million consultations occurring between general practitioners and their patients in the UK every working day and a large number also taking place at a hospital level. Their success or otherwise depends not only on the doctors' clinical knowledge and technical skills, but also on the nature of the social relationship that exists between doctor and patient.

This chapter first considers the doctor–patient relationship in historical terms, and identifies ways in which views of the causes of disease and diagnosis influence the nature of the medical task and relationship between doctor and patient. It then examines the societal expectations of doctors and patients and differing types of relationship that may occur in current medical practice and approaches to treatment decision-making.

HISTORICAL CHANGES IN DOCTOR–PATIENT RELATIONSHIPS

Historical changes in the nature of the doctor–patient relationship have been linked with changes in forms of medical knowledge that provide a frame of reference for medical activities and shape relationships with patients. Jewson (1976) identified three types of medical practice that were each associated with a particular type of relationship between doctor and patient in western Europe over the period 1770–1870. He referred to these as bedside medicine, hospital medicine and laboratory medicine. A major change since then with implications for the doctor–patient relationship is the practice of patient-centred medicine.

■ From bedside to laboratory medicine

Bedside medicine of the late eighteenth century was associated with the definition of disease in terms of its external and subjective manifestations rather than its internal and hidden causes. Diagnosis therefore involved extrapolation from patients' self-report of the course of the illness. Practitioners were also concerned with the functioning of the total bodily system rather than with a particular organ or tissue, and all aspects of the emotional and spiritual life of the patient were viewed as relevant. It was also believed that each individual had his own unique pattern of bodily events that the physician had to discern in each case. Emphasis was therefore given to achieving a personal rapport in the consultative relationship and the exchanges of confidences. This personal relationship was underpinned by the physician's situation as dependent on fees paid by a small number of patients (patrons) drawn from members of the ruling class. Physicians therefore gave considerable emphasis to pleasing their patients, who held a dominant position within a consultative relationship that was based on a personal empathy between the parties, and aimed to elicit and respond to the sick person's confidences and subjective experience of their symptoms.

A dramatic transformation of medical knowledge occurred in the first four decades of the nineteenth century and led to what Jewson termed 'hospital medicine'. This involved the beginnings of a centralized approach to medicine and development of professional consensus regarding diagnosis and therapy. These activities were based on greater pathological knowledge, with diagnosis being based on physical examination of observable structures through the use of stethoscopes and other ways of viewing the body, rather than relying on verbal analysis of subjectively defined sensations and feelings. Symptoms were therefore demoted from the status of defining characteristics of disease to that of secondary indicators of disease. As experiential aspects of disease became of lesser importance, the focus of medical knowledge moved away from the sick person as an individual, to the application of specific diagnostic procedures to identify general categories of disease. Although hospitals were becoming an increasingly important site of medical practice their patients were predominately poor and destitute people who therefore had little opportunity to exercise control, thus increasing distance between the sick person and medical expert. These changes in the approach to diagnosis and in the organisation and professionalisation of medical practice meant that the focus shifted from satisfying the patient to achieving recognition from medical peers.

A third phase was ushered in by developments in histology and experimental physiology, leading to what Jewson termed 'laboratory medicine'. This approach to the practice of scientific medicine emphasized the use of objective laboratory tests to identify morbid physiological processes and thus increasingly removed the patient from the medical professional's field of saliency. This period also saw the development of increasing specialization, and of requirements that practice conformed to the consensus of medical opinion regarding objective measures and processes.

This brief account identifies how historical changes in medical knowledge and practice resulted in shifts in the doctor–patient relationship. In particular they led to reduced significance being given to understanding the patients' subjective perceptions of their illness and a greater reliance on investigations and formal tests. These changes in clinical practice were also associated with organizational changes in the profession of medicine that involved a shift from doctors as individual entrepreneurs dependent on their patients to doctors as specialists within a complex organizational and professional system.

Patient-centred medicine

Since the 1980s there has been a shift from the biomedical model of the previous hospital medicine to what is referred to as 'patient-centred' medicine. This involves a combined biological, psychological and social perspective, often referred to as a biopsychosocial perspective, that gives renewed emphasis to the more personal and subjective aspects of illness and a focus on the whole person. However a patient-centred approach not only views the patient as providing information that facilitates diagnosis and treatment but also as a partner in the consultation and actively engaging in decisions about interventions or management (Box 4.1).

The development of a patient-centred approach has been influenced by changes in views of disease and patient management. This includes a greater awareness that disease and illness are not necessarily coterminous. For example, people who do not feel ill may nevertheless have some classifiable disorder deemed worthy of medical treatment (e.g. hypertension). Conversely, feeling ill and seeking help often bears little relationship to the clinical severity of a condition (see Chapter 3). There is therefore a need to understand patients' own beliefs about their condition and their experience of illness, which may be influenced by their social circumstances and other aspects of their biography and social roles. For example, severe arthritis of the hand may have less impact for an elderly person compared with a younger person, reflecting varying expectations of health and functioning with age, and may have a greater impact for a musician compared with a teacher given the differing impacts on normal role performance.

A second change encouraging a patient-centred approach is the changing pattern of disease from acute to chronic conditions, approximately a quarter of all primary care patient visits now being for chronic illnesses that require regular encounters with the medical system for the duration of the patient's life. Such conditions involve a changed role for medical care from curing to primarily monitoring, coping with symptoms and prolonging decline. Patients with chronic conditions also frequently need to adapt to disability and to be actively involved in managing treatment and other lifestyle changes on a

---

BOX 4.1   Key aspects of a patient-centred consultation

- Biopsychosocial perspective (willingness to become involved in the full range of difficulties patients bring to their doctors and not just their biomedical problems)
- Patient-as-a-person (understanding the individual's experience of his or her illness)
- Sharing power and responsibility (mutual participation of patient and doctor)
- Therapeutic alliance (creating a situation in which the patient feels able to be involved in treatment decisions)
- Doctor-as-a-person (doctor is aware of and responds to patient cues)

From Mead & Bower (2000).

long-term basis that emphasizes the importance of collaborative care, with the patient viewed as a partner in this process, with choices often depending on patients' own views, priorities and circumstances (Campbell & McGauley 2005).

Evidence-based medicine

A development that parallels but contrasts with patient-centred medicine is the growth of evidence-based medicine (EBM). Traditionally clinical experience guided the choice of treatment, with a drug that 'worked' in clinical practice being viewed as an effective treatment, often leading to differing views of the effectiveness of the same intervention. A trend has therefore been to establish objective evidence of the value of different treatments using a randomized controlled trial. This new knowledge of effectiveness is then disseminated through clinical guidelines and protocols, leading to a new evidence-based medicine (EBM) that is based on data from trials rather than individuals' everyday practice (Armstrong 2002). The cost of some drugs has also led to new national guidance of cost effective treatments, and is complemented by guidance and protocols developed at a practice level. Thus increasingly individual doctors practise in a situation of increased professional and managerial control that may conflict with and constrain the practice of patient-centred medicine.

SOCIAL ROLES OF DOCTORS AND PATIENTS

This section presents an overview of the general societal expectations of the roles of doctors and patients and considers the conflicts in the doctor's role arising both from personal values and from doctor's roles as patient advocates, agents of social control and managers of scarce healthcare resources.

Parsons' model of the sick role and doctor's role

Parsons (1951) was one of the earliest sociologists to examine the relationship between doctors and patients. This arose from his theoretical concern with the question of how society is able to function smoothly and respond to problems of deviance. Parsons regarded social functioning as partly achieved through the existence of roles (of father, teacher, shop assistant, and so on), that are each associated with socially prescribed patterns of behaviour. We are, therefore, all aware of how people are likely to behave when they occupy these roles, and of their expectations of us when we occupy the complementary role of child, pupil or customer, which enables interaction to occur fairly smoothly.

Parsons regarded illness as a form of social deviance because it impairs normal role performance. If normal role performance is impaired on a large enough scale this will put the smooth functioning of society at risk (e.g. families caring for children, educational system, transport system, etc.). Parsons believed that the social mechanism that controls illness in society is through the socially prescribed roles for doctors and patients. These roles were described as facilitating interaction and ensuring that both parties work together to return people to a state of health and normal role performance as quickly as possible. In addition an important societal function of the doctor is as a 'gatekeeper' who officially legitimates and controls the amount of illness in society.

Parsons' description of the roles of doctor and patient is presented as an 'ideal type' model. This abstracts and presents what are regarded as the fundamental features of a particular social organization or social role and is an important method of analysing and describing very complex social phenomena. Parsons focused on the roles of the sick person and doctor in the management of acute illness (or acute exacerbations) and was writing in the era of hospital medicine. He depicted the role of sick people as involving four general expectations. First, sick people are allowed, and might even be required, to give up some of their normal activities and responsibilities, such as going to work or playing football. Second, they are regarded as being in need of care. These two expectations and privileges are, however, contingent on the sick person fulfilling the third obligation of wanting to get well as quickly as possible, and the fourth of seeking professional medical advice and cooperating with the doctor (Table 4.1).

Parsons pointed out that the specific expectations of the sick person, such as the number and type of activities the person is expected to give up, are influenced by the nature and severity of the condition. For example, not all illness requires people to relinquish their normal social roles and occupy the status 'sick', and much minor illness is coped with without recourse to the doctor and does not require any changes to a person's everyday life (see Chapter 3).

Parsons saw the role of the doctor as complementary to the role of patient. Just as the patient is expected to cooperate fully with the doctor, so doctors are expected to apply their specialist knowledge and skills for the benefit of the patient, and to act for the welfare of the patient and community rather than in their own self-interest. Doctors are also expected to be objective and emotionally detached, and to be guided by the rules of professional practice. Conformity with these general expectations is an essential requirement for carrying out the tasks of diagnosis and treatment, especially when this involves the need to know intimate details about the patient that are not usually shared between strangers, or the conduct of an intimate physical examination. Parsons also viewed

TABLE 4.1 Parsons' analysis of the roles of patients and doctors	
Patient: sick role	**Doctor: professional role**
Obligations and expectations:	
1. Must want to get well as quickly as possible.	1. Apply a high degree of skill and knowledge to the problems of illness.
2. Should seek professional medical advice and cooperate with the doctor.	2. Act for welfare of patient and community rather than for own self-interest, desire for money, advancement etc.
	3. Be objective and emotionally detached (i.e. should not judge patients' behaviour in terms of personal value system or become emotionally involved with them).
	4. Be guided by rules of professional practice.
Rights:	
1. Allowed (and may be expected) to shed some normal activities and responsibilities (e.g. employment and household tasks).	1. Granted right to examine patients physically and to enquire into intimate areas of physical and personal life.
2. Regarded as being in need of care and unable to get better by his or her own decisions and will.	2. Granted considerable autonomy in professional practice.
	3. Occupies position of authority in relation to the patient.

Reprinted with permission from The Free Press from Parsons (1951).

doctors as enjoying considerable autonomy in executing their professional skills and occupying a position of authority in relation to the patient.

Parsons viewed the sick role as a temporary social role that has been instituted by society with the aim of returning sick people to a state of health and restoring them to fully functioning members of society as quickly as possible. The sick role is also regarded as a universal role, in that its obligations and expectations apply to all sick people with acute illness, whatever their age, gender, ethnicity, occupation or status in other spheres. However, people with a chronic illness, although often needing to consult the doctor regularly, are generally expected to try to achieve their maximum level of functioning and to occupy the status 'sick' only if they experience a change in their usual health.

Parsons' analysis was important in identifying sickness as having social dimensions and describing how the institutionalized roles of sick person and doctor function to reduce the potentially disruptive effects of illness in society. This is partly achieved through the role of the doctor in officially legitimating illness and acting as a gatekeeper to the sick role, thus preventing inappropriate occupancy and enjoyment of the privileges of the sick role, such as time off work or financial benefits, when this is not justified by the patient's medical condition. In addition, the expectations placed on both doctors and patients ensure that people who are officially sanctioned as sick are returned to a state of health and normal role performance as quickly as possible.

The ambivalent responses often displayed by the public and medical staff to conditions such as alcoholism, overdoses, and AIDS are explained by their unwillingness to view such conditions purely as sickness requiring treatment and therefore to grant such people the privileges of the sick role. Others have noted that users of cancer genetic services with a high risk of breast cancer occupy a 'liminal position betwixt the healthy and the sick' (Scott et al 2005).

▥ Conflicts in the doctor's role

Personal values. Whereas Parsons emphasized the consensual nature of the roles and relationships between doctors and patients, in reality, tensions and strains often exist. One set of tensions arises from conflicts between doctors' own values and those of some of their patients. This is particularly likely to occur in relation to abortion, homosexuality, AIDS and other conditions or behaviours invested with moral evaluations. Conflicts may also occur between maintaining the confidentiality of the doctor–patient relationship and disclosing information to a patient's parent or spouse. This raises the question of whether medical confidentiality is absolute, or whether there are any situations when interests are best served by passing on information about a patient. For example, are there are any circumstances in which a doctor at a clinic should disclose that a patient has acquired immunodeficiency syndrome (AIDS), or is positive for HIV, when this is against the patient's wishes? Such situations frequently pose dilemmas for doctors and raise questions concerning their primary duties and responsibilities, as well as possibly presenting conflicts in relation to their own beliefs and values. There are powerful arguments to support the view that priority should be given to maintaining the confidentiality of the doctor–patient relationship, as this has the benefit of preserving patients' trust in doctors and their willingness to consult and discuss their problems freely in the future. Destroying this trust undermines the very foundation of the relationship between doctor and patient.

Social control function. Doctors often experience conflicting demands in terms of their requirement to act in the best interests of their patients and their duty to serve the interests of the state. As Parsons recognized, doctors serve the state as agents of social control in their role as gatekeepers to the sick role with authority to determine who is 'healthy' and who is 'sick', but also have an obligation to act in the best interests of individual patients. When patients request, or even demand, a sick note, problems may arise for the doctor in determining whether disease exists and if the designation of 'sick' and privileges of the sick role can be justified. Approximately 1 million people in the UK report sick each week, with back pain being the major reason for time off work. However it is often difficult for doctors to determine its cause or severity except by relying on patients' reports. This leads to problems in evaluating the legitimacy of claims to the sick role and undertaking the most appropriate actions for their patient while also performing their societal function in ensuring that people do not malinger or occupy the sick role inappropriately (Hussey et al 2004). Other examples of potential role conflicts for doctors include whether to inform patients who are thinking of being tested for human immunodeficiency virus (HIV) of the potential problems of being diagnosed as a carrier for insurance premiums when they are aware that this might discourage testing.

Clinical and managerial control. Doctors increasingly experience differing expectations and potential conflicts arising from the requirement to treat individual patients to the best of their ability and adopt a patient-centred approach to care, while being required to ration scarce resources of staff time, beds and medical equipment and to follow evidence-based protocols (May et al 2005). In addition, a particular problem presented by EBM is to translate evidence-based knowledge derived from large populations into an individual plan for a specific patient.

MODELS OF DOCTOR–PATIENT RELATIONSHIPS

The doctor–patient relationship occurs in a wider context of practice that influences the autonomy or managerial control experienced by doctors. However the relationship between individual doctors and patients in the consultation has been depicted in terms of the relative power and control of doctors and patients, leading to four possible types of relationship (Table 4.2). Most consultations tend towards one type, although in reality these different models often do not exist in pure form.

■ Classification of relationships: power and control

A paternalistic (guidance–cooperation) relationship involves high physician control and low patient control. This accords with Parsons' model where the doctor is dominant and acts as a 'parent' figure who decides what he or she believes to be in the patient's best interest. This traditionally characterized medical consultations based on the biomedical disease model. However it continues to be important, especially in relation to emergency

TABLE 4.2	Types of doctor–patient relationship		
		Doctor control	
Patient control		Low	High
Low		Default	Paternalism
High		Consumerist	Mutuality

Reprinted with permission from Sage Publications.
Source: Stewart & Roter (1989, p. 21).

situations where the doctor often needs to take control and make decisions. Many patients also derive considerable comfort from being able to rely on the doctor in this way and being relieved of burdens of worry and decision making, especially if they are experiencing considerable pain. However, whereas a guidance–cooperation model traditionally characterized medical consultations, especially in the primary care setting, relationships based on mutuality are now increasingly common.

A relationship of mutuality is characterized by the active involvement of patients as more equal partners in the medical consultation. This type of relationship has been described as a 'meeting between experts', in which both parties participate as a joint venture and engage in an exchange of ideas and sharing of belief systems. The doctor brings his or her clinical skills and knowledge to the consultation in terms of diagnostic techniques, knowledge of the causes of disease, prognosis, treatment options and preventive strategies, and patients bring their own expertise in terms of their experiences and explanations of their illness, and knowledge of their particular social circumstances, attitudes to risk, values and preferences.

A consumerist relationship describes a situation in which power relationships are reversed; the patient takes the active role and the doctor adopts a fairly passive role, acceding to the patient's requests for a second opinion, referral to hospital, a sick note, and so on. This most often characterizes relationships in private consultations (fee for service) where the patient has greater autonomy and power through their payment of the doctor (direct or via insurance) who in turn desires to attract and retain consumers. However it has been found that doctors' perceptions of patient pressure are a strong independent predictor of referral and prescribing behaviours (Little et al 2004).

A relationship of default describes a consultation that lacks sufficient direction as patients continue to adopt a passive role even when the doctor reduces some of his or her control. This can arise if patients are not aware of alternatives to a passive patient role or are timid in adopting a more participative relationship.

Influences on the relationship

Different types of relationship, and particularly those characterized by paternalism and mutuality, can be viewed as appropriate to different conditions and stages of illness. However, considerable variation exists that cannot be explained entirely in terms of the patient's medical condition.

A key influence on the nature of the doctor–patient relationship is the doctors' perception of their role and appropriate relationship with patients. Studies have shown that individual doctors tend fairly consistently towards either a doctor-centred (paternalist) or patient-centred consultation style. A doctor-centred style focuses on the biomedical model and involves a tightly controlled consultation with the use of closed questions and relatively little opportunity for patients' participation. In contrast, a patient-centred consultation style involves greater emphasis on listening and eliciting the patients' beliefs, experiences and preferences through the use of open questions (Zandbelt et al 2006). A mutual participation relationship accompanied by a patient-centred consultation style of practice is becoming increasingly common, with current medical training emphasizing the social and psychological aspects of illness and importance of communication skills.

A second influence on the consultation is patients' own expectations of the doctor–patient relationship and their willingness to ask questions. Patients who are most likely to expect a participative relationship are generally younger and have a high social and educational level. However patients' desire to participate in the consultation generally increases over the course of an illness as they gain more knowledge and understanding of their condition. Patients who are passive and unquestioning during initial hospital consultations, therefore usually initiate questions themselves and take a more participative approach by the second or third consultation, with the stage of the disease episode and medical care often being of more importance in patients' desire to actively participate in the consultation than their individual characteristics (Coulter 2002).

Thirdly, structural aspects of the consultation influence interaction between doctor and patient. This includes the wider context of the consultation including how the doctor is paid (fee-for-service, salary or capitation payment), and tensions between achieving patient-centred care and professional and managerial directives that increasingly influence practice (Jones et al 2004). Doctors may also sometimes give greater emphasis to preserving and strengthening the doctor–patient relationship and use available time to respond to patients' psychosocial needs rather than following practice protocols, in terms for example of secondary prevention or changing drug regimes (Summerskill & Pope 2002).

At a micro level consultation is influenced by whether it is an initial meeting or the patient and doctor already have an established relationship, and the influence of time pressures. Doctors commonly cite a shortage of time as a barrier to greater involvement of patients in the consultation and their use of fairly tightly controlled interviewing methods. There is some evidence that discussion of patients' views does not necessarily lead to longer consultations and may also save time in the longer term through resolution of misunderstandings (Belle Brown 2003), although there are relatively few data on the time demands involved in providing adequate information for shared decision-making and achieving concordance.

TREATMENT DECISION-MAKING

The traditional emphasis of communication in the consultation was to understand patients' symptoms, their beliefs about the illness and its impact on their lives. Recently increased attention has been given to communication in relation to treatment decision-making, which again is characterized by greater patient involvement.

Approaches to decision-making

Three main models of treatment decision-making are: *professional choice, shared decision-making* and *consumer choice* (Table 4.3). The professional choice model accords with the

TABLE 4.3	Models of treatment decision-making in a doctor–patient dyad		
Analytical stages	**Professional choice**	**Shared decision**	**Consumer choice (informed)**
Information exchange:			
Flow	One way (largely)	Two way	One way (largely)
Direction	Doctor to patient	Doctor & patient	Doctor to patient
Type	Medical	Medical & personal	Medical
Amount	Minimum legally required	All relevant for decision-making	All relevant for decision-making
Deliberation:	Doctor alone or with other doctors	Doctor and patient (plus potential others)	Patient (plus potential others)
Deciding on treatment to implement	Doctors	Doctor and patient	Patient

traditional paternalist relationship and regards the patient predominantly as a biomedical body and the doctor as medical expert as solely responsible for treatment decisions. Patients are therefore expected to adopt a fairly passive role and merely cooperate with the doctor's advice and treatment. However, decision-making increasingly involves greater patient involvement, with a shift to shared decision-making between doctor and patient. This approach is associated with a relationship of mutuality and acknowledges that both medical knowledge and the patient's beliefs and experiential knowledge are needed to manage the illness successfully. This involves initial sharing of information, taking steps to build a consensus about the preferred treatment and reaching agreement (consensus) on the treatment to implement (Box 4.2). A third approach is the consumer choice model that views the patient as an autonomous decision-maker. This requires that initially the doctor communicates information on all relevant options and their benefits and risks to enable the patient to make an informed treatment decision. Information transfer is therefore seen as the key responsibility and only legitimate contribution of the doctor to the decision-making process, with deliberation and decision-making being the sole prerogative of the patient. Consumer choice is most often associated with a consumerist relationship. However, there are many instances where patients decide on a broad course of action before entering the surgery, such as their desire for a referral, and press the doctor to cooperate with their wishes (Morgan et al 2006).

In practice, the three models of treatment decision-making do not necessarily exist in pure form. One reason is the existence of intermediate approaches. For example, a variant of the professional choice model is what is sometimes referred to as the 'professional as agent' model. This describes a situation where the doctor makes the treatment decision informed by fairly detailed knowledge of the patient's preferences for future health states, life choices, and so on, rather than this decision being purely based on the doctor's professional knowledge and personal choices. Secondly, the clinical encounter may be characterized by a hybrid of elements of more than one model. For example, a consultation may initially be characterized by a two-way information exchange between doctor and patient. However, if problems arise in achieving a shared decision, the clinician might then use the power imbalance in the relationship to persuade the patient to follow his or her advice, often with the promise of a subsequent review of the situation. Similarly, a doctor who favours a shared decision-making model may think, as the interaction proceeds, that the patient has gained enough confidence and gathered enough information to make the decision on his or her own, with the process therefore shifting from a shared to an informed model.

The increasing patient involvement in treatment decisions is endorsed by formal NHS policies that now require that patients are given a choice of hospitals for referral, encouraged to participate as partners in treatment decisions and increasingly involved as users in contributing to the development of services (NHS Executive 1996). This changed

---

BOX 4.2	Four requirements for shared decision-making

1. Both doctor and patient are involved in the decision-making process
2. Both parties share information
3. Both parties take steps to build a consensus about the preferred treatment
4. An agreement (consensus) is reached on the treatment to implement

Based on Charles et al (1999).

position of patients reflects wider medical and social changes. A major medical change is the increasing prevalence of chronic illness in the population, which requires that patients manage their illness and treatments on a long-term basis, and in turn is facilitated by ensuring that the patient understands and endorses the approach to their treatment. Social drivers for change include media coverage of medical scandals that have raised awareness of the need for accountability and encouraged a questioning of professional authority (Stevenson 2004). Patients are also increasingly knowledgeable about health matters through access to health information from the media, Internet and other sources, and may sometimes become an 'expert' in situations where primary care doctors may only have a general understanding of the disorder. In addition, social values increasingly endorse individual autonomy and responsibility and the development of a more equal relationship with professionals.

Despite the formal endorsement of greater patient choices there is evidence that the explicit mention of equally reasonable treatment options is still often neglected in medical consultations (Gatellari et al 2002). This may reflect the doctor's practice style and knowledge of the treatments available for a specific diagnosis, a lack of medical information about the options, organizational constraints of time and cost, etc. or constraints on autonomy and choice associated with clinical and practice guidelines.

Concordance with prescribing

The report of the Royal Pharmaceutical Society of Great Britain (Marinker 1997) introduced the term 'concordance' to describe an approach to prescribing that aims to achieve a therapeutic alliance between doctor and patient, with the goal of achieving the best use of medicines compatible with what the patient desires and is capable of achieving.

Concordance accords with a patient-centred approach to care and shares many similarities with shared decision-making. However, concordance focuses specifically on prescribing decisions. In addition, it not only emphasizes the importance of the open exchange of information and participation of both doctor and patient but also gives primacy to the patient's view, with the most important determinations agreed to be those that are made by the patient (Box 4.3). An important duty of the doctor is therefore to ensure that patients' choices are informed and based on an understanding of prevailing

---

BOX 4.3 Concordance

Definition
'Concordance is based on the notion that the work of the prescriber and patient in the consultation is a negotiation between equals and that the aim is a therapeutic alliance between them. This alliance may, in the end, include an agreement to differ. Its strength lies in a new assumption of respect for the patient's agenda and the creation of openness in the relationship, so that both doctor and patient together can proceed on the basis of reality and not of misunderstanding, distrust or concealment.'

Aim
'The intention is to assist the patient to make as informed choice as possible about the diagnosis and treatment, about the benefit and risk and to take full part in the therapeutic alliance. Although reciprocal, this is an alliance in which the most important determinations are agreed to be those that are made by the patient.'

Source: Marinker 1997 (p.8, p.12).

evidence and risks. A further difference is that a concordant approach does not necessarily require that the patient adopts a key role in decisions. For example, decisions involving professional choice (i.e. doctor makes decisions based on knowledge of patient's views) can still be categorized as concordant if this is the approach that the patient prefers. Shared concordance can therefore be achieved without shared decision-making. If a situation occurs where the doctor and patient have differing preferences and views they may also agree to differ, with the concordat reached then being reviewed at subsequent consultations and changes agreed.

A major driver for the development of concordance as an approach to prescribing was the recognition that, on average about 50% of patients with chronic conditions do not take their treatment as prescribed (Marinker 1997). Major reasons are because they do not share the doctors' view of the appropriateness of the drugs prescribed, or are worried about immediate side-effects or possible long-term harmful effects of the drugs. All medicine taking involves a balance of risk between the damage of the disease process unmodified by medication and the potential damage that may be inflicted by the medicine. Whereas the traditional approach was to impose a medical decision that the patient could challenge only through non-compliance after leaving the consultation, the aim of concordance is to achieve a mutually agreed treatment plan based on patients' informed assessment of risks and benefits. This is based on the assumption that if patients are actively involved and committed to the treatment this will lead to higher rates of adherence and greater improvement in symptoms and physiological function.

Concordance (and shared decision-making more generally) is most feasible and least problematic in areas of 'clinical equipoise' where, from a clinical standpoint, there are several viable and equally appropriate or effective treatment alternatives from which the patient may select according to personal preference, as for example for atrial fibrillation, prostate disease and menopausal symptoms. However problems may arise in situations where patients may wish to be prescribed an expensive new medicine, whereas the prescriber is required to allocate resources to treatments where the benefits are clearer, which may lead to doctors suppressing information about some treatment options. In addition, in some cases a patient may reject potentially life-saving therapy, such as immunosuppressant therapy following renal transplantation, despite the doctor informing them of the risks. However, it can be argued that concordance is a philosophy of care that guides practice, rather than necessarily being implemented in every situation. Open discussion of issues and understanding of the views of doctor and patient is also desirable compared with the traditional patients' passive acceptance of 'doctors' orders', often accompanied by subsequent dissatisfaction and non-compliance.

▓ Patients' preferences for participation

The emphasis on shared decision-making and achieving 'concordance' raises questions of whether and when patients desire to participate in this way. This has been found to depend partly on a patient's state of health; patients in crisis situations or who feel weak or distressed may often prefer to have decisions made for them rather than being more actively involved. Differences in desire for involvement also reflect the complexity of treatment choices. For example, studies of patients with breast cancer and with colorectal cancer identified 20% of the former and 4% of the latter preferring an active role in terms of making their own treatment decisions, with 17% of patients with colorectal cancer and 28% of patients with breast cancer preferring to share responsibility with the doctor for deciding which treatment was best for them. However, 78% of patients with colorectal cancer and 52% with breast cancer preferred to leave the decision to the doctor, although generally wanting the doctor to consider their opinion (Beaver et al 1999). The higher proportion of patients with breast cancer wishing to be actively involved in decision-making might reflect both the clear treatment choices involved with little impact on survival and the younger age of these patients.

Patients' differing desires for involvement identify a key challenge for health professionals of being sensitive to an individual patient's needs. However, even if patients do not wish to actively participate in treatment decisions they generally still desire information about their condition and treatment. For example, Jenkins et al (2001) found that 87% of hospitalized cancer patients interviewed desired all the information about their disease, good and bad. The 13% who stated that in general they preferred to leave disclosure of details up to the doctor tended to be older patients (over 70 years of age) but they still wanted to know certain specific details.

It is often assumed that patient participation and choices in treatment decisions will lead to increased demands on services. However, evidence suggests that the influence of patients' choices on healthcare utilization varies in different situations. For example, studies of cardiovascular conditions suggest that patients are more averse to drug treatment than health professionals and would prefer higher thresholds for beginning antihypertensive treatment, because patients give less value to the benefits of this treatment compared with doctors and are more distressed about side-effects. Similarly, studies conducted in the USA, where surgical rates are relatively high, indicate that some informed patients with mild symptoms resist prostatectomy and hysterectomy in situations where specialists advocate these procedures. In contrast, patients often wish to receive prescriptions for upper respiratory tract infections in situations where doctors regard this as inappropriate (Montgomery & Fahey 2001). A greater patient voice and shared decision-making does not, therefore, necessarily increase demands on services and can ensure that resources are employed more appropriately and increase the effectiveness of care.

DOCTORS' COMMUNICATION SKILLS

Patients entering a medical consultation are often concerned about the possible nature and diagnosis of their condition or treatment, or alternatively may worry about consulting 'inappropriately' and bothering the doctor unnecessarily. Patients therefore generally try to fulfill the role of a cooperative, polite and respectful patient that conforms with Parsons' depiction of social expectations of patients, and unless actively encouraged by the doctor may not ask questions, voice concerns or indicate disagreement. Doctors therefore often believe that patients are satisfied with the communication they received during a consultation as it is difficult for patients to convey dissatisfaction. However, a qualitative study based on 35 patients aged 18 years and over consulting 20 general practitioners, found that only four of the 35 patients voiced all their concerns during the consultation (Barry et al 2000). The most common unvoiced concerns were worries about possible diagnosis and what the future holds, ideas about what is wrong, side-effects, not wanting a prescription, and information relating to social context such as housing, work or social networks. Concerns that were not raised often led to specific problem outcomes, such as major misunderstandings, unwanted prescriptions, non-use of prescriptions and non-adherence to treatment. Much clinically inappropriate prescribing has been attributed to doctors' desire to please their patient, together with mistaken assumptions of what patients wanted or were expecting from the consultation and a failure to elicit patients' views (Britten et al 2004).

Patients' perceptions of inadequacies of communication arise partly from what doctors communicate (content skills). This refers to the substance of questions and the information gathered, including the emphasis given by doctors to understanding the patient's perspective (ideas, concerns, expectations, impact of condition on everyday life, etc.), and the treatments they discuss. The content of communication is influenced by a number of practical and situational factors (time available, initial or subsequent visit, NHS or private patient) but most importantly by how doctors perceive the nature of the medical task and their relationship with patients.

There are also questions of how doctors communicate (process skills). This refers to how they discover the history or provide information, the verbal and non-verbal skills they use, how they develop a relationship with the patient, and the way they organize and structure the communication, including the emphasis given to actively listening to patients, facilitating and encouraging their questions, and discussion of worries and concerns. Process skills relate to five stages and tasks of the consultation (Box 4.4). The skills required to achieve each of these stages are now taught in specialist communication courses and involve skills in verbal communication, including the use of open questions where possible, facilitating, probing and listening, as well as sharing information in a comprehensible manner and negotiating a mutually acceptable treatment plan. Also of importance is non-verbal communication. By maintaining eye contact, looking attentive, nodding encouragingly and using other gestures, the doctor can provide positive feedback to the patient and facilitate his or her participation, whereas continued riffling through notes, twiddling with a pen or failing to look directly at the patient convey disinterest and result in patients failing to describe their problems or to seek information and explanation. Similarly, the patient's body language and eye contact can convey whether he or she is feeling tense, anxious, angry or upset. Indeed, it is estimated that in a normal two-person conversation the verbal component carries less than 35% of the social meaning of the situation, and that 65% or more is carried by the non-verbal components such as eye contact, gaze, facial expression and posture. Physical proximity and the relative positions of doctor and patient in the consulting room also influence interaction, with communication encouraged by seating of equal height and the lack of a physical barrier between participants.

The current emphasis on shared decision-making places new demands on doctors' communication skills, with the need for doctors to transfer technical information to patients about treatment options, risks and their probable benefits in as unbiased, clear and simple a way as possible. This is a particular challenge in situations where the availability of reliable evidence is limited, or when decisions need to be made within the time constraints of a normal consultation. Doctors may also need to help the patient to conceptualize and weigh the risks versus the benefits, to share their treatment recommendations with the patient and/or affirm the patient's treatment preference, while at the same time

---

BOX 4.4   Communication skills and steps to be achieved in the consultation

1. Initiating the session (establishing the initial rapport and identifying the reason(s) for the consultation)
2. Gathering information (exploring the problem, understanding the patient's perspective, providing structure to the consultation)
3. Building the relationship (developing rapport and involving the patient)
4. Explanation and planning (providing the appropriate amount and type of information, aiding accurate recall and understanding, achieving a shared understanding and planning)
5. Closing the session

From Silverman et al. (1998).

being careful not to impose their own values about the best treatment onto the patient. Specialist training programmes are being introduced to respond to these challenges and enhance doctors' skills and competencies in these areas. Direct doctor–patient communication is also increasingly complemented by the availability of decision-aids that are designed to help people make choices among screening or treatment options, through providing information on options and outcomes plus information on probabilities of outcomes tailored to personal health risk factors. This helps patients to clarify values and guides the steps of decision-making. There is also increasing availability of interactive and multimedia systems that can enable people to receive information and advice tailored to their own specific health needs (e.g. NHS Direct online www.nhsdirect.uk).

CHANGES IN THE DOCTOR–PATIENT RELATIONSHIP

The doctor–patient relationship is currently undergoing major changes. Although patient-centred medicine is the accepted model of care, there is currently considerable variation in its implementation, particularly in the extent to which doctors involve patients as active partners and seek to achieve concordance or shared decision-making. For the future there may be increased tensions between the goals of patient-centred medicine and evidence-based practice, as patients become increasingly knowledgeable and 'expert' in their illness, with greater expectations of informed decision-making, but this is accompanied by an increased emphasis on evidence-based medicine and concerns to implement guidelines.

Ongoing changes in the structure of medical practice include the increasing size of general practices and greater involvement of nurses, health visitors, counsellors and other health professionals in the provision of primary care. The tradition of personal continuity in terms of a long-term and continuing relationship between an individual general practitioner and his or her patient is therefore becoming less common and patients increasingly receive care from different members of the primary care team. Meetings between health professional and patient therefore often form more of an 'encounter' than a long-term relationship. Patients are also increasingly treated for multiple conditions that may involve 'shared care' between the hospital and general practice. The involvement of multiple professionals and care across the primary-secondary interface presents new challenges of information transfer, communication and teamwork so as to provide patients with a well-coordinated and seamless service, with risks to continuity of care most commonly occurring at points of transition such as discharge from hospital (Naithani et al 2006).

A further development is the expanding use of telemedicine as a means of delivering health care. This offers increasing possibility for patients to engage in teleconsulting, often from their own homes, thus expanding access to care. However, it also presents new challenges in establishing a relationship between individual patients and healthcare providers and facilitating their communication.

References

Armstrong D 2002 Clinical autonomy, individual and collective: the problem of changing doctors' behaviour. Social Science and Medicine 55:1771–1777

Barry CA et al 2000 Patients' unvoiced agendas in general practice consultations: qualitative study. British Medical Journal 320:1245–1250

Beaver K, Bogg J, Luker KA 1999 Decision-making role preferences and information needs: a comparison of colorectal and breast cancer. Health Expectations 2:266–276

Belle Brown J 2003 Time and the consultation. In Jones R, Britten N, Culpepper L et al (eds) Oxford textbook of primary medical care. Oxford University Press, Oxford, 190–193

Britten N, Stevenson F, Gafaranga J et al 2004 The expression of aversion to medicines in general practice consultations. Social Science and Medicine 59:1495–1503

Campbell C, McGauley G 2005 Doctor–patient relationships in chronic illness: insights from forensic psychiatry. British Medical Journal 330:667–670

Charles C, Whelan T, Gafni A 1999 What do we mean by partnership in making decisions about treatment? British Medical Journal 319:780–782

Coulter A 2002 The autonomous patient: ending paternalism in medical care. The Nuffield Trust, London

Gattellari M, Voigt KJ, Butow PN, Tatersall HN 2002 When the treatment goal is not cure: Are cancer patients equipped to make informed decisions? Journal of Clinical Oncology 20(2):503–513

Hussey S, Hoddinott P, Wilson P et al 2004 Sickness certification in the UK: qualitative study of views of general practitioners in Scotland. British Medical Journal 328:88–92

Jenkins V, Fallowfield L, Saul J 2001 Information needs of patients with cancer: results from a large study in UK cancer centers. British Journal of Cancer 84(1):48–51

Jewson ND 1976 The disappearance of the sick-man from medical cosmology, 1770–1870. Sociology 10(2):225–244

Jones IR, Berney L, Kelly M et al 2004 Is patient involvement possible when decisions involve scarce resources? A qualitative study of decision-making in primary care. Social Science and Medicine 59:93–102

Little P, Dorward M, Warner G et al 2004 Importance of patient pressure and perceived medical need for investigations, referral and prescribing in primary care: nested observational study. British Medical Journal 328:444–448

Marinker M (Chairman of Working Party) 1997 From compliance to concordance: achieving shared goals in medicine taking. Royal Pharmaceutical Society of Great Britain, London

May C, Allison G, Chapple A et al 2004 Framing the doctor-patient relationship in chronic illness: a comparative study of general practitioners' accounts. Sociology of Health and Illness 26(2):135–158

Mead N, Bower P 2000 Patient-centredness: a conceptual framework and review of the empirical literature. Social Science and Medicine 51:1087–1110

Montgomery AA, Fahey T 2001 How do patients' treatment preferences compare with those of clinicians? Quality and Safety in Health Care 10:39–43

Morgan M, Jenkins L, Ridsdale L 2006 Patients' pressure for referral for headache: a qualitative study of general practitioners referral practices British Journal of General Practice 57(534): 29–36

Naithani S, Gulliford M, Morgan M 2006 Patients' perceptions and experiences of continuity of care in diabetes. Health Expectations 9:118–129

NHS Executive 1996 Patient partnership: building a collaborative strategy. Department of Health, Leeds

Parsons T 1951 The social system. Free Press, Glencoe, IL

Scott S, Prior L, Wood F, Gray J 2005 Repositioning the patient: the implications of being 'at risk'. Social Science and Medicine 60(8):1869–1879

Silverman J, Kurtz S, Draper J 1998 Skills for communicating with patients. Radcliffe Press, Oxford

Stevenson F 2004 The patient's perspective. Chapter 3 in C Bond (ed) Concordance. Pharmaceutical Press, London

Stewart M, Roter D (eds) 1989 Communicating with medical patients. Sage, London

Summerskill WSM, Pope C 2002 'I saw the panic rise in her eyes, and evidence-based medicine went out of the door'. An exploratory qualitative study of the barriers to secondary prevention in the management of coronary heart disease. Family Practice 19(6):605–610

Zandbelt LC, Smets EMA, Oort FJ et al 2006 Determinants of physicians' patient-centred behaviour in the medical specialist encounter. Social Science and Medicine 63:899–910

70

CHAPTER

5

Hospitals and patient care

Myfanwy Morgan

Many hospitals not only engage in patient care but also serve as centres of education and training for doctors, nurses and other health workers, and provide a setting for research. A patient admitted to hospital thus enters a complex organization with a variety of goals, and with a well-developed system of rules and procedures for coordinating the different activities and the large numbers and categories of staff. This chapter examines the changing patterns of hospital use and patients' experiences of hospital care. It also considers the importance of staff attitudes and the ways in which nurses' perceptions of their role influence the process and outcomes of care.

PATTERNS OF HOSPITAL USE

■ General hospital patients

There has been a steady reduction in the total number of hospital beds in all established market economies. In the NHS this decline started in the late 1960s and has continued: there were 297 000 beds for all specialities in England in 1987–8 and a 65% decline to 194 000 beds in 1997–8, with a further decrease to 176 000 beds in 2005/06 (59% of 1987/8 figure). This decline in the numbers of hospital beds has occurred across all specialities and age groups. However, it has been associated with increased activity in terms both of numbers of outpatient attendances and inpatient admissions. The latter has been made possible by substantial reductions in length of stay, which have occurred for all specialities, age groups and diagnoses. For example, in the 1940s patients admitted to hospital for myocardial infarction had a length of stay of 5–7 weeks, compared with an average of 4 days today. Similarly, groin hernia repair required a length of stay of about 6 weeks in the 1940s; this reduced to an average of 4.9 days in 1985, and today 51% of groin hernia repair is performed as day surgery. Indeed, a major change in addition to reduced lengths of stay is the considerable increase in procedures performed as day surgery; rates of day surgery increased from 1355 operations in 1984 to over 3 million day case operations in 2005/06, accounting for 28.5% of all episodes with an operation (http://www.hesonline.nhs.uk).

The substantial reduction in lengths of hospital stay has occurred partly as a result of changes in medical views regarding recovery following surgery or major illness. For example, long periods of bed rest used to be regarded as therapeutic, whereas mobilization as soon as possible following surgery is now viewed as beneficial. Clinical developments, including more effective pain control, the availability of new diagnostic tests that reduce the need for long periods of observation, and the development of less invasive medical technologies and surgical procedures, such as laparoscopic techniques and the use of lasers and lithotripsy to replace conventional open surgery, have also reduced recovery time and needs for skilled nursing care and increased opportunities to conduct many procedures as day surgery. In addition, changes in the ways of financing hospital services provided powerful economic incentives to increase the throughput of patients, encouraging both reduced lengths of stay and the expansion of day surgery. Formerly, NHS hospitals received a global budget to cover their activity that was based on the size and composition of their catchment population and rates of hospital use. Hospitals therefore had little incentive to increase patient admissions and throughput. Indeed, a high throughput of patients could lead to risks for hospitals (or particular units) of having a budget overspend; a situation referred to as the 'efficiency trap'. However, new methods of funding mean that the revenue received by a hospital or unit is related to the number of cases treated. As a result, there are incentives to expand day case procedures and reduce lengths of stay.

Despite the aim that patients should only occupy hospital beds while requiring acute care, there is a continuing problem of delayed discharge, particularly among elderly patients with complex needs. Delayed discharge often arises as a result of delayed transfers, where patients deemed to be medically well enough for discharge are unable to leave because arrangements for the continuing care they need have not been finalized. It is estimated that delays among older people with complex needs cost the health service about £170 million a year, the equivalent of 1.7 million hospital beds. Over a third of people affected have delays of more than one month (Bryan et al 2006). This problem of delayed transfers is not confined to the UK but is also encountered in other countries, including Israel, Sweden, Norway, New Zealand and the USA (Vetter 2003). It arises from delays at each stage in the organization of continuing care – assessment by healthcare professionals (primarily occupational therapists) of patients' physical and psychological needs in relation to their domestic circumstances, and assessment of social care needs for personal care and household tasks by care managers, which involves both consideration of the availability of informal care by family and friends and patients' financial circumstances, and hence their eligibility for public support. Once decisions on destination and support have been made, there is a need to find appropriate domiciliary or long-term care providers that accord with the client's individual needs and preferences and available resources. Major barriers and sources of delay in this process have been identified as the shortages of health and social care professionals, inadequate resources available to social services to provide care and confusion of responsibilities between health and social care agencies giving rise to poor coordination. Novel schemes to expedite transfers include hospital-at-home schemes, short-term care home placements and dedicated multi-disciplinary community teams for particular groups of patients, such as people who have suffered a stroke. From January 2004 there has also been provision to impose fines of £120 per day on social service departments that are unable to orchestrate discharge packages within 48 hours of an older person being declared fit to leave an NHS facility.

Psychiatric patients

Psychiatric care is characterized by an even more marked change in service provision and patterns of hospital use. The policy of closing the large Victorian psychiatric hospitals resulted in a very great reduction in the numbers of psychiatric beds. However, the beds available again cater for increasing numbers of admissions. Whereas patients admitted to a psychiatric hospital in the 1940s and early 1950s often spent many years in hospital they are now generally discharged within one month, and most patients are admitted for much shorter periods.

A major change in the provision of care for psychiatric patients has been the gradual closure of the traditional large psychiatric hospitals that provided long-term custodial type care for up to 1000 patients at any one time. This process of hospital closure began in the 1950s with the adoption of a policy of 'deinstitutionalization' and 'community care', and increased in momentum during the 1980s. As a result, care for psychiatric patients now mainly occurs outside the hospital, with short periods of admission to psychiatric wards in general hospitals if required for diagnosis and treatment. Patients are then discharged back to the 'community' to live in their own homes, in hostels or other supported accommodation, or with relatives. This marked shift in the pattern of psychiatric care has occurred in most countries and has been attributed to the interaction of attitudinal, clinical and economic factors, although views differ of the relative importance of each of these influences.

Some people regard the introduction of the major tranquillizers in the mid-1950s as the key factor making community care possible, by enabling people to be treated and aggressive behaviour controlled outside the hospital setting. Others argue that this exaggerates the therapeutic achievement these drugs represent and identify several hospitals that adopted the policy of early discharge well before the new drugs were introduced. They suggest that a more important factor was the prior change in ideas regarding mentally ill people. Patients, rather than being regarded as violent and dangerous and therefore requiring long-term custody and care, were therefore increasingly perceived as having treatable conditions and able to live in the community. Moreover, changes in psychiatric practice emphasized patients' assessment and ability to perform Activities of Daily Living (ADLs), which could best be assessed and developed within a normal setting.

A third explanation of the new emphasis on community care was the increasing humanitarian concerns about the harmful effects of long periods spent in large psychiatric hospitals. Particularly influential was a book ('Asylums') by Erving Goffman (1961), based on his own observational study of a large psychiatric hospital in the USA. Goffman identified these hospitals as performing a disabling function and causing 'institutionalization' among patients. This condition is characterized at a psychological level by patients' lack of interest in leaving the institution, and their general apathy and lack of concern about what is going on around them. Institutionalized patients also demonstrate disturbed and regressive behaviour, including an inability to make choices and decisions, to plan activities or to undertake simple everyday tasks. They can also lose interest in and neglect their own appearance and develop mumbled speech and characteristic shuffling gait. Goffman (1961) attributed these patient characteristics and behaviours to organizational processes within the institution, especially the high level of depersonalization that occurred in the interests of organizational efficiency. For example, patients were subjected to what he described as 'batch processing', which refers to a situation where individuals were all treated alike and performed activities such as getting up, bathing and eating according to an institutional schedule with little scope for individual choices, preferences and decision-making. Personal possessions were also kept to a minimum to make it easier for staff to cope with large numbers of patients, and there was often little regard for privacy. As a result, patients frequently lost their normal self-identity, took on a passive role and became dependent on the institution, with institutional pressures being particularly strong for patients who experienced long lengths of stay and had little contact with the outside world. Recognition of the harmful effects of the institutional environment based on the work of Goffman and others, together with a number of scandals regarding the neglect and ill treatment of patients in psychiatric hospitals and other long-stay institutions, is identified as an important pressure towards a policy of deinstitutionalization on humanitarian grounds.

It is now widely acknowledged that changes in views of mental illness, the availability of new drugs and humanitarian concerns all played a role in the changes in psychiatric care. In addition, economic factors are identified as playing a significant role in creating a climate favourable to the adoption of a policy of community care. This centred on the need to renovate the large psychiatric institutions built in the Victorian era, with their considerable running costs. A policy of community care was therefore seen as reducing costs to the health service as well as achieving other desired goals. However, the overall cost of community care depends on the level of services provided. Community care is cheaper if care largely relies on family carers, but can be more expensive than institutional care if it involves a considerable provision of small residential units and high levels of domiciliary services (see Chapter 16).

The policy of deinstitutionalization, involving the move from institutional to community care, has been of benefit to large numbers of psychiatric patients who previously would have spent many years in a custodial style of care. Follow-up studies of long-stay psychiatric patients resettled in the community indicate that, when carefully planned and adequately resourced, community care is beneficial to most individuals and has minimal detrimental effects on society (McCourt 2000). Planned short hospital stays have also been shown to be as effective as longer periods of hospitalization with no increases in readmission (Johnstone & Zolese 1999). However, there are continuing concerns about whether the needs of some groups are being met adequately in the community. This is because the reduction in hospital beds has not been accompanied by a corresponding increase in residential places in other settings, with the hospital still being responsible for about 80% of the overall mental health budget and long-term care has mainly involved moving people from hospital and community-based residential services into their own homes. This occasionally results in media reports of instances of violent and aggressive behaviour among psychiatric patients living in the community and of high levels of homelessness among people with mental illnesses.

Although the substantial reductions in available beds for psychiatric patients have, as in the acute sector, been accompanied by higher rates of admission, there are also concerns about high levels of delayed discharges. A postal survey sent to English mental health trusts and Primary Care Trusts with responsibility for providing mental health services identified 4% to 20% of beds affected by delayed discharge over the survey period, with variations by speciality. Common reasons for delays were awaiting assessment and awaiting placement in residential accommodation or a domiciliary package of care. (Lewis & Glasby 2006) As a result of the pressure on psychiatric beds, people admitted as unplanned emergencies, frequently compulsorily under the Mental Health Act, often occupy acute admission wards intended for short stays for purposes of diagnosis and treatment. Many wards also include disruptive patients with histories of violence who are not accepted in hostel accommodation and are difficult to place (Quirk & Lelliott 2004). As a result there are problems of a lack of easy access to beds for short-term management of crises. This pressure on available beds is particularly intense in Inner London, often leading to high thresholds for admission and a concentration on acute wards of the most 'difficult' and disruptive patients, especially young men with schizophrenia.

ORGANIZATION OF CARE AND INSTITUTIONAL PERMEABILITY

■ Characteristics of permeability

A study of three acute psychiatric wards in England involving observational data supplemented by 26 tape-recorded interviews with patients, patient advocates and staff identified these wards as being dynamic environments with a lot of activity and spatial movement. The authors suggested that the reality of everyday life in such wards conformed to what they term the 'permeable institution' (Quirk et al 2006). In contrast to the closed environment of psychiatric hospitals in the 1950s and 1960s, there was evidence of permeability associated with:

1. *Ward membership is temporary or 'revolving'*, with the ward population changing rapidly and relationships are therefore usually transitory. The patient group may also include those on extended leave, sometimes to free up beds for new admissions. Discharged patients or patients from other wards or day care services also often visit to either socialize with other patients or to use the ward facilities. The staff group is equally fluid, with the core ward nursing team changing with each shift, and the use of agency or bank staff, and student nurses on short-term placements, resulting in many shifts including nurses who are strangers;

2. *Contact with the outside world is maintained*, with many patients having daily contact with families and friends, with wards being either open to visitors throughout the day or at the discretion of the nurse in charge. Patients also often maintain contact with the outside world by personal mobile phones and may sometimes use this contact to enlist family and friends to intervene with staff on their behalf. They also frequently maintain contact with 'outside' professionals such as social workers, and may leave the ward on periods of unsupervised leave;

3. *Institutional identities are blurred*, with both nursing staff and patients wearing informal clothes and distinctions in dress between nursing staff and patients being fairly subtle. Patients and ward staff usually address one another by their first names, although consultants continue to occupy a hierarchical position.

■ Consequences and control of permeability

Permeability is identified as having both good and bad consequences. On the positive side, patients maintain many of their pre-admission identities and retain a degree of autonomy and links with the outside world, thus reducing risks of institutionalization and the consequent problems of coping on discharge. On the negative side, problems may occur through patients having continued responsibility for managing relationships, their housing situation and personal finances etc. outside the hospital. There may also be problems on the ward of safety and security caused by unwanted people coming onto the ward, with drug use and drug dealing also observed in an Inner-London ward. Much staff time is therefore taken up with managing these adverse effects of permeability.

The degree of permeability of a ward or psychiatric unit can be regulated to prevent some potentially adverse consequences. For example, CCTV cameras can be trained on entry and exit points, individual patients put under special observation or transferred to a locked unit, and visitors asked to leave if disruptive behaviour, drug dealing or other problems are suspected. Patients on wards with a high degree of permeability and risks of aggressive behaviour by other patients may employ proactive strategies to actively avoid risky situations or individuals, including seeking staff protection, soliciting the protective involvement of another patient, or employing more active strategies such as calming down people who look about to become aggressive. They may also aim to get discharged or sometimes escape. However, people who are acutely unwell tend to rely on nursing staff and other patients to assess and manage risk on their behalf rather than engage in proactive risk management strategies (Quirk et al 2004).

Quirk and colleagues (2006) suggest that institutional care is now characterized by degrees of permeability rather than degrees of totalitarianism. They note that staff often experience challenges and dilemmas on a daily basis as they attempt to provide the differing functions of a modern psychiatric ward within a permeable institution. Some problems for nursing staff are:

- how to respect the freedom of movement of informal patients while detaining those held involuntarily under mental health legislation;

- how to provide acceptable accommodation for those whose stay is prolonged and containment and acute care for those just admitted in a crisis;

- how to prevent informal patients who have freedom of movement from engaging in criminal or antisocial activity; and

- how to prevent the intrusion from outside of damaging or antisocial influences while helping patients to maintain links with the outside world in preparation for discharge.

STAFF ATTITUDES AND PATIENT CARE

Provision of rehabilitative care

The provision of a rehabilitative environment within hospitals is particularly important on wards for elderly people and those with mental illness problems. However, achieving this approach to care depends on both the availability of sufficient staff and on favourable staff orientations and approaches to care. The effects of staff attitudes and goals were demonstrated by an observational study of stroke patients cared for on a specialist stroke unit (SU), an elderly care unit (ECU) and a general medical ward (GMW) (Pound & Ebrahim 2000). There was no difference in staffing levels between the SU and ECU but the typical interaction between nurses and patients differed between these sites (Table 5.1). What the researchers referred to as 'emotional labour' consisted of interactions that were gentle, warm, respectful and attentive and which involved a personal rather than a standardized response. This occurred most frequently in ECUs. ECUs were

TABLE 5.1	Summary of typical interaction between nurses and stroke patients				
Setting (patient per nurse)	Emotional labour observed	Failures of emotional labour observed	Standardized interaction observed	Rehabilitation nursing observed
SU (1.8)	Occasionally	Nearly always	Rarely	Rarely
ECU (1.7)	Nearly always	Rarely	Occasionally	Always
GMW (2.9)	Rarely	Rarely	Nearly always	Never

From Pound & Ebrahim (2000).
SU, stroke unit; ECU, elderly care unit; GMW, general medical ward.

also characterized by greater frequency of 'rehabilitation nursing', which meant that nurses encouraged patients to wash, dress and go to the toilet independently where possible and spent the extra time with patients that this necessitated. By contrast, nurses on SUs were more likely to perform these tasks for patients and, although kindly in their approach, were often observed to treat patients as non-persons to whom things were done. The ECU was also characterized by greater communication and involvement of nurses in working with physiotherapists to carry over patients' physiotherapy activity to the wards and emphasized a holistic approach to care. A key factor contributing to these different patterns of care was identified as the greater formal training in rehabilitation among nurses in ECUs, which encouraged a rehabilitation philosophy and approach in the unit. Nurses working in ECUs also appeared to have accepted their low status and to regard emotional labour as an important aspect of their nursing role. By contrast, nurses working on SUs were concerned to enhance their professional status by undertaking an extended clinical/technological role. They therefore focused on functional and technical aspects of care that were regarded as enhancing their status, such as testing for swallow reflexes, inserting nasogastric tubes and so on. The findings of this research suggest that a greater emphasis on rehabilitation nursing in stroke units might enhance the positive effects of the specialized medical treatment provided by these units. However, achieving this depends on the attitude of members of staff and their perception of their role, with caring and emotional work with patients generally being less valued than technological skills on most wards within the acute hospital, although highly valued in hospice settings and wards where the primary goal is that of palliative and supportive care.

The notion of emotional labour described by Pound & Ebrahim (2000) forms one aspect of what Strauss et al (1982) described as the 'sentimental' work undertaken by health professionals. This comprises different forms of interaction that together make up a patient-centred approach to care. Strauss et al identified seven types of sentimental work based on observations they conducted in six hospitals over a period of 2 years (Box 5.1). Aspects of sentimental work include:

- A style of communication that seeks to create a partnership with patients in the medical task (interactional work)

- The provision of emotional support to patients through their hospital experience to promote patients' well-being and facilitate the conduct of medical procedures (trust work, composure work and biographical work)

- Maintaining patients' sense of identity in the face of illness and experience of impersonal care (identity work, rectification work).

BOX 5.1   Typology of types of sentimental work undertaken among hospital patients

1. Interactional work and moral rules: following taken-for-granted rules regarding behaviour (e.g. listening carefully, not breaking in abruptly on the speaker, not shouting, not being brusque or breaking in on privacy). Orienting and preparing the person you are working 'on', explaining the options, decisions or overall work, and getting consent to doing anything to their body and pacing work in relation to patients' energy and their capacity for enduring pain.
2. Trust work: establishing trust through demonstrating competence and showing concern for patients' physical, interactional and personal sensibilities through talk, reassuring touching, subtle gestures, etc.
3. Composure work: giving reassuring words and gestures to help patients through a painful or frightening experience.
4. Biographical work: eliciting information about the patients' social circumstances, support and lifestyle to aid medical diagnosis and decisions such as the pacing of prescribed therapy, as well as facilitating relationships between nurses and patients.
5. Identity work: an extension of biographical work that involves helping patients maintain and improve a sense of identity in the face of illness. This includes long conversations with terminally ill patients to keep spirits up and further a patient's closure on his or her life, or to prepare people for their post-hospital lives.
6. Awareness of context work: this refers to staff withholding information that they believe patients will find difficult to handle. However, the practice is now of greater disclosure and recognition that non-disclosure is an unstable situation because patients move to suspicion or full awareness of the situation.
7. Rectification work: this occurs when patients express aggrievement or a sense of insult during or following the flouting of interactional rules, or when their composure has been shattered. It involves 'picking up the pieces' and reassuring patients that they really are people despite being treated as a non-person (e.g. following some visits to machined sites for diagnosis or therapy or following some ward rounds).

From: Strauss et al (1982).

Strauss and colleagues note that sentimental work occurs mainly at the margins of the main line (medical-nursing, technical) of action in acute hospital settings and, although assisting the achievement of these tasks, is often not recorded. However, if the ideology of the ward or unit emphasizes sentimental work, interaction involving caring and emotional labour is accorded greater value and priority by staff, rather than being excluded or devalued in professional–patient interactions.

Increasing emphasis is now given in medical and nurse training to patient partnership, empowerment and choice, and thus to implementing the various dimensions of sentimental work. However, this approach to care is by no means universal, even within settings that are formally concerned with rehabilitation and care. For example, a study of five hospital wards caring for older people identified staff as often performing nursing tasks on patients without asking their permission rather than promoting patients' independence and feeling of being in control of their own lives. They also often failed to encourage patients to make choices and to participate actively in their own care, or to provide patients (and their relatives) with information about future care options and answer their questions clearly, with the least empowering ward being an elderly care rehabilitation ward (Faulkner 2001). Achieving personalized care and a rehabilitative environment for chronically ill patients takes time and training. It also requires sufficient numbers of qualified staff and the valuing by staff of these aspects of care.

Accident & Emergency services

One aspect of professional–patient relationships is the tendency in some situations for staff to evaluate patients in both social and medical terms. In particular, the considerable range of patients attending Accident & Emergency (A&E) departments, and their varying medical needs, provides considerable opportunity for such evaluation. A classic study that was conducted in three A&E departments (Jeffrey 1979) identified a group of patients depicted by junior doctors as 'good' patients in terms of their medical condition. These patients presented with conditions that allowed junior A&E staff to practise and develop the clinical skills necessary to pass professional examinations or to practise their chosen speciality, or were acutely ill patients (e.g. head injuries, cardiac arrests, road traffic accidents) who tested the general competence and maturity of staff in coping with their rapid early treatment. At the other end of the continuum were patients described in negative social terms and categorized as 'rubbish' (dross, etc.). These consisted of four main groups of patients – people presenting with 'trivia', drunks, regular overdoses and tramps. Each of these groups was regarded as having broken the unwritten rules of appropriate patient behaviour.

Patients presenting at A&E departments with medical 'trivia' are viewed as having a condition that is neither due to trauma nor is urgent and therefore not a legitimate demand on an A&E service. Levels of such 'inappropriate' use are estimated to range from about 6% to over 40% of attendances, which reflects both differences in areas and the characteristics of populations and differences in professional views and definitions of inappropriate attenders (Murphy 1998). Studies examining why patients attend A&E departments for what is deemed medical 'trivia' suggest that this occurs among people not registered with a GP and also because individuals feel unable to evaluate the medical seriousness of the condition, especially in relation to the illness of a very young child. The choice of A&E attendance rather than primary care usually reflects the more immediate access (i.e. lack of a booked appointment system) and provision of an out-of-hours service, together in many cases with the expectation of more specialist hospital level care (Sanders 2000). Whereas previously the aim was to change the behaviours of people designated as inappropriate attenders at A&E departments, current policies have responded by the establishment of minor injuries units and general practitioner and nurse specialists within A&E departments to treat medically trivial conditions. A national nurse-led telephone advice system (NHS Direct) now also provides information and advice as to whether medical care is necessary. There is, however, some evidence that NHS Direct nurses may often encourage presentation at hospital in their concern not to overlook a serious problem.

PATIENTS' EXPERIENCES AND INVOLVEMENT

Stress and anxiety

Admission to hospital is routine for hospital staff but forms a major event in people's lives and is often a source of considerable anxiety and stress. For patients, the fact that 'something is wrong,' requiring diagnosis, treatment or both, often forms a source of anxiety in itself. For some patients there are further uncertainties about whether they will be cured, left with a physical disability or faced with an early death. Patients are also frequently apprehensive about the discomfort and pain they might experience in undergoing diagnostic or operative procedures, and often worry about having an anaesthetic. In addition, the actual experience of being a patient in hospital is often stressful. Particular sources of stress include a lack of privacy, lack of familiarity with the different categories of staff and with the general routines of the ward, problems of being disturbed on the ward and not being able to sleep, and not being given sufficient information about their medical condition or treatment. Patients about to be discharged might also worry about how they will manage at home. For young children, admission to hospital and separation from their parents and familiar surroundings can be particularly traumatic. As a result, there is now greater emphasis and provision for parents to spend long periods of time on the ward and in some cases to participate in their child's care.

Recognition of the high level of stress that is often experienced by hospital patients has led to a greater emphasis on preparing patients (and children) for hospital admission through written information and personal communication to explain their treatment and hospital stay. This patient preparation has been demonstrated to have positive effects on measures of anxiety, pain and satisfaction among patients undergoing surgery or treatments such as radiotherapy (Shuldham 1999). It is also of particular importance for day surgery, as this requires that patients are admitted and discharged on the same day and manage their recovery at home. Increasing use is now made of audio tapes and cassettes to provide patients with information about their condition and treatment options. There is also greater emphasis on ensuring that information is 'patient-centred', and reflects the priorities and needs of patients rather than those of the health professionals. The sick person's reaction to being in hospital in terms of anxiety, worry, fear and depression, also draws attention to the importance of 'emotional labour' by hospital staff, which acknowledges that the object of medical work is alive, sentient and reacting. Work done with or on human beings needs to take into account their response to that work, and is therefore accompanied by the provision of information, support and comfort that responds to individual patient needs.

▓ Patient and user involvement

A major shift in health policy is the requirement, as set out in 'The NHS Plan' (Department of Health 2000), that Hospital Trusts and other parts of the NHS take account of the public's and users' views in developing the service, and that patients are fully involved in decisions about their own care as active partners with professionals.

The incorporation of a public/user voice is seen as an essential element at every level of the service, acting as a lever for change. This is being implemented through a variety of fora set up to elicit the views of local groups and communities, including the appointment of patient/user/public representatives to key committees concerned with the quality and service development at both national and local levels, and supporting them in this process. This has led to new ways of organizing aspects of the service, including redesigning processes in clinics to increase their efficiency and acceptability, and developing rapid access and integrated care schemes. There has also been an increase in patient information materials (leaflets, booklets, videos, etc.) that aim to respond to patients' own questions and concerns and help patients with a specific condition to understand what the disease is, and its parameters, stages of treatment, what is likely to happen to them and the options available. This includes the availability of websites that enable patients to learn what the experience of a particular illness is really like for patients and their carers through hearing about the experiences of others based on their own descriptions (www.dipex.org/). Patients admitted to NHS hospitals are also now accorded greater rights, including the right of access to their health records, participation in treatment decisions and full disclosure of treatment options as part of informed consent. These measures taken together aim to increase the acceptability and efficiency of services and to address major causes of dissatisfaction among hospital patients regarding communication about their condition and treatment, and a perceived lack of information about the hospital and its routine which contribute to patients' feelings of stress.

THE CHANGING ORGANIZATION OF CARE

Like any large organizations, hospitals are in a continuous process of evolution and change. They were founded as institutions for the care of the sick poor, who were removed from the community because of infectious disease, but became the major site of clinical practice and the location of technologies for diagnosis and treatment. A current trend is for lengths of stay to decline and for care to increasingly move outside the hospital. This is exemplified by the expansion in minor surgery undertaken by general practitioners, the substantial increases in day surgery, the availability of home dialysis and fetal monitoring, developments in specialist clinics in primary care and consultant outreach sessions, and the increasing emphasis on treating chronic conditions in the community. As part of the modernization of the NHS and its provision for older people set out in *The NHS Plan* (Department of Health 2000) and the *National Service Framework: Older People* (Department of Health 2001) a new range of services has been developed, collectively known as 'intermediate care', that aim to prevent unnecessary hospital admissions, facilitate earlier discharges and reduce premature admission to long-term care. Although previously various forms of residential care and non-residential services have existed (e.g. day hospital, day centre and domiciliary services), current policies aim to expand this provision and ensure that services are integrated across primary care, community health services, social care, housing and the acute sector (Martin et al 2007).

Changes in the organization of care have been accompanied by increasing numbers of nurses, physiotherapists, midwives and other health professionals working in the community. Some hospital consultants also hold specialist outreach sessions for diabetes, ophthalmology and other conditions. Much care therefore involves different professional groups working in the community and may also require a hospital consultation or short periods of hospital care. Current trends suggest that the hospital will become the centre of a vertically integrated system in which acute beds play only a modest role. This change in function and blurring of the primary/secondary interface has implications for clinical training and medical work, as well as for patients' experiences of medical care. In particular, it emphasizes the importance of good coordination between primary and secondary services, and communication between staff and between staff and patients. This has led to increasing emphasis on patients' experience of 'continuity of care' in terms of a 'seamless service'. This goes beyond personal continuity in terms of the provision of continuing care from a single individual and increasingly requires informational and management continuity, with discrete healthcare events being experienced as coherent, connected and consistent with the patients' medical needs and personal context (Box 5.2). For patients and their families, the experience of continuity is the perception that providers know what has happened before, that different providers agree on a management plan, and that a

---

BOX 5.2   Three types of continuity of care

Informational continuity – the use of information on past events and personal circumstances to make current care appropriate for each individual.
Management continuity – a consistent and coherent approach to the management of a health condition that is responsive to a patient's changing needs.
Relational continuity – an ongoing therapeutic relationship between a patient and one or more providers.

Source: Haggerty et al (2003) p. 1220.

provider who knows them will care for them in the future. For providers, the experience of continuity relates to their perception that they have sufficient knowledge and information about a patient to apply their professional competence and the confidence that their care inputs will be recognized and pursued by other providers. Critical points in terms of continuity of care occur at discharge from hospital and movement between services, especially the movement between children's services and adult services.

References

Bryan K, Gage H, Gilbert K 2006 Delayed transfers of older people from hospital: causes and policy implications. Health Policy 76:194–201

Department of Health (DoH) 2000 The NHS plan: a plan for investment, a plan for reform. Cmnd 4818-1. HMSO, London

Department of Health 2001 National service framework for older people. Department of Health, London

Faulkner M 2001 A measure of patient empowerment in hospital environments catering for older people. Journal of Advanced Nursing 34(5):676–686

Goffman E 1961 Asylums. Doubleday, New York

Haggerty JL, Reid RJ, Freeman GK et al 2003 Continuity of care: a multidisciplinary review. British Medical Journal 327:1219–1221

Jeffrey R 1979 Normal rubbish: deviant patients in the casualty department. Sociology of Health and Illness 1:90–107

Johnstone P, Zolese G 1999 Systematic review of the effectiveness of planned short hospital stays for mental health care. British Medical Journal 318:1387–1390

Lewis R, Glasby G 2006 Delayed discharge from mental health hospitals: results of an English postal survey. Health & Social Care in the Community 14(3):225–230

Martin GP, Hewitt GJ, Faulkner TA, Parker H 2007 The organization, form and function of intermediate care services and systems in England: results from a national survey. Health & Social Care in the Community 15(2):146–154

McCourt CA 2000 Life after hospital closure: users' views of living in residential 'resettlement' projects. A case study in consumer led research. Health Expectations 3:192–202

Murphy AW 1998 'Inappropriate' attenders at accident and emergency departments. 1: definition, incidence and reasons for attendance. Family Practice 15(1):23–32

Pound P, Ebrahim S 2000 Rhetoric and reality in stroke patient care. Social Science and Medicine 51:1437–1446

Quirk A, Lelliott P, Seale C 2004 Service users' strategies for managing risk in the volatile environment of an acute psychiatric ward. Social Science & Medicine 59:2573–2583

Quirk A, Lelliott P, Seale C 2006 The permeable institution: An ethnographic study of three acute psychiatric wards in London. Social Science & Medicine 63:2105–2117

Sanders J 2000 A review of health professional attitudes and patient perceptions on 'inappropriate' accident and emergency attendances. The implications for current minor injury service provision in England and Wales. Journal of Advanced Nursing 31(5):1097–1105

Shuldham C 1999 A review of the impact of pre-operative education on recovery from surgery. International Journal of Nursing Studies 36:171–177

Strauss A et al 1982 Sentimental work in the technological hospital. Sociology of Health and Illness 4(3):254–278

Vetter N 2003 Inappropriately delayed discharge from hospital: what do we know? British Medical Journal 326:927–928

6

Living with chronic illness

David Locker

Since the early 1970s sociologists have increasingly turned their attention to the issues and challenges involved in chronic illness and disability. Studies of people with disabilities were common before this time, but were predominantly concerned with psychological factors and their role in the rehabilitation process.

During the 1970s considerable effort was invested in developing appropriate measures of chronic illness and disability, estimating the prevalence and severity of disability, assessing the needs of people with disabilities and identifying gaps in service provision for these individuals and the families who cared for them. In the 1980s more attention was paid to the experience of living with chronic illness and disability (Anderson & Bury 1988, Conrad 1987). Numerous studies are now available that describe in some detail what it is like for individuals and families to live with a long-term, disabling disorder. The rationale underlying this work is that 'a sound, effective and ethical approach to chronic illness must lie in awareness of and attention to the experiences, values, priorities and expectations of (these people) and their families' (Anderson & Bury 1988). This means that a detailed understanding of the impact of chronic illness and disability on daily life is necessary for the providers of medical and social services to offer appropriate care and support.

This recent emphasis on chronic illness reflects the fact that chronic disabling disorders, rather than acute infectious diseases, are the major cause of mortality in industrial societies and present a significant challenge to the medical-care system (see Chapter 1). Even where chronic conditions are not fatal, they are major sources of suffering for individuals and families. As Verbrugge & Jette (1994) indicate, people mostly live with rather than die from chronic conditions. Given that the populations of western societies are ageing (see Chapter 11), it is predicted that the proportion of consultations in medical practice devoted to the psychosocial and other problems of daily living associated with chronic illness will increase. As a result, there will be a fundamental shift in medical practice from 'cure' to 'care' (Williams 1989).

The emergence of an interest in chronic illness also coincided with an increase in government provision for people with disabling disorders. In the UK, 1970 saw the passing of the Chronically Sick and Disabled Persons Act, which made it mandatory for local authorities to identify people with disabilities, to determine their needs and to provide services to meet those needs (Topliss 1979). In 1974, a Minister for the Disabled was appointed with specific responsibilities for the group. These developments led to an increase in services and financial benefits for people with disabilities and those who cared for them, although these were somewhat eroded during the late 1980s.

A further development which stimulated a greater awareness of the needs and priorities of people living with chronic illness was the emergence of the 'disability movement' (Conrad 1987). This consisted of groups dedicated to self-help and political action. The former offered help and support through the sharing of individual experience, while the latter used the political process to secure fundamental rights and to promote independent living. The aim here was to ensure that people with chronic disabling disorders would themselves define their needs and the most appropriate way of providing for them, rather than having these imposed by putative 'experts' and professionals. Such political activism contributed to the UK Disability Discrimination Act of 1995 and the creation in 2000 of the Disability Rights Commission whose aim is to stop discrimination against people with disabilities and to promote equal opportunities. The 1995 Act was extended in 2002 with new employment rights and rights of access becoming law in 2004.

CHARACTERISTICS OF CHRONIC ILLNESS

The term 'chronic illness' encompasses a wide range of conditions affecting almost all body systems. Cancer, stroke, end-stage renal disease, poliomyelitis, multiple sclerosis, rheumatoid arthritis, psoriasis, epilepsy and chronic obstructive airways disease are common examples. The most fundamental characteristic of chronic illnesses is that they are long-term and have a profound influence on the lives of sufferers. Some are fatal and some are not; some are stable with a certain prognosis, others may show great variation in terms of their day-to-day manifestations and their long-term course and outcome. In the majority of cases medical intervention is palliative; it seeks to control symptoms but cannot offer a cure. Consequently, maximizing the welfare of these individuals and their families means maintaining or improving the quality of daily life rather than attempting to eradicate the disease process itself.

Some of the problems encountered by people with a chronic disabling disorder stem directly from the symptomatic character of their illness. In this respect, every chronic condition is somewhat distinct. For example, the person with rheumatoid arthritis must cope with chronic pain, the person with respiratory disease must live with breathlessness and an inadequate oxygen supply, and the person with end-stage renal failure must cope with the demands of a dialysis machine. In other respects the problems faced by people with chronic illnesses may be common to all, irrespective of the nature of their condition. Unemployment or reduced career prospects, social isolation and estrangement from family and friends, loss of important roles, changed physical appearance and problems with self-esteem and identity are experienced by many such individuals. Another fundamental characteristic of chronic conditions is that these assaults on the body, daily activities (encompassing home, work and leisure) and social relationships (including relationships with self and others) must be managed in the course of everyday life. When chronic illness becomes severe, daily life may be entirely consumed in coping with its symptoms, the medical regimens intended to control it and its social consequences (Locker 1983).

Prevalence of chronic illness and disability

A number of surveys of national and local populations have been undertaken in order to estimate the prevalence of disability. These have produced somewhat different results, largely because different definitions and measures of disability have been employed. A national study in the UK, the Survey of Disability in Great Britain undertaken in 1985 by the Office of Population Censuses and Surveys (OPCS), found that 14.2% of the adult population were disabled (OPCS 1988). Rates increased substantially with age and were higher among women than men. Other studies have reported that the most common causes of significant disability are neurological, musculoskeletal and respiratory diseases such as stroke, multiple sclerosis, Parkinson's disease and rheumatoid arthritis. The most recent estimates of disability in the UK come from the Health Surveys for England. In 2000–01 18% of those aged 16 years and over reported having a disability with 5% having severe disability. For those 75 years and over, 51% of women and 43% of men reported being disabled (Hirani & Malbut 2002). Similarly, it has been estimated that about 35 million Americans, or one in seven, have disabling conditions sufficiently severe to interfere with daily life. One factor increasing the prevalence of some types of disability is medicine's increasing success at averting the death of many people with developmental abnormalities such as spina bifida and the consequences of accidents such as spinal cord resection. HIV/AIDS has also been transformed from an invariably fatal condition into a chronic illness by the advent of therapies which control the replication of the virus responsible for the disease.

Studies of disability probably underestimate the prevalence of chronic illness. Conditions such as diabetes, psoriasis and epilepsy may not be identified by conventional measures of disability. Consequently, the percentage of the population living with a chronic condition is likely to be higher than the 14.2% identified by the OPCS survey. One estimate derived from work by the Royal College of Physicians suggested that just over one-fifth of the population was subject to some type of chronic illness.

More recent surveys have provided data on the prevalence of specific conditions among specific age groups. These confirm the difference between estimates of the prevalence of chronic conditions and estimates of the prevalence of disability. For example, a survey of a sample of the population aged 45 years and over living in the north of England found a prevalence of stroke of 17.5 persons per 1000. However, the prevalence of stroke-related dependence was lower at 11.7 persons per 1000 (O'Mahoney et al 1999). Similarly, projections based on national data collected in 1997 suggest that by 2020 60 million persons in the USA will be affected by arthritis, with 11.6 million being limited by this condition (Morbidity and Mortality Weekly Report 2001). These data also indicated that the prevalence of persons with arthritis had increased by approximately 750 000 persons per year since 1990. Other evidence from the USA suggests that from 1982 to 1999 there was an overall reduction in the prevalence of disability among elderly people (Manton & Gu 2001) and further declines have been observed in the most recent study. In 2004–2005 19% of people 65 years and over were disabled, compared to 26.5% in 1982. It is also the case that the annual rate of decline has accelerated from 0.6% in 1984 to 2.2% in 2004–2005 (Manton et al 2006). European data also indicate a reduction in the prevalence of disability in more recent cohorts of elderly women (Winblad et al 2001). In the UK, small falls in rates of disability have been observed for the period 1995–2000. Nevertheless, the ageing of the population will most likely mean an increase in the numbers of people living with a disabling condition even though the prevalence is falling.

Impairment, disability and handicap

A systematic approach to thinking about chronic illness is to be found in the International Classification of Impairments, Disabilities or Handicaps (ICIDH), a manual which classifies the consequences of disease (Badley 1993, Wood 1980). In order to better understand these consequences, it offers three concepts: impairment, disability and handicap. Impairment is concerned with abnormalities in the structure or functioning of the body or its parts, disability with the performance of activities, and handicap with the broader social and psychological consequences of living with impairment and disability. Because it is dependent on the social context in which it occurs, handicap can best be understood by sociological enquiry. Formal definitions of these terms are given in Box 6.1.

The three concepts are also organized into a model or theoretical framework which relates these dimensions of experience to each other (Fig. 6.1).

This model has caused some confusion, especially since some have interpreted the arrows to indicate time; so that an individual with a chronic condition moves along the sequence and inevitably becomes handicapped. In fact, the arrows mean 'may or may not lead to'. Disability may result from impairment and handicap may result from disability, but this is not necessarily so. The examples given in Box 6.2 illustrate this point. Moreover, there is no necessary relationship between the severity of impairment and the severity of disability and/or handicap that results. For example, a study of people with multiple sclerosis found that the psychosocial handicaps they suffered were not related to the severity of the underlying disease (Harper et al 1986). Similarly, a study of individuals with chronic respiratory disease found that clinical measures of lung function were not good predictors of disability, and there was considerable variability in the extent of handicap associated with a given level of disability (Williams & Bury 1989a, b).

Although the ICIDH scheme has been widely used it has been subject to some criticism, particularly in the US, where alternative schemes have been developed and adopted (Nagi 1991, Verbrugge & Jette 1994). At the heart of the problem is the use of the term handicap and the way in which is has been defined. In the USA the term handicapped has

---

> **BOX 6.1**   ICIDH Definitions
>
> - **Impairment**: an impairment is any loss or abnormality of psychological, physiological or anatomical structure or function.
> - **Disability**: a disability is a restriction or lack (resulting from an impairment) of ability to perform an activity in a manner or within the range considered normal for a human being.
> - **Handicap**: a handicap is a disadvantage for a given individual, resulting from an impairment or a disability, that limits or prevents the fulfilment of a role that is normal (depending on age, sex and social and cultural factors) for that individual.

> **BOX 6.2** Interrelations of impairment, disability and handicap
>
> - An individual with arthritis (disease) will have pain and swelling in involved joints which will be stiff and limited in their range of motion (impairment). Consequently, there may be difficulty in carrying out activities such as walking or climbing stairs (disability). This may disadvantage the individual in terms of mobility around the community or finding a job, which in turn may lead to social isolation of relative poverty (handicap).
> - People with extreme short sight or diabetes are impaired but because these conditions can be corrected with devices or drugs, they would not necessarily be disabled in terms of any limitations in the activities they perform. However, in certain circumstances they may be handicapped by their conditions. For example, short sight may prevent access to certain occupations and diabetes may impose a burden on the individual because of dietary restrictions and the need for regular insulin injections.
> - A person with a severe facial disfigurement which is present at birth or the result of an accident would be impaired. They would not experience any limitations in the tasks or activities of daily life and would not be disabled. However, they may be handicapped in the sense that social attitudes towards physical attractiveness could lead to low self-esteem and difficulty in forming romantic relationships.
> - A person with cerebral palsy may have a range of impairments including problems with speech or use of the limbs. These could lead to disabilities in many activities including mobility around the community, difficulties with self-care and difficulties with communication. As a result, the individual could be handicapped in a number of areas of life. Alternatively, recognition of the person's intellectual abilities could open opportunities for a high status professional career with a high income. In turn, this would facilitate autonomy and choice.
>
> Adapted from Badley (1995).

87

been used to describe people in a pejorative way and is now generally avoided. In addition, the term carries the implication that the problems people experience are intrinsic, that is, the product of personal deficiencies and failings. Finally, because the definition of handicap uses the word 'role', which generally refers to activities and tasks, some have found the distinction between disability and handicap unclear.

One way around these difficulties is to think of handicap in terms of disadvantage and deprivation. For example, an individual who uses a wheelchair may be at a disadvantage in seeking work compared to the able-bodied simply because many workplaces have steps, stairs and wash-rooms or other facilities inaccessible to a wheelchair. As a consequence individuals may be deprived of jobs commensurate with their education and skills, or may become unemployed and deprived of the income, social contacts and other benefits that accrue from work. Even less-tangible problems such as the mental burden and low self-esteem that may accompany chronic illness can be understood in these terms: the individual is deprived of peace of mind and a sense of self-worth.

This example highlights a crucial aspect of handicap. It does not stem from the individual but from the environments in which he/she must live. An alternative definition which

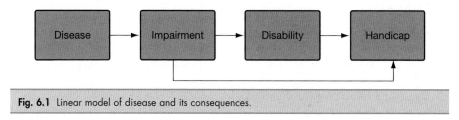

Fig. 6.1 Linear model of disease and its consequences.

makes this explicit states that handicap consists of 'the opportunities that a person has missed because of barriers in the environment' (Halbertsma 1989). In fact, a review of recent definitions of handicap found that they all contained reference to the environment (Badley 1995). In this context, environment refers not only to the physical environment, but also to material, social and attitudinal environments.

Medical and social models of disability

The above comments regarding the concept of handicap are intended to highlight the difference between medical and social models of disability. This distinction arose out of criticisms of the ICIDH model by people who were active in organizations and movements that aimed to secure basic civil rights for people with disabilities. In the medical model, disability is defined as a deviation from biomedical norms of structure and function and the disadvantages that disabled people experience are seen as the direct and inevitable consequence of their impairments and disabilities (Bickenbach et al 1999). Consequently, disability is a problem of a person best addressed by medical intervention to cure the disease or help the person adjust to their limitations. The social model sees the problems experienced by people with disabilities as being the direct product of the physical, social and attitudinal environments referred to above. The problem is not that disabled people cannot meet the demands of everyday life; rather, the problem is a failure of the environment to adjust to the needs and desires of people with disabilities. Political action and social change are necessary to ensure the full participation of people with disabilities in all areas of social life (WHO 1999).

While the ICIDH model attempted to offer a non-medical account of disablement, the language it used to describe the links between impairment, disability and handicap, its description of the nature of handicap and its failure to focus on the key role played by the environment meant that it embodied many of the features of the medical model (Bickenbach et al 1999).

A revised model: functioning, disability and health

An early modification to the ICIDH model emphasized the need to view handicap as emerging out of external factors that interact with disease/impairment/disability. One attempt to describe these factors made reference to the physical environment, the social situation of the person and the resources available to them (Badley 1987). In a more recent contribution, Verbrugge & Jette (1994) provided a more elaborate classification, including both personal and environmental factors in the process which links impairment/disability and their outcomes (Box 6.3). The importance of these factors is that they provide avenues for interventions that aim to improve the quality of life of persons so affected.

In response to criticisms of the original ICIDH model, a more comprehensive modification has recently been developed by the World Health Organization (Halbertsma et al 2000). This is called the International Classification of Functioning, Disability and Health known as ICF (WHO 1999). This has moved away from being a 'consequences of disease' model, to a 'components of health' model. Its key components are *body structures and functions* and impairments in structure or function; *activities*, which are tasks or activities undertaken by a person and difficulties or limitations an individual may have in executing those activities; and *participation*, which consists of involvement in life situations in the context of where an individual lives. Participation restrictions are problems a person may experience with respect to involvement in life situations. Each of these components, and

---

BOX 6.3   Factors influencing the disablement process

Extra-individual factors
- Medical care and rehabilitation (surgery, physical therapy, speech therapy, counselling, health education, job retraining, etc.)
- Medication and other therapeutic regimens (drugs, recreational therapy, aquatic exercise, biofeedback meditation, rest/energy conservation, etc.)
- External supports (personal assistance, special equipment and devices, day care, respite care, meals-on-wheels, etc.)
- Buildings, physical and social environment (structural modifications at home/job, access to buildings and public transport, health insurance and access to medical care, laws and regulations, employment legislation, social attitudes, etc.)

Intra-individual factors
- Life-style and behaviour changes (overt changes to alter disease activity and impact)
- Psychosocial attributes and coping (positive affect, emotional vigour, locus of control, cognitive adaptation to disability, personal support, peer support groups, etc.)
- Activity accommodations (changes in kinds of activities, ways of doing them, frequency or length of time doing them)

Reprinted with kind permission from Elsevier Science Ltd from Verbrugge & Jette (1994).

---

the relationships between them are influenced by *contextual factors*; that is, *personal and environmental factors* of the kind described in Box 6.3. This scheme attempts to integrate the medical and social models of disability into a broader biopsychosocial model that gives due recognition to the significance of the environment in influencing functioning and overall health and well-being.

THE MEANING OF CHRONIC ILLNESS

From a sociological point of view and from the point of view of those living with a chronic illness, the disadvantage and deprivation they experience is, perhaps, the important consideration. This is because such experiences are closely allied with the quality of life. Arguably, within the right environments, the quality of life of many people with impairments and disabilities would not be much different from that of those without.

Because of its significance, two issues concerning disadvantage and deprivation warrant further attention: first, their multidimensional character; and second, the significance of material and social resources in managing the problems created by chronic illness. As mentioned above, many of these problems have their origins in the interaction of individuals with their environments.

Dimensions of disadvantage and deprivation

Whereas early sociological approaches to chronic illness and disability drew on the theory of the sick role (Parsons 1951) (see Chapter 4), labelling theory (Lemert 1967) and Goffman's analysis of stigma (Goffman 1963) (see Chapter 13), more contemporary approaches have used detailed case studies to understand what it means to live with a chronic disabling disorder. This 'experience of illness' perspective is to be found in numerous books and scholarly papers published over the last 20 years and all have disadvantage, deprivation and quality of life as their central concern.

Stated simply, the meaning of chronic illness is to be found in its practical and symbolic consequences (Blaxter 1976, Bury 1988). These consequences take the form of problems which people with chronic disabling conditions and their families must solve if they are to attain a quality of life of minimal tolerability.

For example, one study of people with rheumatoid arthritis found that all faced the following problems: managing the symptoms of the disease and the medical treatments designed to control them; problems with the practical matters of everyday living, such as self-care, household management and mobility around the home and community; problems with respect to finding work or maintaining a meaningful role in the work-force; economic problems following unemployment; and problems in social relationships and family life (Locker 1983). The emotional burden of being chronically ill, its psychological consequences in the form of depression and frustration and feelings of vulnerability were prominent among this group of people, as was the necessity of adapting to a more limited life. The participants in this study also encountered what might be termed cognitive problems. That is, they were faced with the task of making sense of the onset of chronic illness and sought answers to the unanswerable question 'Why me?'. In addition, they were constantly engaged in efforts to make sense of the day-to-day variation in levels of pain and stiffness in an attempt to establish order in their world and render their unpredictable existence predictable. As many studies have revealed, a significant aspect of being or caring for a person with a disability is the 'daily grind'; the never-ending and unrewarded practical and psychological work involved in coping with these problems on a daily basis. A more detailed account of some of these issues is presented below.

▮ The significance of resources

A crucial factor which has an influence on how, and the extent to which, the problems associated with chronic illness and disability are managed is the resources to which individuals have access. These resources may take many forms; time, energy, money, social support, appropriate housing, formal services which foster independence rather than exacerbate dependence and knowledge and information are perhaps the most important. Psychological resources and dispositions are also important. The magnitude and range of resources available to individuals and families, and the coping strategies of which they form a part, influence how well the consequences of chronic conditions are managed.

In a sense, the fact that personal and social resources must be allocated to solving mundane practical matters is part of the handicap that flows from chronic illness. Money may have to be used to pay someone to clean the house and do the shopping rather than being used to make life more enjoyable. As chronic illness progresses, it is sometimes the case that available resources shrink. Physical resources may decline as a result of the worsening of the disease, money may decline when the individual becomes unemployed and his/her spouse gives up work to adopt a full-time caring role, and social support may be eroded as friendship networks or families collapse under the strain of chronic illness. In these instances, life becomes nothing more than the work and effort of solving illness-related problems and getting through the day.

The concept of resources is a crucial one. On the one hand, it provides one of the mechanisms which link disability, disadvantage and deprivation; while on the other, it draws attention to the unequal distribution of resources in society and the ability/inability of individuals from different socio-economic groups to maintain a satisfactory existence in the face of chronic illness. In this way, it links personal concerns with wider social and political issues. People from working-class backgrounds, women, ethnic minorities and those who live in deprived urban communities are likely to be the most vulnerable in the face of chronic illness.

It is also the case that the illness experience can vary with historical period and culture. As Bury (1988) has indicated, chronic illness has two levels of meaning. One is to be found in the kinds of problems described above. The other is to be found in the significance or connotations that particular conditions carry, and the extent to which a given condition renders an individual culturally incompetent, that is, unable to perform ordinary activities in socially appropriate ways. The extent to which an individual is devalued by chronic illness will also be influenced by what the illness means in its particular cultural environment. For example, chronic obstructive airways disease is 'linked in the public mind to smoking (so) that the image of a wheezing, coughing, breathless old man is often greeted with little sympathy' (Williams & Bury 1989b: 609). This lack of sympathy may reflect a lack of attention to, and resources invested in, those suffering from the disease. Similarly, AIDS is closely allied in public thinking to devalued and socially stigmatized groups such as male homosexuals and i.v. drug users, and behaviours which predispose the person to disease transmission. In this sense, AIDS constitutes a major assault on privacy. To reveal AIDS does not just reveal the presence of a disease, it reveals much more about identity and life-style. In this way, the handicapping nature of chronic illness flows also directly from social and cultural values.

MAJOR THEMES IN RESEARCH ON THE EXPERIENCE OF ILLNESS

It is not possible to convey the realities of living with chronic illness within the confines of a short chapter such as this. However, some impression can be gained of its pervasive effects by a brief discussion of some of the major themes evident in research on the experience of illness. Conrad (1987) has identified a number of such themes. Five are mentioned here; another, stigma, is the subject of Chapter 13.

▓ Uncertainty

Many chronic conditions are surrounded by uncertainty. This may begin at the time when the individual first notices that something is wrong and may continue throughout the entire course of the illness. Many chronic illnesses have a slow and insidious onset and emerge in the form of vague symptoms that persist for years before diagnosis (prediagnostic uncertainty). With multiple sclerosis the delay between appearance of symptoms and diagnosis may be as long as 15 years (Robinson 1988). During this time sufferers are convinced that something is wrong, but often find their complaints dismissed by medical practitioners as trivial or as evidence of malingering or hypochondria. This can be a very trying time for the individual and his/her family. When a diagnosis is finally obtained, it often comes as a relief; it legitimates the person's complaints and experiences and brings to an end conflicts with others over the reality of the symptoms (Robinson 1988).

However, uncertainty may follow the diagnosis itself. This is often so with respect to predicting the course and outcome of the disease (trajectory uncertainty). Coupled with the uncertainty which can surround day-to-day fluctuations in symptoms (symptomatic uncertainty), this can severely disrupt family life. It makes both short- and long-term planning impossible and often means that living arrangements have to be constantly revised. Managing this uncertainty by whatever means available can become a major component of daily life.

A good example of uncertainty is provided by rheumatoid arthritis (RA). The symptoms of this disease, joint pain and stiffness, are highly unpredictable. The location and severity of the pain varies from day to day, and may even change during the course of a day. What seems to be a 'good day' in the morning may become a 'bad day' by the afternoon. This variability and unpredictability means that people with RA find it difficult to make sense of their symptoms and to contain them within acceptable boundaries. Many attempt to impose a degree of certainty on their existence by trying to identify events which precede acute phases or particularly painful days. Cold or damp weather and physical and emotional stress are frequently seen as the cause of pain and avoided as far as possible. However, a 'bad day' for which no apparent reason can be found leaves sufferers confused and adds to their distress (Locker 1983).

Family relations

There is clear evidence that chronic illness can place intolerable strains on families. This can arise because of the necessity to provide high levels of care and support, the emotional connotations of giving and receiving help and changes in family roles and relationships. Even where families are able and willing to provide help, the person with a chronic disabling condition may feel that he or she is a burden and may refuse the assistance that is needed. It is also the case that particularly distressing symptoms, such as chronic pain, may lead the individual to withdraw from family life altogether. In some instances, both individual and family become isolated from the wider world. Marital breakdown is not uncommon in these instances.

MacDonald (1988) provides insights into the effects of chronic illness on marital and family relationships in her study of people living with the sequelae of rectal cancer. Two-thirds of the people she interviewed had a colostomy, with the remainder having been treated by excision of the cancer and anastomosis. Most of the individuals reported a loss of sexual capacity and a decline in the quality of the marital relationship. This was partly due to the physical effects of surgery and partly due to feelings of shame and embarrassment. These feelings of stigma were most marked among younger men, who reported that the consequences of surgery and fears for the future had created a barrier between them and their wives.

The consequences of surgery also had a profound effect on social relationships in general. Again, shame and embarrassment about noise and odours from the stoma, worries about offending others and feelings of self-disgust caused many to avoid social contacts and to lead a far more restricted life.

Biographical work and the reconstitution of self

All chronic disabling conditions pose a threat to identity and self-concept. One of the reasons for this is that the onset of chronic illness often constitutes a 'biographical disruption' (Bury 1982) and calls into question both past and future. It necessitates a fundamental rethinking of both biography and self-concept. Williams (1984) argues that people with chronic illness must indulge in a process he calls 'narrative reconstruction', in which the individual's biography is reorganized in order to account for the onset of illness. This identification of cause, which draws on lay theories concerning the aetiology of illness, is part of the process of coming to terms with chronic illness. It gives meaning and order to the individual's world.

Charmaz (1987) has described how chronically sick people are involved in a constant struggle to lead valued lives and maintain definitions of self which are positive and worthwhile. This can be difficult; cultural definitions of disability devalue the individual and interactions with others may constantly undermine the individual's sense of self-worth. Charmaz (1987) considers the 'loss of self' to be a powerful form of suffering experienced by the chronically ill.

However, the extent to which the onset of a chronic condition, even when sudden, disrupts a life previously lived depends upon the context in which it occurs. In a study of older people who were in the process of recovery from strokes, their age and the existence of other chronic conditions that they dealt with prior to the stroke meant that the illness was treated as just another event in a life already limited in various ways, rather than an event that had a profound impact on their lives and identities (Faircloth et al 2004). In their accounts of the illness, stroke became a 'normal component of old age'. While previous studies indicate that stroke constitutes a biographical disruption, many of these involved younger, professional people whose illness experiences were quite different from the more elderly people studied by Faircloth and colleagues.

Managing medical regimens

People with chronic disabling disorders must learn to manage their symptoms and manifestations during everyday life. The person with rheumatoid arthritis, for example, rapidly learns how much activity is possible before pain rises to intolerable levels. Daily life is then planned and organized in ways that allow the individual to accomplish a few valued activities before pain intercedes and he or she is forced to rest. The individual must also learn to manage the medical regimens prescribed to control symptoms. These can include diet, drugs or the use of advanced technologies such as a dialysis machine. In some instances the treatment can be as bad as the disease, consuming time, energy and financial resources and requiring hard work (Jobling 1988). The whole life of the chronically sick person can become organized around treatment.

An illuminating example is provided by a study of people with postpolio respiratory impairment, whose capacity to breathe had deteriorated to such an extent that permanent connection to a positive-pressure ventilator by means of a tracheostomy became necessary (Locker & Kaufert 1988). This highly efficient form of mechanical ventilation substantially improved physical and psychological health, allowed for far greater mobility than older technologies and transformed the quality of everyday life. However, the use of this machine meant that the individual concerned, and those providing care and support, had to learn a wide range of skills in order to manage the machine, including recharging batteries, suctioning tubing and maintaining the humidification system. Because this machinery often malfunctioned, usually without warning, it had to be carefully monitored and strategies had to be developed to cope with sudden failure. The potential for respiratory crises left both sufferers and family members feeling vulnerable and insecure. As a consequence, the machine, and tending to the needs of the machine, became a central focus of everyday life.

A less dramatic example is provided by a study of people with psoriasis, a disfiguring skin disease (Jobling 1988). 'Treatment' involves strict conformity over weeks, months or even years, to a programme of repetitive daily bathing, rubbing and scrubbing. This is followed by anointment with oils, creams, pastes or ointments, some of which may involve a noxious smell. Regular exposure to the sun's rays, or at least an equivalent produced by a machine, is another component. All of this may take up several hours a day.

It is often the case that any prescribed regimen is substantially altered by the person concerned. This allows them to exert control over their illness and to maximize their well-being by avoiding some of the negative aspects of medical treatments.

Information, awareness and sharing

For the person with a chronic illness, information is a significant resource for managing daily life. It reduces uncertainty, helps the individual to come to terms with the illness and allows for the development of strategies for managing the illness in everyday life. Nevertheless, many people with chronic conditions express dissatisfaction with the amount of information they are able to obtain about their disorder. Difficulty with communication is a major problem in the relationships between people with chronic illnesses and their doctors. Many rectal cancer patients interviewed by MacDonald (1988) were dissatisfied with what they were told about their operation, and some felt inadequately prepared for dealing with the colostomy and its effects. Some reported not knowing what a colostomy was, even at the time of surgery, and many complained of inadequate follow-up care from their family doctor.

Given these problems in communication, information may be culled from a variety of sources: from books and publications, from self-help groups or from others with the same or similar illnesses. This information provides the basis for action and the feeling that it is possible to do something about and have some control over the illness.

THE EXPERT PATIENT

As the issues discussed above indicate, many people with chronic conditions are involved in a constant process of decision-making and management with respect to their illness. The outcome of this process is a body of knowledge and experience that has recently been formally acknowledged in the notion of the expert patient (Donaldson 2003). As Lorig (2002) states: 'Expert patients are those who take responsibility for the day to day decisions about their health and who work with healthcare providers as collaborators and partners to produce the best possible health given the resources at hand. Expert patients are not only consumers of health but also producers of health'. To maximize their capacity as producers, patients may need education to equip them for this role especially if their condition is of recent onset. In the USA, this education has been provided via chronic disease management programmes. These consist of short courses involving a series of meetings led by lay tutors who are themselves chronically ill. The courses focus on disease-related problem solving and provide practical skills such as goal-setting and other skills such as enhancing patients' self-efficacy, that is their confidence that they can successfully self-manage their illness. Such programmes, funded through the National Health Service, are being implemented in the UK with the intention of reducing disability and healthcare costs. There is some evidence that these self-management programmes improve health outcomes and lower healthcare utilization (Bodenheimer et al 2002), although the evidence is often not as robust as it needs to be (Taylor & Bury 2007).

THE DOCTOR–PATIENT RELATIONSHIP IN CHRONIC ILLNESS

Patients with chronic disabling disorders can be difficult for a medical practitioner to treat. This is only partly due to the fact that medicine often has relatively few interventions which make a real difference to the patient's condition. It also arises because the medical gaze is frequently a narrow one, concerned predominantly with disease to the exclusion of its social and emotional consequences for patients and families. Moreover, the complexity of many chronic conditions, a lack of knowledge on the part of the physician concerning the individual's illness and the fact that hospitals are largely organized around the care of acute rather than chronic diseases make it difficult for the individual to obtain care and support appropriate to their needs (Albrecht 2001, Bury 1997).

Anderson & Bury (1988) indicate the need for 'a reorientation of the focus for care from repairing damage caused by disease to education and understanding for living with chronic illness'. In this sense, information, advice and support are among the most important interventions a doctor has to offer, their goal being to help the patient live as normal and satisfying a life as possible within family and community. Such help needs to be approached with care and sensitivity; patients need to be offered choices, not have them made by others on their behalves. This means ensuring that individuals are helped to be independent and not encouraged into dependency.

By giving due attention to the particular problems associated with a chronic condition, the care that is offered to both the sufferer and the family can be made more appropriate and relevant to their social and emotional concerns. This presupposes that the professional is fully aware of the many meanings of chronic illness, the burdens carried by the individual and those who provide informal support, and the contextual factors which shape these meanings and burdens. This, in turn, highlights the issues of communication and information (see Chapter 4) and the importance of a free exchange of information between doctors and those with a chronic illness. Each has much to teach the other in working together to maximize the individual's quality of life. This collaborative care approach recognizes that while professionals may be experts about disease, patients are experts about their own lives. In order to capitalize on this expertise health professionals must change their perspective and embrace a new role – that of healthcare partner in which patients are helped to help themselves (Lorig 2002).

References

Albrecht G 2001 Rationing care to disabled people. Social Heath and Illness 23:654–677

Anderson R, Bury M (eds) 1988 Living with chronic illness: the experiences of patients and their families. Hyman Unwin, London

Badley E 1993 An introduction to the concepts and classifications of the international classification of impairments, disabilities and handicaps. Disability and Rehabilitation 15: 161–178

Badley E 1995 The genesis of handicap: definition, models of disablement and role of external factors. Disability and Rehabilitation 15:53–62

Badley EM 1987 The ICIDH: format, application in different settings, and distinction between disability and handicap. International Disability Studies 9:122–128

Bickenbach J, Chatterji S, Badley E, Ustun T 1999 Models of disablement, universalism and the classification of impairments, disabilities and handicaps. Social Science and Medicine 48:1171–1187

Blaxter M 1976 The meaning of disability. Heinemann, London

Bodenheimer T, Lorig K, Holman H, Grumbach K 2002 Patient self-management of chronic disease in primary care. JAMA 288:2469–2475

Bury M 1982 Chronic illness as biographical disruption. Sociology Health and Illness 4:167–182

Bury M 1988 Meanings at risk: the experience of arthritis. In: Anderson R, Bury M (eds) Living with chronic illness: the experiences of patients and their families. Hyman Unwin, London

Bury M 1997 Chronic illness and disability. In: Health and illness in a changing society. Routledge, London

Charmaz K 1987 Struggling for a self: identity levels of the chronically ill. Research in the Sociology of Health Care 6:283–321

Conrad P 1987 The experience of illness: recent and new directions. Research in the Sociology of Health Care 6:1–31

Donaldson L 2003 Expert patients usher in a new era for the NHS. British Medical Journal 326:7402

Faircloth C, Boylstein C, Rittman M et al 2004 Sudden illness and biographical flow in narratives of stroke recovery. Sociology, Health and Illness 26:242–261

Goffman E 1963 Stigma. Prentice Hall, Englewood Cliffs, NJ

Halbertsma J 1989 The ICIDH: A study of how it is used and evaluated. A review of the application of a classification relating to the consequences of disease. Zoetermeer: WCC Standing Committee on Classification and Terminology of the National Council of Public Health

Halbertsma J, Heerkens Y, Hirs W et al 2000 Towards a new ICIDH. Disability and Rehabilitation 22:144–156

Harper A, Harper D, Chambers L et al 1986 An epidemiological description of physical, social and psychological problems in multiple sclerosis. Journal of Chronic Diseases 39:305–310

Hirani V, Malbut K 2002 Health Survey for England 2000. Disability among older people. Stationery Office, London

Jobling R 1988 The experience of psoriasis under treatment. In: Anderson R, Bury M (eds) Living with chronic illness: the experiences of patients and their families. Hyman Unwin, London

Lemert E 1967 Human deviance, social problems and social control. Prentice-Hall, Englewood Cliffs, NJ

Locker D 1983 Disability and disadvantage: the consequences of chronic illness. Tavistock, London

Locker D, Kaufert J 1988 The breath of life: medical technology and the careers of people with post respiratory poliomyelitis. Sociology, Health and Illness 10:24–40

Lorig K 2002 Partnerships between expert patients and physicians. Lancet 359:814–815

MacDonald L 1988 The experience of stigma: living with rectal cancer. In: Anderson R, Bury M (eds) Living with chronic illness: the experiences of patients and their families. Hyman Unwin, London

Manton K, Gu X 2001 Changes in the prevalence of chronic disability in the Unites States black and non-black population above age 65 from 1982 to 1999. Proceedings of the National Academy of Sciences of the USA 98:6354–6359

Manton K, Xiliang G, Lamb V 2006 Change in chronic disability from 1982 to 2004–5 as measured by long term changes in function and health in the U.S. elderly population. Proceedings of the National Academy of Sciences of the USA 103:18374–18379

Morbidity and Mortality Weekly Report (MMWR) 2001 Prevalence of arthritis – United States, 1997. Morbidity and Mortality Weekly Report 50:334–336

Nagi S 1991 Disability concepts revisited: implications for prevention. In: Pope A, Tarlov A (eds) Disability in America: toward a national agenda for prevention. National Academy Press, Washington DC

Office of Population Censuses and Surveys 1988 OPCS Surveys of disability in Great Britain: the prevalence of disability among adults. HMSO, London

O'Mahoney P, Thomson R, Rodgers H, James O 1999 The prevalence of stroke and associated disability. Journal of Public Health Medicine 21:166–171

Parsons T 1951 The Social System. Free Press, New York

Robinson I 1988 Reconstructing lives: negotiating the meaning of multiple sclerosis. In: Anderson R, Bury M (eds) Living with chronic illness: the experiences of patients and their families. Hyman Unwin, London

Taylor D, Bury M 2007 Chronic illness, expert patients and care transition. Social Science and Medicine 29:27–45

Topliss E 1979 Provision for the disabled. Martin Robertson, London

Verbrugge L, Jette A 1994 The disablement process. Social Science and Medicine 38:1–14

Williams G 1984 The genesis of chronic illness: narrative reconstruction. Sociology, Health and Illness 6:175–200

Williams S 1989 Chronic respiratory illness and disability: a critical review of the psychosocial literature. Social Science and Medicine 28:791–803

Williams S, Bury M 1989a Breathtaking: the consequences of chronic respiratory disorder (unpublished paper)

Williams S, Bury M 1989b Impairment, disability and handicap in chronic respiratory illness. Social Science and Medicine 29:609–616

Winblad I, Jaaskelainen M, Kivela S et al 2001 Prevalence of disability in three birth cohorts at old age over time spans of 10 and 20 years. Journal of Clinical Epidemiology 54:1019–1024

Wood P 1980 The language of disablement: a glossary relating to disease and its consequences. International Rehabilitation Medicine 2:86–92

WHO 1999 ICIDH-2: International classification of functioning and disability. Beta-2 draft, short version. World Health Organization, Geneva

Dying, death and bereavement

Graham Scambler

The facts and circumstances of death have varied historically and geographically. Before concentrating on contemporary Britain, it is worth putting recent British experience into a broader global perspective. In 1955, the average life expectancy at birth worldwide was 48 years; by 1995 it had risen to 65 years. The World Health Organization (WHO 1998a) predicts that it will rise to 73 years by 2025, by which date it is also anticipated that no country will have an average life expectancy of less than 50 years. Reductions in infant mortality and in early childhood deaths are primarily responsible for this (see Chapter 1). However, a marked diversity remains between continents and countries. Table 7.1 documents the age structures of populations and life expectancy at birth globally.

Some 16 countries actually experienced a decline in life expectancy at birth between 1975 and 1995 (WHO 1998a). This applies to a number of Eastern European countries: for example, in the Russian Federation life expectancy for males fell dramatically from 64 in 1985–1990 to 57 in 1994; for females the fall was from 74 to 71. These declines appear to reflect increases in particular causes of death, influenced by deteriorating public service provision as well as by falling material standards of living. Middle-aged men have suffered the most severe decline, with increases in deaths from cardiovascular disease, accidental poisonings, suicide and, most strikingly, homicide (so that by 1993–4 Russia surpassed the USA as the country with the highest homicide rate). In Uganda, where AIDS is the leading cause of death for young adults, life expectancy at birth declined from a peak of 56 to 41 in 1995–2000 (Seale 2000).

TALKING ABOUT DEATH

The inescapable fact of death provides one of the principal parameters of the human condition. As Lofland (1978) writes, 'it can neither be 'believed' nor 'magicked' nor 'scienced'

| TABLE 7.1 | Age structures of populations and life expectancy globally |

	Distribution (%) by age group (1996)			Life expectancy at birth (1995–2000)
	0–14 years	15–64 years	65+ years	
Africa	43.7	53.2	3.2	53.8
America	28.8	63.2	8.0	72.4
Asia	31.5	63.1	5.4	66.2
Europe	18.9	67.1	14.0	72.6
Oceania	25.9	64.5	9.6	73.9
World	31.1	62.3	6.6	65.6

Adapted from WHO (1998b).

away'. Increasingly, through the twentieth century to the present, physicians and other healthcare workers in countries like Britain have been called upon to give often prolonged treatment and support to the terminally ill and their families. A higher proportion of people than ever before experience 'slow' as opposed to 'quick' dying; that is, dying has typically become a more protracted process. The reasons for this have been well documented and are summarized in Box 7.1. For obvious reasons, this change has enhanced the salience of communication around death. It is ironic, therefore, that many historians have maintained that death over the last century or so has become more and more 'unmentionable'. Aries (1983) characterizes modern – demythologized and secularized – death as invisible death: 'we ignore the existence of a scandal that we have been unable to prevent; we act as if it did not exist, and thus mercilessly force the bereaved to say nothing. A heavy silence has fallen over the subject of death'. According to Aries, death has grown fearful again, imbued with all its 'old savagery'.

| BOX 7.1 | Conditions facilitating 'quick dying' in the pre-modern era and 'slow dying' in the modern era |

Conditions facilitating quick dying

Low level of medical technology

Late detection of disease-(or fatality-) producing conditions

Simple definition of death (e.g. cessation of heart beat)

High incidence of mortality from acute disease

High incidence of fatality-producing injuries

Customary killing or suicide of, or fatal passivity towards, the person once he or she has entered the 'dying' category

Conditions facilitating slow dying

High level of medical technology

Early detection of disease-(or fatality-) producing conditions

Complex definition of death (e.g. irreversible cessation of higher brain activity)

High incidence of mortality from chronic or degenerative disease

Low incidence of fatality-producing injuries

Customary curative and activist orientation toward the dying with a high value placed on the prolongation of life

Reproduced with permission of Sage Publications Inc. from Lofland (1978).

Countering this view that the denial of death is now ubiquitous, however, Seale (1995) has pointed to evidence that 'scripts' for proclaiming 'heroic self-identity in the face of death' are currently being promoted by many professional 'experts' and appropriated by growing numbers of lay people. His contention is that these scripts, less 'masculine' and more 'feminine' in orientation than their predecessors, redefine 'heroic death' as involving a struggle to gain knowledge, opportunities to demonstrate courage, and a state of emotional calm or equilibrium in which dying people and carers alike participate. The emphasis is on care, concern and emotional expression. Some deaths, Seale admits, cannot be written into such scripts; for example, those of the very old, the mentally confused and sudden unexpected deaths. And there are rival scripts: there are those, for example, who prefer the benefits of continuing the everyday project of the self oblivious of oncoming death, with others sharing the burden of awareness in an attempt to protect the dying person from the strain of knowing. But Seale conjectures that what he terms 'scripts of heroic death' are gaining ground.

Walter (1994) is another to resist the notion that death has become taboo in modern society, even referring to a recent 'revival of death'. He sees this revival as comprising two different strands. The first or 'late modern' strand is motivated by professional experts – including palliative care nurses, bereavement counsellors and so on, as well as doctors – seeking control over death and dying. The second or 'post-modern' strand reflects the responses of ordinary people seeking to express their emotions without hindrance or instruction. There is a contradiction between these two strands. The late modern strand of death's revival aims to bridge the gap between private experiences and public discourses by the sponsorship and dissemination of knowledge that makes private experiences of death part of public discourses about death. In this way, experts exert control over their clients' private experiences. In bereavement counselling, for example, the trained expert, representing the public, recognizes and legitimizes the emotions of the bereaved while at the same time protecting the public from these emotions by providing secure and secluded contexts for their expression. The post-modern strand of the revival of death, however, rejects the professional preoccupation with neatly delineated stages, instead celebrating the heterogeneity of death, dying and bereavement and insisting that people be free to die and grieve in their own ways and to give expression to their emotions as they see fit. The post-modern strand invites private feelings into the public sphere not so they can be controlled and legitimized by experts but to demand they be taken seriously in their own right. This articulation of diversity has the effect of challenging the public discourses about death and the cultural authority of the expertise underpinning them.

In another publication, Walter (1996) distinguishes between the dominant perspectives on death to be found in 'traditional', 'modern' and 'postmodern' societies. In this context traditional societies are taken to be pre-industrial, including hunter-gatherer, nomadic and agrarian societies. Modern societies are societies that have undergone processes of industrialization and subscribe to notions of progress via the use of science and technology, dating in Europe from the mid-sixteenth century. Post-modern societies are associated with the latter part of the twentieth century, when modern values are said to have become fragmented and open to popular dispute. Box 7.2 summarizes Walter's historical types of death. It can be seen that for him religion forms the basis of meaning in traditional societies; that religion is usurped by medical science in modern societies; and that in post-modern societies the dominance of either religion or science has given way to a greater emphasis on the individual, in the process privileging psychology and sense of self. It can be seen that Walter's earlier reference to the tension between late modern and post-modern revivals of death, dying and bereavement can be situated within this framework.

BOX 7.2	Changing perspectives on death in traditional, modern and postmodern societies		
	Traditional death	**Modern death**	**Post-modern death**
Authority	Tradition	Professional expertise	Personal choice
Authority figure	Priest	Doctor	The Self
Dominant discourse	Theology	Medicine	Psychology
Coping through	Prayer	Silence	Expressive feelings
The traveller	Soul	Body	Personality
Bodily context	Living with death	Death controlled	Living with dying
Social context	Community	Hospital	Family

Walter (1996).

Howarth (2007) acknowledges the usefulness of Walter's framework while noting that his division beteeen traditional, modern and post-modern societies lends itself to over-simplification. More significantly, she argues that Walter's stress on a resurgent post-modern authority of the self actually amounts to little more than an attempt to re-assert the authority of science via psychology. Psychology, she argues, is becoming the fore-most discipline for understanding mortality since it is the point of scientific access to the emotions and the self. While it is true that contemporary culture is more fragmen-ted and diverse than hitherto, it is a mistake to overlook the mix of traditional, modern and post-modern in the present. Timmermans (2005) is sceptical about a new focus on psychology, maintaining that medicine itself has re-asserted its cultural authority in relation to the emotions and the self through what he calls 'death brokering'. This refers to medicine's activities to render individual deaths culturally appropriate. Doctors' inter-ventions in the contemporary era, he argues, are geared to postponing death for as long as is biologically and normatively feasible. When death eventually occurs, they help negotiate a culturally acceptable passing; and after death, they rationalize the inevitabil-ity of its occurrence with a statement on its causes. It is medical experts who broker the often frightening and ambiguous aspects of death and dying.

Independently of differences between analysts and commentators, it is not surprising that deciding whether to tell someone he or she is dying continues to be regarded as prob-lematic for health workers. When asked, most people anticipate that they would want to be told if they were dying; physicians are themselves unexceptional in this respect. But how much credibility should be attached to such responses? Can young, healthy indivi-duals accurately predict how they will feel as death approaches?

Cartwright et al (1973), who interviewed relatives of a national sample of people who had died in the preceding year in Britain, were told by relatives that 37% of those dying knew as much, and a further 20% 'half knew'. Nearly three-quarters of the relatives felt they had themselves known. It was also apparent from this study that the relatives received more information from all sources than did the people who were dying. Less information was forthcoming if death occurred in a hospital than if it occurred at home; in both contexts, however, the general practitioner was the key informant. Herd (1990), in a study of terminal care in a semirural part of Britain, also found principal lay carers to be less aware and knowledgeable about what was happening if death took place in hospital than if it took place in the home. A more recent study by Seale & Cartwright (1994), however, suggests a changing picture. In 250 accounts from lay relatives, friends and others who knew people in a random national sample of adult deaths, 54% reported that both parties had been aware that the person was dying. In 36% of situations the respondent knew, but the dying person did not; in 8% neither knew; and in 1% the respondent did not know, although the deceased did.

Awareness of dying

Glaser & Strauss (1965) found there to be four common types of 'awareness context' in relation to the dying. They define 'awareness context' as: 'what each interacting person knows of the patient's defined status, along with his recognition of others' awareness of his own definition'. The four types are summarized in Box 7.3. Some commentators have assumed that 'closed', 'suspected' and 'mutual pretence' awareness contexts are intrinsically undesirable and that health workers, especially physicians, are exclusively to blame for the fact that they frequently exist. As a study by McIntosh (1977) suggests, however, such assumptions can be naive and misleading. McIntosh interviewed both patients and physicians. Most patients he spoke to suspected malignancy. The majority sought information from members of the hospital team but, according to McIntosh's estimate, two out of every three did not 'really' want their diagnostic suspicions confirmed and fewer still 'really' wanted to know their prognosis. They sought exclusively information that would reinforce an optimistic conception of their condition: uncertainty afforded hope. Most patients also felt – somewhat unrealistically, given McIntosh's documentation of physicians' predisposition not to disclose – that they would be told everything if they asked.

Timmermans (1994) has suggested that Glaser and Strauss's 'open awareness context' requires refinement 'to include the diversity of viewpoints of family members and patients'. He delineates three types of open awareness. The context of 'suspended open awareness' occurs when patients and their relatives simply ignore or 'deny' the information. This can arise in three sets of circumstances. First, it can be a transitory feature after the disclosure of the terminal condition and prognosis. Disbelief here is an initial reaction to cope with the shock of disclosure – 'the open awareness context is nascent: the news has been given but its radical consequences have not been fully assimilated'. Second, disbelief can become a permanent and preferred state, with even the reality of the underlying condition being called into question. And third, patients can come to question or doubt

---

BOX 7.3   'Awareness contexts' in relation to dying

1. Closed awareness: the patient does not recognize his or her impending death, although everyone else does
2. Suspected awareness: the patient suspects what others know and attempts either to confirm or to invalidate these suspicions
3. Mutual pretence awareness: each party defines the patient as dying but each 'pretends' that the other has not done so
4. Open awareness: health workers and patient are each aware that the latter is dying, and they act on this awareness fairly openly

Reproduced with permission of Aldine Press from Glaser & Strauss (1965).

the outcomes of their conditions in situations of unexpected deterioration or improve-ment. The context of 'uncertain open awareness' occurs when patients and relatives do not dismiss the possibility of death but 'prefer the uncertainty of not understanding exactly what is going on'. The context of 'active open awareness' occurs when hope for recovery is abandoned and patients and their families understand the full ramifications of the impending death and try to find ways of coming to terms with it.

Mamo (1999) suggests that the analyses of both Glaser & Strauss and of Timmermans disregard the importance of emotions, arguing that they fail to address 'the complexity of emotional management and the existence of emotional surges in the context of dying'. She maintains that cognitions and emotions are in fact intertwined: 'awareness emerges and sub-sides in a complex web of emotions and cognition'. She commends further study, in particular of the multiple ways in which emotional work is performed by dying patients and their families.

As McIntosh found, physicians are not always ready to communicate openly. In a Canadian study of 118 encounters during which 17 male surgeons disclosed the results of biopsies to women with breast cancer, Taylor (1988) found that each surgeon appeared to have adopted a favoured 'strategy' that he used routinely, thus 'bypassing the individuality of each case'. Four techniques were discerned. The first – communication – was deployed by some surgeons when they were in a position to make a reasonable and definite prognosis of the condition in terms comprehensible to the patient. Many surgeons claimed to use this technique, but in fact few did. Only 10% of the 118 disclosures were of this type. The second – admission of uncertainty – was used by a small minority of surgeons when no clinical prog-nosis was justified; 15% of the disclosures took this form. The third technique – dissimulation, or the pronouncement of a prognosis that could not be clinically substantiated – occurred when surgeons were reluctant to share the extent of their uncertainty with their patients; 30% of the disclosures fell into this category. The final technique – evasion – or 'the failure to communicate a clinically substantiated prognosis', was used by a number of surgeons who preferred not to respond directly to patients' questions. 'For those surgeons whose patients asked direct questions to which the appropriate technical response might reveal a low chance of long-term survival, repressing information was a favoured policy.' Not infrequently, replies to specific questions drew on general statistics not easily applicable to the individual case. In 45% of disclosures surgeons used evasion as a means of coping with direct questions posed by women.

If one thing is clear it is that there is no easy, general answer to the question 'To tell or not to tell?'. Hinton (1967) offers physicians the following counsel:

> 'Although it is not an infallible guide as to how much the dying patient should be told, his apparent wishes and questions do point the way. This means that the manner in which he puts his views should he closely attended to – the intonations and the exact wording may be very revealing. It also means that he must be given ample opportunity to express his ideas and ask his questions. If the questions are sincere, however, then why not give quite straight answers to the patient's questions about his illness and the outcome? It makes for beneficial trust.'

A study by Hinton (1980) highlights the importance of giving dying patients the oppor-tunity to talk. He interviewed 80 patients with terminal cancer at a mean of 10 weeks before death; 66% told him that they recognized they might or would soon die, 8% were non-committal, and 26% spoke only of improvement. Some patients spoke of dying to either their spouse or the staff and not to the interviewer, but they tended to say less to their spouse than to the interviewer and less still to members of the staff. This tendency is illustrated in Fig. 7.1. Hinton concludes that people are often ready to share their awareness if someone is prepared to listen.

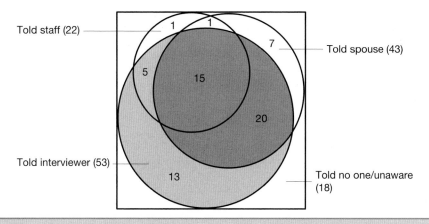

Fig. 7.1 Awareness of the possibility of dying as shown by different people by 80 patients with terminal cancer. The square represents the 80 patients and the three shaded circles their communicated awareness to staff, spouse and interviewer.
(Reproduced with permission from Hinton 1980.)

■ Stages of dying

How people come to terms with the prospect of imminent death depends on many factors (Hinton 1984). Of obvious importance is the nature of the physical and mental distress experienced. A number of national surveys have been conducted, relying on data from surviving relatives or others. Table 7.2 lists the main symptoms experienced by people dying from cancer, heart disease and stroke from a large national study in Britain in 1990. Pain, nausea and vomiting, difficulty swallowing, constipation and pressure sores seem more prevalent for people dying of cancer. Breathlessness is a particular problem for people with heart disease. Mental confusion and incontinence affect more people dying from strokes. In general, cancer caused a large number of symptoms and a larger proportion of these

TABLE 7.2	Symptoms experienced in the last year of life in Britain (1990)		
	Cancer %	**Heart disease %**	**Stroke %**
Pain	88	77	66
Breathlessness	54	60	37
Nausea and vomiting	59	32	23
Difficulty swallowing	41	16	23
Constipation	63	38	45
Mental confusion	41	32	50
Pressure sores	28	11	20
Urinary incontinence	40	30	56
Bowel incontinence	32	17	37
N =	2063	683	229

From Addington-Hall (1996).

were defined as 'very distressing' for the dying person; but the duration of symptoms for cancer was less than for other conditions (Addington-Hall et al 1998). It has regularly been found that, when compared with lay carers, health workers tend to underestimate patients' symptoms and to overestimate the success of treatment (Herd 1990).

Among the many factors that can influence how individuals cope with terminal illness are age, family intimacy and support, and religious convictions. There is enormous individual variation and hence unpredictability in any given case. Kubler-Ross (1970) has claimed, however, that people who know they are dying typically pass through five 'stages' (Box 7.4).

Several writers have criticized Kubler-Ross's specification of discrete stages of dying, usually on the grounds that it represents an overgeneralization based on subjective data. Certainly Kubler-Ross's stages should not be regarded either as unidirectional or as sequential.

BOX 7.4   Stages of dying

First stage: denial and isolation

Many people, on being told they are dying, experience a temporary state of shock. When the numbness disappears, a common response is: 'No, it can't be me'. One's own death is all but inconceivable. 'Denial' is usually a temporary defence but some take it further, perhaps 'shopping around' for a more amenable clinical opinion (only three of the 200 patients in Kubler-Ross's study attempted to deny the approach of death to the very end). A deep feeling of 'isolation' is normal at this stage.

Second stage: anger

When the initial stage of denial can no longer be maintained, it is often replaced by feelings of anger, rage, envy and resentment. The question 'Why me?' is posed. The anger can be displaced and at times projected onto the environment almost at random (although it can, of course, be justified as well as unjustified). The hospital team, especially the nursing staff, frequently bear the brunt of these outbursts.

Third stage: bargaining

The third stage of 'bargaining', Kubler-Ross argues, has only rarely been acknowledged. The point is that terminally ill people will sometimes negotiate – openly with health workers or secretly with God – to postpone death: postponement will be the reward for a promise of good behaviour. For example, many patients in the study promised to donate parts of their bodies to medical science if the physicians undertook to use their knowledge of science to extend their lives.

Fourth stage: depression

When terminally ill patients can no longer deny their illness, when they are compelled to endure more surgery, when they grow weaker, the numbness or stoicism or anger gives way to a sense of great loss. This 'depression' can be reactive; for example, a woman with cancer of the uterus might feel she is no longer a woman, or what Kubler-Ross calls preparatory, that is, based on impending losses associated with death itself.

Fifth stage: acceptance

The final stage of 'acceptance' is one in which dying patients commonly find a sort of peace, a peace that is largely a function of weakness and a diminished interest in the world. 'It is as if the pain has gone, the struggle is over...'. Kubler-Ross adds that this is also the time during which the family usually needs more help, understanding and support than the patient.

Reproduced with permission of Tavistock Publications from Kubler-Ross (1970).

PLACE OF DEATH

Those, like Aries, who argue that death has become increasingly invisible during the twentieth century attach considerable significance to the fact that, since the 1930s and 1940s, death has been substantially removed from the community or 'hospitalized'. In the hospital, according to this thesis, death is no longer an occasion of ritual ceremony over which the dying person and his or her kin and friends hold sway. The physicians and hospital team are the new 'masters of death', of its moment as well as its circumstances. This interpretation of changing events is once again open to criticism. Seymour (1999) has shown, for example, that the common representation of the medicalized, hospitalized death as antithetical to an idealized 'natural death' is simplistic. She found that the next of kin tended to see death as 'natural' when medical technology delivered outcomes they expected, appeared amenable to human manipulation and intention, was accessible to their understanding, and seemed to 'fit' with the wider context of the dying person's life. There is no doubt, however, that the hospitalization of death has continued; two-thirds of deaths in Britain now occur in hospitals, compared with only a half in 1960 (Seale 2000).

There is a growing feeling that the hospital is too frequently an inappropriate place in which to die. In his essay on 'The Loneliness of Dying', Elias (1985), who is fully aware of how emotionally taxing, as well as rewarding, a death in the family home can be, nevertheless stresses that in modern hospitals 'dying people can be cared for in accordance with the latest biophysical specialist knowledge, but often neutrally as regards feeling; they may die in total isolation'. Most hospitals are designed to provide for acute illness, and terminally ill people in acute wards can both disturb other patients and members of ward staff and be disturbed by them; most hospitals do not set aside a whole or part of a ward for dying patients because they are anxious to avoid the stigma of a 'death ward'. Several alternative locations exist in Britain, including special units within conventional hospitals, but the most discussed are the home and the hospice.

■ The home

For many health workers and lay persons alike, despite the statistical trend to hospitalization, the home remains the 'natural' and 'proper' place in which to die. As Bowling & Cartwright (1982) discovered, however, the care of dying people at home imposes severe physical, financial and psychological strains on relatives. In Herd's (1990) study, 74% of lay carers (four out of every five of them female relatives) mentioned 'emotional strain' as a problem, and 51% mentioned 'physical strain'. Table 7.3 ranks those aspects of home care that Herd's lay carers defined as 'worrying'. Lay carers are also likely to find their own activities restricted: Bowling & Cartwright report 26% describing their activities as 'severely restricted' and a further 19% as 'fairly restricted'. The extent to which professional and other support is at hand is likely to be contingent upon ad hoc factors affecting local planning and provision. Currently, hospitalization in Britain is a function of the absence of local planning and provision. There are shortages of helpers ranging from Macmillan nurses to home helps and providers of meals-on-wheels.

■ The hospice

The hospice movement was founded in the mid-nineteenth century and was largely pioneered in Britain, although inpatient hospices still deal with only 4% of dying people, and generally with those dying from cancer. The favoured pattern in Britain is to build small units in the grounds of general hospitals, using their facilities but remaining administratively independent. The range of care provided in a hospice is intermediate between that of a

TABLE 7.3	Worrying aspects of home care identified by lay carers	
		Number (%) of respondents
Anxiety about medication		26 (49)
Inability to leave patient unattended		22 (42)
Not knowing what to expect		18 (34)
Inability to help		15 (28)
Fear of being alone when death took place		11 (21)
Anxiety about what to do when death took place		5 (9)
Anxiety about calling the doctor		3 (6)
Other		5 (9)

Reproduced with permission from Herd (1990).

long-stay hospital and that of an acute hospital. The staffing ratios are similar to those of an acute hospital, but the call for diagnostic and other 'support' services is much less. The average length of stay is also closer to that of patients in an acute hospital than that of patients in a long-stay hospital, and costs are in keeping with this.

Central to the philosophy of the hospice is the view that the whole professional caring team should work in unison to develop the skills the dying person needs. Howarth (2007) lists six core tenets of the hospice model: that it provides *holistic care*; that it involves *interdisciplinary teams*; that it is *non-hierarchical*; that it is *not rule-bound*; that hospice work should be viewed as *vocational*; and that it should be committeed to *research and education*. Dramatic improvements in care originated in hospices in the last quarter of the twentieth century, for example, in standards of palliative medicine; hospice teams have reduced levels of uncontrolled pain to 8% and less (Parkes 1984). It should not be assumed, however, that, given the choice, everybody would opt for death in a hospice. In one study, which compared the care given in four radiotherapy wards of an acute hospital, in a Foundation Home visited by two general practitioners and in a hospice (Hinton 1979), little difference was found between the acute hospital and the Foundation Home, but there was some evidence that patients were less depressed and anxious in the hospice and preferred the more frank communication available there. It was also found, however, that patients gave most praise to the outpatient system of care, despite experiencing more anxiety or irritability at home. The author concluded: 'treatment cannot be judged solely by the mental quiet it brings; freedom or hope may be preferred even if they bring worry'. It has been found that home-centred patients tend to experience more pain than hospital-centred patients, and their relatives more stress; but it does not follow that, even knowing this, patients and their relatives would necessarily choose to leave home. It should not be concluded that because adequate support for home care is rarely available the hospitalization of death should be accelerated.

Another more recent and small-scale study, however, has challenged the 'mantra' that 'home is best'. Following their study of the preferences of cancer patients and their carers, Thomas and colleagues (2004) showed that some patients positively opted for hospice care. The principal reasons cited for this choice were: limitations imposed by the informal care resources or living circumstances; the drive to protect loved ones and to relieve them of the burden of care; the wish to sustain personal dignity once loss of bodily control has occurred; the attraction of 'safe' professional treatment and care in the face of pain and other distressing symptoms; and witnessing the exceptionally caring qualities of the hospice relative to most forms of hospital care. What the findings of the studies

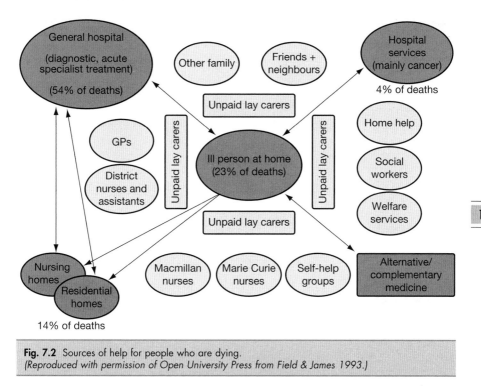

Fig. 7.2 Sources of help for people who are dying.
(Reproduced with permission of Open University Press from Field & James 1993.)

reported here suggest is that it is extremely difficult to specify particular criteria of the 'good death'; indeed their bureaucratic specification, like lack of family means or local resources, can remove the freedom of individual preference.

Figure 7.2 summarizes the sources of help available to people who are dying in Britain.

PATTERNS OF DEATH AND BEREAVEMENT

Sudnow (1967) has drawn a distinction between biological and social death. The problem of how to define biological death has been resolved by the medical profession for the time being in favour of the irreversible cessation of higher brain activity. Sudnow uses the term 'social death' in a general sense to refer to how organizations deal with different modes of dying and death. More specifically, social death is marked, within the hospital setting, by that point at which a patient is treated essentially as a corpse, although still perhaps biologically alive. He gives an example of social death preceding biological death. A nurse on duty with a woman she explained was 'dying' was observed to spend 2 or 3 minutes trying to close the woman's eyelids. After several unsuccessful attempts she managed to shut them and said, with a sigh of relief, 'Now they're right'. When questioned, she said that a patient's eyes must be closed after death, so that the body will resemble a sleeping person. It was more difficult to accomplish this, she explained, after the muscles and skin had begun to stiffen. She always tried to close them before death. This made for greater efficiency when the time came for ward personnel to wrap the body. It was a matter of consideration toward those workers who preferred to handle dead bodies as little as possible.

Mulkay (1993) interprets the concept of social death more broadly. Social death might precede biological death, as in Sudnow's example, or, alternatively, social existence might continue long after death, 'for example, when distraught parents visit the grave of a dead child and talk and write to that child about their previous life together and about the reunion to come' (Clegg 1988). The defining feature of social death, then, is the cessation of the individual person as an active agent in others' lives. Mulkay argues that the profile of social death has changed considerably over the last century as a result of people's collective responses to changes in the social distribution of biological death, changes in the social setting of death, and changes in the clinical nature of death. Consider the elderly, for example. Mulkay suggests that the start of the 'death sequence' in our society occurs, particularly for men, at the time of retirement from work. This is a key transition, when people's participation in social life significantly diminishes – independently of personal variations in state of health – owing to the socially recognized approach of death. From retirement on, elderly people in Britain are typically channelled away from the principal arenas of social activity and their ties with the wider society progressively weakened in anticipation of their biological end (Williams 1990). With admission to a hospital or, increasingly, a residential or nursing home, where the bureaucratic 'neglect of the patient as a person' (Field 1989) converges with the physical, emotional and communicative withdrawal of the living from those on the death sequence, the death sequence of society at large is repeated in microcosm.

◼ Trajectories of dying

Glaser & Strauss (1968) distinguish seven 'critical junctures' in what is sometimes called the 'career' of the dying patient:

1. the definition of the patient as dying

2. staff and family then make their preparations for the patient's death, as the patient might do if he or she knows that death is near

3. at some point there seems to be 'nothing more to do' to prevent death

4. the final descent, which can take weeks, days or merely hours

5. the 'last hours'

6. the death watch

7. death itself.

When these critical junctures occur as expected – as it were, on schedule – then all those involved, including sometimes the patient, are prepared for them. When, however, critical junctures occur unexpectedly, hospital staff and the patient's family alike can be unprepared. If a patient is expected to die quite soon, for example, but vacillates sufficiently often, then both staff and family are likely to find the experience stressful.

Predictability, then, makes the work of hospital teams easier. Miscalculations in forecasting can play havoc with the organization of work. When crises do occur, the staff attempt to regain control as quickly as possible, but sometimes the disruption of work is accompanied by a shattering of what Glaser & Strauss (1965) have called a ward's characteristic 'sentimental mood' or order. They cite an example:

> 'In an intensive care unit where cardiac patients die frequently, the mood is relatively unaffected by one more speedy expected death; but if a hopeless patient lingers on and on, or if his wife, perhaps, refuses to accept his dying and causes 'scenes', then both mood and work itself are profoundly affected.'

Glaser & Strauss (1968) differentiate between a number of patterns of death, 'dying trajectories', paying special attention to the distinction noted earlier between 'quick' and 'slow' dying. Quick dying, they claim, can take three forms: 'the expected quick death'; 'unexpected quick dying, but expected to die'; and 'unexpected quick dying, not expected to die'. They report that, in general, unexpected quick deaths are more disturbing for staff and families than expected quick deaths. Even expected quick deaths, however, can give rise to distinctive difficulties. Glaser and Strauss focus on staff–family interaction and note, for example, that the likely presence of the family at the bedside when death occurs requires careful handling by the staff, because a 'scene' will disrupt ward order and worry other patients. Slow dying 'is fraught with both hazard and opportunity'. On the one hand, the dying could take 'too long', be unexpectedly painful or unpleasant, and so on; on the other hand, a slow decline can allow time for wills to be made or families to come together, and can provide the setting for quiet and dignified endings. All these consequences are less likely to occur with quick dying.

End-of-life decisions

End-of-life decisions in medical practice can include euthanasia and physician-assisted suicide (administering or supplying drugs to end a life at the request of a patient); measures intended to end life without an explicit request from a patient; the alleviation of pain or other symptoms with treatments that are considered possibly or certainly to hasten death; and withdrawing or witholding treatments that potentially prolong life (non-treatment decisions) (Seale 2006a). The background to these decisions has become more complex. Definitions of death itself have grown more sophisticated; moreover, definitional processes are beginning to be influenced by 'external factors' like the harvesting of organs. A range of legal, ethical, medical and psychosocial issues have also to be considered. Conducting a postal survey of 857 general practitioners, Seale (2006b) found that in medical practice in the United Kingdom in 2004, the proportion of deaths involving voluntary euthanasia was 0.16%; physician-assisted suicide, 0%; ending of life without explicit consent of the patient, 0.33%; alleviation of symptoms with possibly life shortening effect, 32.8%; and non-treatment decisions, 30.3%. Comparing his data with published results from other countries, Seale infers that doctors in the UK act with relative caution, especially in shortening life by more than a few days. Discussions with patients and relatives about end-of-life decisions occur regularly, but less often than in countries with more 'permissive' legislation (e.g. Netherlands, Belgium or Switzerland). UK doctors are likely to hold discussions with other colleagues. Seale concludes that the relatively low rate of end-of-life decicions involving doctor-assisted dying in the UK, and the relatively high rate of non-treatment decisions, suggests a culture of medical decision-making informed by a palliative care philosophy. It is likely that debate around these issues will grow, possibly with increasingly legalistic or bureaucratic 'solutions' coming to the fore.

Bereavement and mourning

Just as experiences of impending death vary from person to person, so does the experience of losing a relative or friend. Much depends on the nature of the relationship. However, a sudden, unexpected death is often harder to get over than one where there was time to grieve before the occurrence of death: this is known as 'anticipatory' or 'prebereavement mourning'.

In his anthropological study of death in Britain, Gorer (1965) argues that mourners typically pass through three stages:

1. a short period of shock, usually lasting from death until the disposal of the body

2. a period of intense mourning, accompanied by withdrawal of attention and affect from the external world and by physiological changes like disturbed sleep, vivid dreams, failure of appetite and loss of weight

3. a final period of re-established social and physical homeostasis, with sleep and weight stabilized and interest again directed outwards.

Gorer's principal thesis is that, in an increasingly secular Britain, only the first of these three periods is socially acknowledged and surrounded by ceremony and ritual. After the funeral or postfuneral meal, mourners are frequently abandoned to cope alone. To counter this social isolation during a time of continuing need for succour and support (periods 2 and 3), he advocates the creation of new secular rituals to replace now defunct religious ones.

Kamerman (1988) suggests that this twentieth-century process of 'deritualization' has been accompanied by a process of 'rationalization'. By this he means that death has increasingly come to be subsumed under conventions or routines that render it non-intrusive. Responses to death have become more 'business-like'. Both deritualization and rationalization are epitomized by the growing preference for cremation over burial. Approximately two-thirds of bodies are now cremated in Britain.

Advocates of the idea of a revival of death, whose work was discussed earlier in this chapter, have asserted a new emphasis on the emotions and the self and are seeing or predicting an upsurge of consumer demand for individually tailored projects of bereavement and mourning. What they see as novel individualism and greater choice, however, others see as the emergence of niche markets in death, dying and bereavement, stretching from commodities that demonstrate love and loss to distinct and rival schools of bereavement counselling and support. It can sometimes be difficult to distinguish between what individuals choose and what they are invited to choose, or what is effectively chosen on their behalf, by the state legislature, by the marketplace, or indeed by the health and allied professions.

It remains the case that many health students and workers receive minimal preparation for coping with terminal care and bereavement. Glaser and Strauss argue that much non-technical conduct in relation to the dying and bereaved is influenced by common-sense assumptions, 'essentially untouched by professional considerations or by current knowledge from the behavioural sciences'. The argument for the provision of a good grounding in those aspects of care – psychological, social, organizational and ethical – is a strong one. MacLeod's (2001) small ethnographic study of 10 doctors' reflections on learning to care for people who are dying suggests that medical training is still often inadequate and that in practice learning frequently occurs as a result of retrospectively identified 'turning points' or specific encounters with dying patients.

References

Addington-Hall J 1996 Heart disease and stroke: lessons from cancer care. In: Ford G, Lewin I (eds) Managing terminal illness. Royal College of Physicians, London

Addington-Hall J, Altmann D, McCarthy M 1998 Variations by age in symptoms and dependency levels experienced by people in the last year of life, as reported by surviving family, friends and officials. Age and Ageing 27:129–136

Aries P 1983 The hour of our death. Penguin, London

Bowling A, Cartwright A 1982 Life after death: a study of the elderly widowed. Tavistock, London

Cartwright A, Hockey L, Anderson J 1973 Life before death. Routledge & Kegan Paul, London

Clegg F 1988 Decisions at a time of grief. Cambridge University Press, Cambridge

Elias N 1985 The loneliness of dying. Basil Blackwell, Oxford

Field D 1989 Nursing the dying. Tavistock/Routledge, London

Field D, James N 1993 Where and how people die. In: Clark D (ed) The future for palliative care. Open University Press, Buckingham

Glaser B, Strauss A 1965 Awareness of dying. Aldine, Chicago. IL

Glaser B, Strauss A 1968 Time for dying. Aldine, Chicago, IL

Gorer G 1965 Death, grief and mourning in contemporary Britain. Cresset Press, London

Herd E 1990 Terminal care in a semi-rural area. British Journal of General Practice. 40:248–251

Hinton J 1967 Dying. Penguin, London

Hinton J 1979 Comparison of places and policies for terminal care. Lancet ii:29–32

Hinton J 1980 Whom do dying patients tell? British Medical Journal 281:1328–1330

Hinton J 1984 Coping with terminal illness. In: Fitzpatrick R et al (eds) The experience of illness. Tavistock, London

Howarth G 2007 Death and dying: a sociological introduction. Polity, Cambridge

Kamerman J 1988 Death in the midst of life: social and cultural influences on death, grief and mourning. Prentice Hall, Englewood Cliffs, NJ

Kubler-Ross E 1970 On death and dying. Tavistock, London

Lofland L 1978 The craft of dying: the modern face of death. Sage Publications, Beverly Hills, CA

McIntosh J 1977 Communication and awareness in a cancer ward. Croom Helm, London

MacLeod R 2001 On reflection: doctors learning to care for people who are dying. Social Science & Medicine 52:1719–1727

Mamo L 1999 Death and dying: confluences of emotion and awareness. Sociology of Health & Illness 21:13–36

Mulkay M 1993 Social death in Britain. In: Clark D (ed) The sociology of death. Blackwell, Oxford

Parkes C 1984 'Hospice' versus 'hospital' care: a re-evaluation after 10 years as seen by surviving spouses. Postgraduate Medical Journal 50:120–124

Seale C 1995 Heroic death. Sociology, Health and Illness 29:597–613

Seale C 2000 Changing patterns of death and dying. Social Science and Medicine 51:917–930

Seale C 2006a National survey of end-of-life decicioc made by UK medical practitioners. Palliative Medicine 20:3–10

Seale C 2006b Characteristics of end-of-life decisions: survey of UK medical practitioners. Palliative Medicine 20:653–659

Seale C, Cartwright A 1994 The year before death. Averbery, Aldershot

Seymour J 1999 Revisiting medicalization and 'natural' death. Social Science and Medicine 49:691–704

Sudnow D 1967 Passing on: the social organization of dying. Prentice Hall, New York

Taylor K 1988 'Telling bad news': physicians and the disclosure of undesirable information. Sociology, Health and Illness 10:109–132

Thomas C, Morris S, Clark D 2004 Place of death: preferences among cancer patients and their carers. Social Science and Medicine 58:2431–2444

Timmermans S 1994 Dying of awareness: the theory awareness contexts revisited. Sociology, Health and Illness 16:322–339

Timmermans S 2005 Death brokering: constructing culturally appropriate deaths. Sociology of Health and Illness 39:993–1013

Walter T 1994 The revival of death. Routledge, London

Walter T 1996 Facing death without tradition. In: Howarth G, Jupp P (eds) Contemporary issues in the sociology of death, dying and disposal. Macmillan, Basingstoke

Williams R 1990 A protestant legacy: attitudes to death and illness amon golder Aberdonians. Clarendon Press, Oxford

World Health Organization (WHO). 1998a World Health Report. WHO, Geneva

World Health Organization (WHO). 1998b World Health Statistics. WHO, Geneva

PART 3

Social structure and health

Inequality and social class

Mel Bartley
David Blane

In Bethnal Green in the year 1839 the average age of death in the different social classes was as follows: 'Gentlemen and persons engaged in professions, and their families ... 45 years; tradesmen and their families ... 26 years; Mechanics, servants and labourers, and their families ... 16 years' (Chadwick 1842). The average age of deaths in these social classes was found to vary somewhat from area to area, but similar differences between the classes were found in all areas of Britain.

Chadwick's study provided some of the first evidence that health varies with social class. The population's general level of health has improved dramatically since the first half of the nineteenth century, but subsequent investigations have shown that a relationship between mortality rates and social class remains. This has been repeatedly confirmed and shown to apply equally to morbidity. In 1980, the influential 'Black Report' (DHSS 1980) raised awareness in the medical profession of the extent to which poor health is associated with social class, and pointed out the ways in which social and health policies might be used to improve population health by reducing health inequality. It is important, therefore, to understand both what is meant by 'social class' and why it should be related to health indicators of many kinds. With this in mind, this chapter starts with details of some modern inequalities and of different ways of accounting for them, the most influential of which draws on concepts of social class. It then goes on to examine the relationship between social class and health.

SOME DIMENSIONS OF INEQUALITY IN THE UK

Wealth and income

Wealth, defined in terms of marketable assets, is very unequally distributed. In 2003 the richest 1% of the population aged 18 or over owned 21% of the country's total personal wealth, the richest 10% of the population owned 53% of total wealth and the poorest 50% of the population owned approximately 7%. If the value of housing is omitted from estimates of marketable assets, then the resulting distribution is even more skewed, with the richest 1% owning 34% and the poorest 50% a mere 1% (Office for National Statistics 2007). In 2001–2 one-half of all households in the UK reported having less than £1500 in savings, with 28% reporting no savings at all (Office for National Statistics 2003). It can be argued that the wealth that is owned by the majority of the population is used in an attempt to guarantee the necessities of life, whereas the wealth of the rich also brings with it social power, in the sense of ownership of land and voting rights in the decisions of financial and industrial corporations.

Income, which consists mainly of earnings from employment but also includes investment income and the various state benefits, is more equally distributed than wealth. During the 1970s there was relatively little change in the distribution of income among households, but the 1980s were characterized by a substantial increase in inequality: between 1981 and 1989, whereas average income rose by 27% when adjusted for inflation, the income of the top 10% rose by 38% and that of the bottom 10% by only 7%. Income distribution seemed to stabilize during the first half of the 1990s but in the most recent period for which data are available there appears to have been a further increase in inequality (Office for National Statistics 2001, 2007 i.e. ref above). Access to state facilities such as the education system and health service can also be seen as part of income, as can benefits in kind, which are received on top of earnings from employment. Although those on low incomes derive marginally greater benefit from the former, benefits in kind go disproportionately to those with high incomes and tend to be greatest for those with the highest salaries. Thus, large inequalities in income remain despite the redistribution achieved by mechanisms such as income tax, state benefits and access to state facilities.

Working conditions

The term 'social class' is correctly used to refer to an individual worker's employment relations and conditions. Employment relations vary from those typical of people doing higher level professional and managerial jobs, such as medical consultants and managers of large companies, to, at the other extreme, those typical of people doing the most routine and heavily supervised forms of work such as working in a call centre. Many of the most routine jobs also involve less skilled types of 'manual' work, although much manual work done nowadays is highly skilled and well paid (for example the work of plumbers). An individual's income is strongly tied to the nature of his or her work.

For a number of reasons, the difference in total weekly pay is not as great as the difference in the hourly rate. Routine workers are more likely to work overtime: in 1998, 14% of the average gross weekly earnings of £327 paid to routine manual workers came in the form of overtime, compared with 3% of the average gross weekly earnings of £505 paid to non-manual workers (Office for National Statistics 2000). Routine workers are also more likely to work shifts, which attract additional payment, and to be paid some form of production bonus. As these additional sources of income are likely to vary from week to week, it is more difficult for routine workers and their families to make financially sound plans, a disadvantage that is reinforced by routine workers' greater likelihood of being made redundant. Of considerable financial importance after retirement, routine workers are less likely to be members of an occupational pension scheme than workers in professional, managerial or technical occupations.

Routine work, especially in manual occupations, is usually more physically demanding, noisier and more dangerous than professional, managerial or technical work (Hunter 1975), as well as being more likely to involve the physical and social disruption of shift work. Despite its more hazardous nature, routine work lasts longer than professional manageral and technical work. Routine jobs usually do not require specialist qualifications, so that workers enter the workforce at an earlier age and, as has been noted, their basic working week is likely to be longer and they are more likely to work overtime. In addition, their holidays are shorter, with non-routine workers being more likely to receive in excess of 5 weeks holiday per year. By definition, routine work is also more likely to be repetitive than the work of professionals and managers, to offer little autonomy and to be experienced as boring. Routine workers are subject to closer supervision and tighter discipline; most have to clock-in at work, automatically lose money when late for work, face dismissal if continually late, and many need a supervisor's permission to use the lavatory or obtain a drink outside the set work-breaks.

POVERTY

The inequalities so far documented have been illustrated in terms of routine occupations compared with professional, managerial and technical occupations. Such comparisons are useful because they indicate the direction and size of the general trends, but they can create the misleading impression that the workforce is divided into homogeneous blocks whose members share the same income and living and working conditions and that these, in turn, are clearly better or worse than those of the next block. In reality, there is considerable variation in income and conditions within each block and considerable overlap between them. As a result, there is always room for debate about where it is appropriate to draw lines on this continuous distribution to identify specific groups. This problem complicates the definition of poverty and attempts to identify those who are exposed to poverty first need to be clear about the sense in which the term is being used.

The term 'poverty' has been used in two ways. Absolute poverty refers to a standard of living that cannot sustain life. When the term is used in this sense it could describe, for example, destitute people in the drought-stricken areas of the Sahel. One problem with this definition, however, is its failure to specify how long people can live before their standard of living is judged incapable of sustaining life. As the experience of hunger strikers demonstrates, no standard of living is so low as to kill instantaneously, and low-grade malnutrition might influence mortality only after many years. In addition, because very few people in the rich countries of the world are starving, using the term poverty in its absolute sense fails to address the hardships that are endured by many members of these societies.

'Relative poverty' refers to a standard of living below that which is considered normal or acceptable by the members of a particular society: 'The resources [of those in relative poverty] are so seriously below those commanded by the average individual or family that they are, in effect, excluded from ordinary living patterns, customs and activities' (Townsend 1979). Using the term in this relative sense allows the concept of poverty to be applied to rich societies such as Britain, although for research purposes it does pose the problem of how to establish empirically what is considered normal or acceptable in a particular society. This relative 'poverty line' can be established by means of surveys. A less expensive method, which is frequently used in research, is to equate relative poverty with an income below the level of eligibility for the various state benefits.

Townsend's classic study of poverty in the UK found that 7% of households, containing 3.3 million people, received an income below the state benefits level, and that a further 24% of households, which contained 11.9 million people, were on the margins of poverty, defined as an income less than 40% above the state benefits level. When those in poverty were analysed according to their labour market, personal and other characteristics, the three largest groups were those employed on low wages or in casual work, the disabled and long-term sick and the elderly retired, with the unemployed and one-parent families being the next largest groups (Townsend 1979).

The threshold now generally adopted to define low income in Britain is 60% of median equivalized household disposable income (equivalization here denotes adjustment for size and composition of the household). In fact, this threshold is one of those used in the government's antipoverty strategy. In 1998–9, 18% of the British population lived in households with incomes below this level. This proportion was fairly static during the 1960s, 1970s and early 1980s, fluctuating between 10 and 15%, but it rose steeply from 1985 to peak at 21% in 1992. Children are disproportionately present in low-income households: in 1998–9, 24% of children, or 3.1 million, were living in such households in Britain. There is a clear relationship between work and income. In 1998–9, only 2% of those living in households where all adults were in full-time work were in low-income households, compared with 64% of those in households where the head or spouse were unemployed; 26% of those in households where the head or spouse was aged 60 or over lived in low-income households (Office for National Statistics 2001).

Low income can lead to material and other forms of deprivation. Compared with that of the better paid, for example, the diet of the low paid contains far less fresh fruit, significantly less fresh vegetables, fresh fish and cheese, and more white bread, potatoes, sugar, lard and margarine (MAFF 1989). The Poverty and Social Exclusion Survey commissioned by the Joseph Rowntree Foundation sought to identify the items that a majority of the public perceive to be 'necessities', that is, which all adults should be able to afford and that they should not have to do without. About 28% of people in 1999 said they were unable to afford two or more of these items; 25% were unable to have 'regular savings of £10 a month for rainy days or retirement'; and nearly one-fifth could not afford a 'holiday away from home once a year not staying with relatives'. Other 'one-off' larger items of expenditure that more than 10% could not afford were 'replace or repair broken electrical goods', 'replace worn-out furniture', and 'money to keep home in a decent state of decoration'.

A potential shortcoming of such cross-sectional data is the extent to which they obscure the association between poverty and certain phases of the lifecycle. In societies where incomes are derived primarily from the labour market and where human reproduction predominantly occurs within nuclear families, there is an in-built tendency for an individual's standard of living to be lowest during childhood, active parenthood and old age, and to be highest during the intervening phases. This longitudinal approach has certain advantages: it draws attention to the association between poverty and childhood; it reminds us that those who are not currently living in poverty might have experienced it in the past or might realistically expect to experience it in the future; and it enables us to see that it is often the same individuals whose standard of living will dip below the poverty line during the low phases of the lifecycle. Thus, the child reared in poverty is educationally handicapped and is likely to be an early entrant to the unskilled sector of the labour market, where low wages and insecure employment will make family formation financially difficult and where the lack of an occupational pension scheme will predispose to poverty after retirement. Some idea of the proportion of the population that is likely to experience relative poverty at some stage during their lives is given by combining those who were found to be in poverty with those who were on its margins in the study quoted earlier; that is, 31% of households or 15 million people. Rather than being a marginal problem, therefore, poverty, or the realistic fear of it, is a fact of life for a substantial proportion of the population.

There is a considerable overlap between medical problems and poverty or the phases of the lifecycle where the standard of living tends to dip. The size of this overlap is illustrated by the 75% of prescriptions that are exempt from charges, a figure that can rise to 90% in some areas. The medical consequences of poverty start before birth, with poor maternal nutrition contributing to prematurity and low birth weight. During childhood, poor nutrition inhibits normal growth and development; lack of hygienic facilities predisposes to infestations with scabies, head lice and intestinal worms; damp housing increases the incidence of upper-respiratory-tract infections, which can lead to chronic ear disease, partial deafness and a poor educational record; and lack of play facilities hinders psychological development and increases the risk of accidents.

During active parenthood the health hazards stem from attempts to maximize income. Men and women with financial responsibility for children might seek the premiums attached to shift work, or the 'danger money' associated with hazardous jobs, as well as working overtime, taking a second part-time job on top of their main employment or working in the informal economy where poor health-and-safety conditions predominate. Such strategies increase income, but at the cost of physical exhaustion, risk of accidents, disrupted family life and increased vulnerability to depression in the care-taker alone at home with young children. Other, psychological, effects include exhaustion by the ceaseless struggle to 'make ends meet' and low self-esteem because of failure in this struggle, shame because one's children cannot have the same things as other children and fear lest the furniture is repossessed, the gas or electricity is cut off or one is made homeless because of insufficient money to pay hire purchase instalments, energy bills and rent.

During old age, the health effects of poverty reflect both immediate problems and the accumulation of past effects. Malnutrition ('tea and toast syndrome') and hypothermia are obvious examples, although the large increase in mortality during the winter compared with the summer months is probably a more important effect.

In summary, relative poverty affects a sizeable proportion of the British population. Because of the relationship between poverty and ill health, an even larger proportion of the patients whom doctors treat are likely to be affected in some way by its associated problems.

SOCIAL STRATIFICATION

Many other aspects of inequality could have been examined, in addition to those already discussed, including education, career prospects and leisure activities (Reid 1989). These inequalities tend to go together, so that an individual who is disadvantaged in one area of life is likely to be disadvantaged in others. In the same way, someone who is advantaged in one area of life is likely to be similarly advantaged in others. The term 'social stratification' generally refers to this kind of socially structured inequality, and the concept of social class describes the form that social stratification takes in industrialized societies such as contemporary Britain. Most societies to date have been hierarchically structured in some way. Historical forms of stratification have included, for example, the Hindu caste system and the various estates of feudal society. Some social theorists, drawing on the work of the early German sociologist Max Weber, consider that the stratification of modern industrial societies involves three main dimensions: social class, social status or honour, and the political power of organized groups. Although class, status and power are usually related, so that, for example, unskilled labourers generally have low social status and little political influence, they are analytically distinct and can vary independently of one another. Although it is generally agreed that social class is the most fundamental dimension of stratification, sociologists often differ in their precise definition and treatment of class and there are a number of competing theories.

The theory most widely used in the general population divides society into two stereotyped groups of roughly equal size. The 'middle class' consists of people who earn monthly salaries in non-routine, professional, technical or managerial jobs, borrow money to buy their own homes and encourage their children to get as much formal education as possible. The 'working-class', by contrast, consists of people who earn weekly wages in more routine, often manual jobs, rent their homes, often from housing associations or local councils, and try to get their children started in a secure job as soon as they are allowed to leave school. Most of the population appear to have little difficulty in placing themselves in one or other of these two classes. One study that included an unprompted question about self-rated social class found that 40% of the population spontaneously described themselves as middle class and 48% as working class. The study's subjects were found to have made this distinction chiefly on differences in lifestyle, but they were also influenced by considerations of family background, occupation and wealth (Townsend 1979). Recent social changes might have blurred this distinction somewhat. People from a wide range of occupations now own, or hope to own, their homes, take foreign holidays and drink wine. Likewise, managers and professionals are now no strangers to job insecurity, and must often live in rented accommodation due to the increasing gap between their salaries and house prices. The status of many professional jobs such as teaching has fallen, and the political power of the traditional middle classes in the UK is waning in the face of the growth of a much smaller group of very powerful owners of global financial and industrial companies.

Most academic social scientists tend to favour some version of Weber's class scheme, whereas the lay population, as we have seen, tends to use the working-class–middle-class distinction. Another approach, derived from the work of Karl Marx, is unusual in having advocates in both camps. It divides society into two main social classes on the basis of ownership and control of the land, industry and financial institutions. The 'working class' in Marx's analysis consists of the overwhelming majority of the population, who own only things they can use; and who live by selling their mental or physical labour power. Social changes since Marx's death have required considerable, and often disputed, elaboration of his original analysis. But it is very simple to understand what class you belong to according to Marx. Ask yourself how long you could continue your present lifestyle without a paid job. If the answer is 'not very long', you belong to the working class according to this definition.

For research purposes a more precise and detailed definition of social class is generally necessary. Many scales have been devised to meet this need, although each of these has its own particular strengths and weaknesses. The Registrar General's classification has been the most widely used in medical research. It divides the population into five social classes, I–V, with social class III being further subdivided into non-manual (IIIN) and manual (IIIM). This system of classification is based on occupation, and it groups occupations into social classes according to their skill level and general social standing in the community. Men are allocated to a social class on the basis of their own occupation, married women on the basis of their husband's occupation, children on that of their father and the retired and unemployed on that of their last significant period of employment. Single women are classified on the basis of their own occupation (OPCS 1980).

Certain characteristics of the Registrar General's classification need to be appreciated. Being based on the general social standing of different occupations, it is primarily a measure of status rather than economic class or living standards. As the earlier comments on Weber indicate, however, the link between social status and economic class is sufficiently strong for the classification to act as a reasonable indicator of lifetime earnings and conditions of life. Second, the Registrar General's social classes are not internally homogeneous. Social class II, for example, contains both tenant farmers working a few dozen acres and farmers who own thousands of acres; similarly, it contains both the corner shopkeeper and the senior manager in a multinational company. Third, the Registrar General's classification deals inadequately with women's employment, which, among other things, weakens its power as an indicator of living standards. Married women are classified by the occupation of their husband, although the standard of living of the family's members can be decisively affected by whether or not she has paid employment. It has been calculated that the number of families living in poverty would double if they were deprived of these earnings. Finally, it is possible to question the relevance of an occupationally based classification to a world of flexible labour markets, job insecurity and high rates of non-employment (long term sickness and early retirement as well as unemployment).

Problems such as these have prompted attempts to devise a more satisfactory classification, resulting in the new National Statistics Socio-economic Classification (NS-SEC) (Rose & O'Reilly 1997). The NS-SEC assigns people to social classes based on clear criteria. These are: the extent to which people in a particular job have job security, a career structure with promotion opportunities, incremental pay increases, autonomy to plan their own work schedule, authority over the work of others, whether they are paid a monthly salary rather than weekly or hourly. The basic divisions are between employers, who employ other people and exercise some degree of control and authority over them; employees, who sell their labour and find themselves under the control of employers in the process; and the self-employed, who experience neither. However, employees are further differentiated according to their 'service relationship' and the 'labour contract'. Managers and professionals have a service relationship with their employer that is characterized by a high degree of trust and delegated authority on the part of their employers. Such occupations are typically long-term and compensate for 'service' to the employer through salaries and salary arrangements (like company cars), together with salary increments, pension rights, job security and opportunities for career advancement. The labour contracts of working-class employees, on the other hand, typically specify discrete amounts of labour under close supervision in return for wages calculated on a 'piece' or time basis. Intermediate occupations are characterized by a mixed form of regulation between the service relationship and the labour contract (Bartley 2003, Chandola 2000). Table 8.1 compares the Registrar General's classification with the NS-SEC.

Because the use of the NS-SEC in official statistics and other studies is relatively new, the examples given below of the relationship between social class and health use the older Registrar-General's social classification.

TABLE 8.1	Registrar General's and SEC classifications of social classes	
	Registrar General	**NC-SEC**
I	Professional	1. Senior professionals/senior managers
II	Intermediate	2. Associate professionals/junior managers
IIIN	Skilled non-manual	3. Other administrative and clerical workers
IIIM	Skilled manual	4. Own account non-professional
IV	Semi-skilled manual	5. Supervisors, technicians and related workers
V	Unskilled manual	6. Intermediate workers
		7. Other workers
		8. Never worked/other inactive

N = non-manual; M = manual.

SOCIAL CLASS AND HEALTH

■ UK data

As the quotation from Chadwick in the opening paragraph of this chapter illustrates, it has long been recognized that the various positions in the social hierarchy are associated with different chances of premature death. Good quality data on the relationship between social class and mortality in England and Wales were published each decade for most of the twentieth century. The data reproduced in Table 8.2 are the most recent available, but the general pattern that they reveal has been a constant feature of all the earlier reports. The mortality rates increase in a step-wise fashion as one moves from the

TABLE 8.2	Social class and deaths due to all causes (England and Wales, 1991–3, 1993–5)			
Social class	**Still-birth rate[a]**	**Infant mortality rate[b]**	**Mortality rate (1–15 years)[c]**	**Standardized mortality ratio (men, 20–64 years)[d]**
I	4	4	18	66
II	4	5	16	72
IIIN	5	5	16	100
IIIM	5	6	26	117
IV	6	7	22	116
V	8	8	42	189

Adapted from Drever & Whitehead (1997)
N = non-manual; M = manual.
[a] Number of deaths per 1000 live and dead births; rounded to the nearest integer, 1993–5.
[b] Number of deaths in the first year of life per 1000 live births; rounded to the nearest integer, 1993–5.
[c] Number of deaths per 100,000 population aged 1–15 years; rounded to the nearest integer, 1991–3.
[d] The ratio of the observed mortality rate in a social class to its expected rate from the total population, multiplied by 100, 1991–3.

TABLE 8.3	Social class and major causes of death (England and Wales; 1986–92): age-standardized mortality rates per 100 000			
		Social class		
Cause of death	I/II	IIIN	IIIM	IV/V
Males 35–64 years				
Ischaemic heart disease	160	162	231	266
Lung cancer	35	50	77	80
Cerebrovascular disease	29	27	33	40
Respiratory diseases	13	21	36	48
Females 35–64 years				
Ischaemic heart disease	29	39	59	78
Lung cancer	16	17	34	47
Cerebrovascular disease	14	22	18	34
Respiratory diseases	11	12	23	29
Breast cancer	52	49	46	54

Adapted from Drever & Whitehead (1997).
N = non-manual; M = manual.

Registrar General's social class I to social class V, with the mortality rate of the latter being approximately twice that of the former. This social class gradient in total deaths due to all causes is found among both males and females and within all age groups, although the differences tend to narrow with increasing age.

Certain specific, major causes of death are listed in Table 8.3. For most causes the mortality rates increase as one moves from social class I to class V, so showing the same gradient as deaths due to all causes combined. There are exceptions, however, which show little or no social class gradient; breast cancer in women has been the most prevalent of these, although this pattern appears to be changing. As this suggests, unlike the gradient for deaths due to all causes, the social class gradient for some causes of death changed considerably during the 20th century. Coronary heart disease is the most prominent of these; its mortality rate was highest in social class I and lowest in class V for the first half of the century; this gradient flattened out in the third quarter and reversed in the final quarter, so that its mortality rate is now highest in social class V and lowest in class I.

The data presented so far have been mortality rates, and their use as a measure of health has certain advantages. In the vast majority of cases, death is an unambiguous event that can be recorded with high reliability. Death is also one of the few times that an individual is legally obliged to be seen by a doctor, with the result that the recording of death is virtually complete. Mortality rates, therefore, are reliable and complete measures. Nevertheless, they are not perfect measures of health. The term 'health' implies the absence of disease as well as the absence of premature death (see Chapter 18). As a result, attempts to understand the relationship between social class and health have recently begun to examine the way in which morbidity (illness) varies with social class.

For a variety of reasons, the measurement of morbidity is more difficult than that of mortality. Consulting a doctor could be taken as a measure of morbidity. Manual workers consult doctors more frequently than non-manual workers, but it should not be assumed that this is solely because of differences in health. Differences in consultation rates result from differences in illness behaviour (Chapter 3) as well as differences in morbidity. Indeed, non-manual workers appear to be the more frequent consulters when 'use/need ratios' are used to relate consultation rates to the prevalence of illness in the various social classes. The illnesses that people report when questioned as part of a representative survey appear to avoid this problem with consultation rates, so rates of reported illness could be taken as a second measure of morbidity. Manual workers report more illnesses of all types, especially chronic and limiting long-standing illness, than non-manual workers, with the differences tending to widen in the older age groups (Drever & Whitehead 1997). All measures of self-reported morbidity, however, involve subjective judgements about illness and its severity. The observed class differences on these measures might be due to systematic variation in these judgements. The more physically demanding nature of manual occupations, for example, might mean that illness is less easily tolerated and recognized earlier.

Some studies have used clinical measures of morbidity on samples of the whole population. These studies should provide results that are free from possible contamination by illness behaviour and systematic subjective variation. Among middle-aged men in the British Regional Heart Study, manual workers were more likely to have experienced angina than non-manual workers; similar social class differences were found in obesity and, to a lesser extent, in blood pressure (Pocock et al 1987, Shaper et al 1988, Weatherall & Shaper 1988). Among men and women of working age in the Health and Lifestyle Survey, manual workers were more likely to experience psychological malaise, to have poorer respiratory function and, to a lesser extent, higher blood pressure than non-manual workers (Cox et al 1987). Studies of this type are expensive and therefore rare. An additional disadvantage is that they usually concentrate on one specific disease, so they are unable to provide information about social class differences in overall morbidity. Like all surveys, they also suffer from non-responders, so their results are not based on the complete coverage achieved by mortality data.

In summary, for many decades reliable and complete data in Britain have shown a step-wise gradient in mortality across the social classes, with members of social class V ('non-skilled manual' according to the old Registrar-General's classification) having approximately twice the chance of dying at any particular age as members of social class I ('professionals' according to the Registrar-General's classification). Recently, attention has turned to morbidity, which is a more valid measure of health than mortality, but difficult to measure with comparable reliability and completeness. Social class differences have been found in various measures of morbidity. The size of these differences appears to vary considerably. The lack of a close match between social class differences in mortality and in morbidity is not surprising. Some major causes of death, such as accidents and violence, need not be preceded by illness and disease, and some common serious diseases, such as arthritis and depression, rarely cause death.

International data

British data on health inequalities are richer and longer standing than those from elsewhere. In recent years, however, information on socioeconomic differences in health has become available for many other countries. In most cases, these studies have used measures of social position that differ from the Registrar General's occupational social classes. The number of years of formal education and the level of income are the most frequently used. In general, these alternative measures of socioeconomic position show the same relationship to health as the Registrar General's classes in Britain. Mortality and morbidity rates are lowest in the most advantaged group, highest in the least advantaged group and, in between, increase along a step-wise gradient. Recently, moreover, there has been a discernible tendency for studies yielding cross-country comparisons to show a widening of inequalities in health. The most dramatic widening seems to be occurring in central and eastern Europe, but countries with 'good health profiles', such as the Netherlands, Sweden and Denmark, are also signalling persisting or growing inequalities (Drever & Whitehead 1997).

USA

In 1990, death rates at ages 25–64 years, for males and females combined, were 471 per 100 000 for those who had received 8 years or less of formal education and 264 per 100 000 for those who had received 16 years or more (DHHS 1994). In another large-scale study, the death rates of white males showed an inverse gradient with the level of median family income. At the extremes of the income distribution, those with a median family income of less than $7500 had a death rate of 81 per 10 000 compared with 39 for those with more than $32 500 (Davey Smith et al 1992).

European Union

In the Netherlands in 1981–5, the rate of self-reported chronic illness among people aged 16 years or more was over 50% higher in those who left formal education after primary school than in those who had received a university education (Mackenbach 1993).

In Spain in 1987 the prevalence of chronic illness among women aged 20–44 years was nearly 50% higher in the poorest income group than in the highest income group (Kunst & Mackenbach 1994).

Eastern Europe

In Poland in 1988–9 the death rate among men aged 50–64 years was 22 per 1000 among those who left formal education after primary school and 10 per 1000 among those with a university education (Brajczewski & Rogucka 1993).

Among women in Russia who received primary school and university education a similar, although smaller, difference in death rates has been reported (Davis et al 1994).

Socioeconomic differences in health are therefore not confined to Britain. They have been found in every country that has examined the issue and are probably a feature of all industrialized societies. British efforts to understand this phenomenon are now part of an international endeavour.

INTERPRETATION OF THE RELATIONSHIP BETWEEN SOCIAL CLASS AND HEALTH

The association between social class and health shows that death and disease are socially structured, as opposed to randomly distributed throughout the population, and that they vary in line with the differences in living standards that were documented earlier. However, correlation does not imply causation, and the relationship needs to be examined further. Investigations of health inequality tend to use four 'explanatory models' in the search for greater understanding (Bartley 2003). These are: behavioural, material, psychosocial and life-course models.

Behavioural model

Behavioural explanations involve class differences in behaviours that are health damaging or health promoting, and which, at least in principle, are subject to individual choice. This type of explanation is sometimes called 'behavioural/cultural' because cultures differ quite widely in the types of behaviours they encourage or forbid (for example, eating meat, drinking alcohol). But whether or not the large social class differences in Western populations in things like smoking and diet can usefully be regarded as 'cultural' is more problematic.

Dietary choices, the consumption of drugs like tobacco and alcohol, active leisure-time pursuits and the use of preventive medical services such as immunization, contraception and antenatal surveillance are examples of behaviours that vary with social class and could partly explain class differences in health. Considerable weight is given to this type of explanation by the evidence that has accumulated as a result of medicine's long interest in such issues. But long-term studies following people's behaviour and changes in their health have shown that behaviour explains only about a third of the class differences in illness and mortality. Perhaps more importantly, intervention studies have rarely produced the clear-cut improvements in health that would be predicted by the behavioural/cultural approach. One reason for this is that it is very difficult to change behaviours once and for all. The other reason is that even when reduction in the hazardous behaviours has been achieved, improvements in health have been rather disappointing.

The social and economic context in which health behaviours occur also needs to be recognized. Diet is influenced by both cultural preferences and disposable income. The ability of nicotine to maintain a constant mood in situations of stress and monotony might predispose towards cigarette smoking in repetitive and highly supervised occupations. Other evidence cautions against a one-sided emphasis on behavioural factors. Early in the twentieth century, cigarette smoking was more prevalent among the middle class than the working class, but class gradients in mortality were similar to the present.

Materialist model

Materialist explanations, by contrast, involve hazards that are inherent in the present form of social organization and to which some people have no choice but to be exposed.

The Black Report judged that materialist explanations were the most important in accounting for social class differences in health. The health-damaging effects of air pollution and occupational exposure to physicochemical hazards had already been recognized. More recently, local levels of economic and social deprivation have been identified as powerful predictors of mortality and morbidity. Damp housing has been shown to be associated with worse health, particularly with higher rates of respiratory disease in children. Unemployment has been associated with psychological morbidity and raised mortality among unemployed men and their spouses. Each of these factors could contribute to class differences in health because they are all more likely to be experienced by working class than middle class people.

There is thus a certain amount of evidence to support the materialist type of explanation. But the full importance of material living standards can only be understood over the life course in the longer term. An amount of money that would provide sufficient calories to allow a person to survive for a month is not equivalent to the amount necessary to allow him or her to have a diet that will support health over the long term, or to pay for a clean, dry and warm home, or to cover the expenses involved in avoiding social isolation. Soap, toothpaste, a TV and the ability to entertain friends and family now and then might appear to be 'luxuries'. Yet according to the best evidence we have on a healthy life-style, social isolation (due to being dirty, or being in total ignorance of what everyone else is talking about) is as harmful as poor diet and lack of exercise for long-term health (Morris et al 2002).

Psychosocial model

One of the most widely researched explanations for health inequality is the 'psychosocial model', which argues that explanations for health inequality may need to include what are described as 'psychosocial risk factors'. These include social support, control and autonomy at work, the balance between home and work, the balance between efforts and rewards.

According to this explanatory model, feelings that arise because of inequality, subordination and lack of social support may directly affect biological processes. Rather than laying emphasis on physical hazards, or on behaviour alone, the psychosocial model focuses on the way social inequality makes people feel, and how these feelings may themselves alter body chemistry.

The original ideas behind this line of research were based on the existence of the so called 'fight or flight' response. In the human evolutionary past, the argument goes, violent activity to either counter-attack or flee from a predator or aggressor would follow the arousal of the sympathetic nervous system (Brunner 2000, Steptoe & Willemsen 2002). Adrenaline, fats and sugars are released into the blood to feed muscular effort, and at the same time levels of a clotting factor, fibrinogen, are increased in case of injury. Vigorous physical activity uses up these substances when the individual fights or runs away. If the animal or person survives, the parasympathetic nervous system quickly returns the body to a more normal state. However, under modern conditions, feelings of fear or anger in humans are less often responded to by physical effort, for example when caught in a traffic jam, or being bullied by a superior at work. Even when escape is made, this is done without physical effort. And endurance of prolonged stress over long periods of time is thought by some to lead to an increase in 'allostatic load' (McEwen 1998). The term 'allostasis' means literally 'the ability of the body to keep itself stable' during changes in the external environment. The 'allostatic load' model of psychosocial causes of ill health focuses on what may happen when there are too many changes in too short at period of time, so that the body's attempts to respond produce overload and exhaustion. The idea would lead us to expect, for example, that an objectionable boss would be harder to bear in an environment that was also too hot, cold, or noisy, or when the individual also had a poor diet.

Some evidence can also be found that allostatic overload is more common amongst less socio-economically privileged people. Several studies have shown that people in less advantaged social positions have higher blood pressure, and higher fibrinogen. Social epidemiologists have concluded that there might be a causal pathway by which stressful social circumstances produce emotional responses, which in turn bring about biological changes that increase the risk of heart disease.

LIFE-COURSE MODEL

Until quite recently, research on health inequality tended to ignore the dimension of time, and the accumulation of advantage or disadvantage that is associated with social class. As the earlier sections of this chapter have indicated, inequalities are found in many spheres of life. Social class is the concept that stresses the likelihood that advantage or disadvantage in one sphere, and at one time, will be associated with advantage or disadvantage in others. Those who experienced poor home conditions are more likely to go on and experience occupational disadvantage. Lower paid jobs mean that these are likely to be the same people who have worse housing in more polluted and unfriendly areas. In other words, disadvantages in their various forms are likely to accumulate through childhood and adulthood and into old age. It will not be possible to make a secure judgement about the relative importance of behavioural/cultural, psychosocial and materialist explanations until the effect on health of such combined and accumulating disadvantages has been established.

CONTEMPORARY DEBATES

■ Which explanatory model is the best?

It is now widely agreed that health behaviours, although important, only explain about 30% of the differences in health between the most and the least advantaged social groups. Health professionals have targeted smoking, drinking, diet and exercise for many years, but while levels of life expectancy have increased rapidly, there has been little sign of any decrease in health inquality. If the health disadvantage of the less privileged social groups is to be lessened, other processes than health behaviours need to be understood. To the present time, there have not been very many systematic attempts to match different explanatory models to the data that exist in order to evaluate them against each other. For example, many authorities think that life has become more stressful since the 1950s, but at the same time heart attacks and cardiovascular mortality have rapidly decreased. In fact, the increase in life expectancy has taken place at a time of rapidly increasing material living standards (even if this has been accompanied by rising income inequality), giving some support to the materialist explanation first put forward in the 1980s. A mixture of the materialist and life-course explanations would allow us to also take into account the improvements in conditions of babies and young children. Homes with access to private kitchens and indoor bathrooms were far more available to middle class than working class families in the 1920s and 1930s, but by the 1960s most working class families had these amenities as well. The child of a manual worker in the 1960s was therefore far less likely to grow up with the long term consequences of repeated and chronic infections. Education became more widely available, and after 1964 all children stayed an extra year at school, up to the age of 16. Working on Saturdays became rare, and the majority of occupations came to include paid holidays. Compared to the 1920s and 1930s, unemployment between 1945 and 1979 remained at a very low level. All of these changes would have contributed to lower amounts of time spent exposed to a range of health hazards.

This is not to dismiss the importance of psychosocial factors. Perhaps their most important role is in the understanding of social inequality in health behaviours. After various Government reports in the USA and UK in the 1960s, the public were made aware of the link between smoking and health, but middle class men were far quicker to abandon the habit than working class men, and smoking in women even increased. Research shows that working class people are no less aware of the dangers than middle class people. Male smokers are equally likely to express a wish to give up in all social classes, while younger women tend to balance the risks of smoking against the perceived risk of gaining weight. But both work and social situations in which the individual feels less valued and less in control of events seem to increase the difficulty of controlling any form of addiction. Younger people must weigh up the relative benefits of a 'pleasure' in the here and now against a longer life expectancy at some distant and perhaps uncertain future. These are not material considerations, but relate to how people feel about their present and future. Also, as the classical material hazards such as poor housing and dangers of the industrial workplace become less common (in part because there are so few industrial jobs left), psychosocial hazards may increase in relative importance. No one who has ever experienced it could imagine that going to work each day to face bullying or social isolation can be healthy.

Is a more unequal economy bad for health?

An influential contributor to debates on inequality and health has maintained that the level of income inequality is a crucial determinant of the health of populations in more affluent societies like Britain (Wilkinson 1996). Wilkinson argued that once certain levels of gross national product (GNP) per capita have been reached, the principal determinant of level of health status within a country is degree of income inequality. Once countries A and B have passed through what he calls the 'epidemiological transition', then the population of country A can be twice as rich as that of country B without being any healthier. In short, the populations of rich 'equal' countries have better health profiles than the populations of rich 'unequal' countries. He went on to claim that social cohesion and trust provide the dominant mechanisms linking a country's degree of income equality with health. He argued that there is evidence that where income inequalities are more marked, social divisions tend to be exacerbated; levels of trust and strength of community life tend to be lower; rates of social anxiety and chronic stress tend to be higher; rates of hostility, violence and murder tend to be higher; and there tends to develop a 'culture of inequality' characterized by a more hostile and less hospitable environment. His research has therefore been based on a form of the 'psychosocial model'. But instead of relating stress levels in groups such as social classes to individual health, he relates income inequality in whole populations to the relationships between members of those populations and thereby to average population health. Even for people in more advantaged socioeconomic situations, a highly unequal society is more dangerous for health (Wilkinson 2000).

Wilkinson's general thesis on the nature of the epidemiological transition has been challenged on statistical grounds, and his notion of a 'psychosocial pathway' linking income inequality to health differences has been criticized by a number of commentators.

Scambler & Higgs (2001) offer a different interpretation of Wilkinson's findings by adopting a concept of class that owes much to Marx's perspective mentioned earlier. According to them, countries with a more unequal distribution of income and wealth are simply those in which the social classes with more wealth have more control over the political process which determines the levels of taxation, and the provision of housing, health and social services to those with lower incomes. In other words, it is the concentration of power and associated changes in economic policies that are basic to understanding the increase in income inequality and, ultimately, the 'widening gap' in health inequalities.

THE OVERALL PICTURE

The work of social researchers such as Chadwick and Farr made the Victorians aware of the vicious circle of 'poverty causes disease which causes poverty'. Despite the subsequent development of the welfare state, disabled people and those with chronic diseases are still at risk of relative poverty. This side of the Victorians' vicious circle, however, would now appear less important than the side that stresses the effect of material well-being, or the lack of it, on health. The health inequalities of today are primarily due to the combined effect of class differences in exposure to factors that promote health or cause disease.

This was the conclusion reached by the Department of Health Working Group that produced the Black Report. The Report went on to suggest measures for starting to eliminate health inequalities. There are 37 of these recommendations. A few were designed to ensure better information about class differences in health. Most were carefully targeted at a limited number of issues where class differences in health were thought to be widest and most likely to respond to relatively small sums of money. Disability was the subject of six recommendations designed to break its links with poverty. These covered prevention (fetal screening for neural tube defects and Down syndrome), welfare procedures (a comprehensive disablement allowance), housing (more specialist housing for disabled people) and community-care services (resources shifted towards home-help and nursing services for disabled people). This set of recommendations appears designed to prevent disability where this is presently possible (fetal screening) and, where it is not, to ensure that the lives of working-class people with disabilities are not markedly disadvantaged in terms of income (welfare procedures) and living conditions (housing and community services).

In addition to disability, equally detailed recommendations were made concerning infant and child health, cigarette smoking, occupational health and safety and local authority housing. Particular priority was given to the abolition of child poverty by means of a new infant-care allowance, increased child benefit and the provision of free school meals. These recommendations, in common with the rest of the report, were described by the incumbent Conservative government as 'unrealistic' and the report was published 'without any commitment by the Government to its proposals'. Nevertheless, subsequent research has greatly increased our understanding of the relationship between social class and health.

When the Labour government was elected in 1997 it promptly established an 'Independent Inquiry into Inequalities in Health' (Stationery Office 1998). Even before the Acheson Report, as it was known, was published, a Green Paper entitled 'Our Healthier Nation' (DoH 1998) had stated as one of its aims improving the health of the worst off in society and narrowing what it called 'the health gap'. The Acheson Report itself noted that average mortality had fallen over the previous 50 years, but concluded that 'unacceptable inequalities in health persist' and that 'for many measures of health, inequalities have either remained the same or have widened in recent years'. This applied at all stages of the life course. The Report acknowledged that income, education and employment were fundamental determinants of ill health, as well as the material environment and life-style. Its recommendations went well beyond the remit of the Department of Health, calling for policy development in relation to poverty, income, tax and benefits, education, employment, housing and environment, mobility, transport and pollution, and nutrition. The three main areas defined as crucial are listed in Box 8.1.

BOX 8.1	Crucial areas identified by the Acheson report

1. All policies likely to have an impact on health should be evaluated in terms of their impact on health inequalities.
2. A high priority should be given to the health of families with children.
3. Further steps should be taken to reduce income inequalities and improve the living standards of poor households.

The authors of the Black Report welcomed its successor, drawing attention in particular to the recommendation relating to material factors, which specified the urgent need to reduce income inequalities and improve the living standards of households in receipt of social security benefits (Black et al 1999). However, the Acheson Report has been criticized for not prioritizing its recommendations, for being overly vague and for not costing its suggested policies, and early audits of government responses have been cautious, even pessimistic (Shaw et al 1999). It remains to be seen whether there will be a willingness to act effectively against factors, such as income inequality, which continue to underpin health inequalities in Britain.

References

Bartley M 2003 Health inequality: an introduction to concepts, theories and methods. Polity Press, Cambridge

Black D et al 1999 Better benefits for health: plan to implement the central recommendations of the Acheson Report. British Medical Journal 318:724–727

Brajczewski C, Rogucka E 1993 Social class differences in rates of premature mortality among adults in the city of Wroclaw. American Journal of Human Biology 5:461–471

Brunner E 2000 Towards a new social biology. In: Berkman L, Kawachi I (eds.) Social epidemiology. Oxford University Press, Oxford, p 306–331

Chadwick E 1842 Report on the sanitary condition of the labouring population of Great Britain 1842. Edinburgh University Press, Edinburgh. Reprinted 1965

Chandola T 2000 Social class differences in mortality using the new UK National Statistics Socio-Economic Classification. Social Science and Medicine 50:641–649

Cox BD et al 1987 The health and lifestyle survey: preliminary report. Health Promotion Research Trust, London

Davey Smith G et al 1992 Income differentials in mortality risk among 305,099 white men. European Society of Medical Sociology Conference, Edinburgh, September 1992 (Abstract)

Davis CE et al 1994 Correlates of mortality in Russian and US women: the Lipid Research Clinics Program. American Journal of Epidemiology 139:369–379

Department of Health (DoH) 1998 Our healthier nation: a contract for health. HMSO, London

Department of Health and Human Services (DHHS) 1994 Health United States 1993. National Centre for Health Statistics, Hyattsville, MD

Department of Health and Social Security (DHSS) 1980 Inequalities in health: report of a research working group (The Black Report). HMSO, London

Drever F, Whitehead M (eds) 1997 Health inequalities. National Statistics, London

Hunter D 1975 The diseases of occupations, 5th edn. English Universities Press, London

Kunst AE, Mackenbach JP 1994 Measuring socio-economic inequalities in health. WHO Regional Office for Europe, Copenhagen

McEwen BS 1998 Protective and damaging effects of stress mediators. New England Journal of Medicine 338:171–179

Mackenbach JP 1993 Inequalities in health in the Netherlands according to age, gender, marital status, level of education, degree of urbanisation and region. European Journal of Public Health 3:112–118

Ministry of Agriculture, Fisheries and Food (MAFF) 1989 Household food consumption and expenditure 1988. HMSO, London

Morris JN, Donkin AJM, Wonderling D et al 2002 A minimum income for healthy living. Journal of Epidemiology and Community Health 54: 885–889

Office for National Statistics 2000 Social Trends 30. HMSO, London

Office For National Statistics 2001 Social Trends 31. HMSO, London

Office for National Statistics 2003 Household Savings by household type and amount 2001/2, Social Trends 34

Office for National Statistics 2007 ONS Online http://www.statistics.gov.uk/cci/ nugget_print.asp?ID=2 accessed 18/05/07

131

Office of Population Censuses and Surveys (OPCS) 1980 Classification of occupations 1980. HMSO, London

Pocock SJ et al 1987 Social class differences in ischaemic heart disease in British men. Lancet ii:197–201

Reid I 1989 Social class differences in Britain, 3rd edn. Fontana Press, London

Rose D, O'Reilly K (eds) 1997 Constructing classes: towards a new social classification for the UK. Office for National Statistics, London

Scambler G, Higgs P 2001 'The dog that didn't bark': taking class seriously in the health inequalities debate. Social Science and Medicine 52:157–159

Shaper AG, Ashby D, Pocock SJ 1988 Blood pressure and hypertension in middle-aged British men. Journal of Hypertension 6:367–374

Shaw M, Dorling D, Gordon D, Davey Smith G 1999 The widening gap: health inequalities and policy in Britain. Policy Press, Bristol

Stationery Office 1998 Independent inquiry into inequalities in health (the Acheson Report). HMSO, London

Steptoe A, Willemsen G 2002 Psychophysiological responsivity in coronary heart disease. In: Stansfeld S, Marmot M (eds) Stress and the heart. BMJ Books, London, p 168–180

Townsend P 1979 Poverty in the United Kingdom. Penguin, London

Weatherall R, Shaper AG 1988 Overweight and obesity in middle-aged British men. Journal of Clinical Nutrition 42:221–231

Wilkinson R 1996 Unhealthy societies: the afflictions of inequality. Routledge, London

Wilkinson R 2000 Deeper than neo-liberalism: a reply to David Coburn. Social Science and Medicine 51:997–1000

Women and health

Annette Scambler

This chapter presents a broad sweep of health differences between the genders, starting with life expectancy and mortality data, and moving on to a general discussion of morbidity differences before detailing some issues of health of especial significance to women. A consideration of issues of masculinity and femininity and of mental health connects with material on embodiment, body hatred and eating disorders in young women, and childbirth provides a forum for further consideration of the medicalization and control of women's bodies. To attempt to understand the relationship of gender to health it is first essential to explore the relative social positions of men and women in contemporary society.

GENDER ROLES AND WOMEN'S POSITION IN SOCIETY

We live in a social environment where gender plays a significant role in social status and in access to material resources, health and well-being, and where roles, responsibilities and power are not shared equally between males and females. It is tempting, when looking at gender, to focus on the enormous range of changes that undoubtedly occurred over the course of the 20th century, with women now found in every sphere of society. We have had a female Prime Minister and women at the head of unions and major business, leisure, academic and professional organizations. Women now comprise over half the entrants to medical school and are entering the legal profession in large numbers. It would be very easy to paint a picture of women in the process of equalling or even displacing the existing male captains of industry. That would be a simplistic view. Although there have been significant shifts in gender norms in society, such changes have occurred within a complex web of power and advantage that still leaves women light years away from even material parity with men.

Some evidence is required here and a good place to start is with the seat of government itself. As of 2005, after the Labour Party's third general election victory, there was a complement of 646 MPs, of whom 126 were female. That is just under 20% of the total, although over half the population is female. However, prior to Labour's 1997 victory, only 9% of MPs were female. The doubling of the female contingent in 1997 to just over 18% was largely due to the introduction of women-only shortlists by the Labour Party, to counter a male bias in the selection process, but this policy had to be abandoned after legal challenges under the Sex Discrimination Act. After the 2001 election, when the number of women elected dropped for the first time in 20 years, the Sex Discrimination (Election Candidates) Act of 2002 was passed allowing political parties to adopt positive measures to boost the number of women elected to both the national and regional parliaments and assemblies. That this measure is still needed almost 100 years after women first gained a partial vote in 1918, speaks volumes. Despite this development, in the early years of the Labour government women were not high on the agenda. The minimum wage had to be won in the European Court, despite the fact that 80% of those to benefit would be women. As of October, 2006 the minimum wage stood at a princely £5.35 per hour and around 70% of beneficiaries are still women. Despite the rhetoric around childcare support for women, only 25% of children under eight in England and Wales have access to childminding, full-day care or out of hours care (ONS 2006b). There have been more recent positive moves towards equality, but it would be naïve to suggest that more female MPs, alone, will effect the needed changes. In terms of power, only 25% of cabinet members were women after the 2005 election; they made just over 18% of the House of Lords, only 24% of MEPs, and just over a quarter of local councillors in England (Women and Equality Unit, January, 2006). Women comprise less than 1% of senior ranks in the armed services, only 10% of senior police officers, only 9% of senior judiciary, only one in nine university vice chancellors, only three in ten headteachers at secondary and FE level, and just a quarter of top management in the Civil Service (EOC 2006). Some dedicated work is going on within the lower levels of government, however, and the 'Gender Equality Duty' came into force in April, 2007. This requires all public authorities in England, Wales and Scotland to promote gender equality and eliminate sex discrimination, and to demonstrate that they do so themselves. The remit is broad and covers everything from access to flexi-hours to provision of public transport to health service availability, etc. However, as we are about to see, gender norms are deeply entrenched, and the Duty only relates to the public sector, not the private.

■ Changes in family size and structure

Since the 1970s marriage has been declining and divorce rising. Between 1971 and mid 2006, the percentage of households comprising 'traditional families' – composed of parents and dependent children – declined from over a third to just less than one quarter, and lone-parent households with dependent children doubled to 7%, nine out of ten of them female headed. Nearly a quarter of all dependent children now live in lone-parent families, 90% of them with their mothers (Social Trends 2007). By 2005, the average age of first marriage in England and Wales had risen to 29 for women and 32 for men (a rise of 6 years over a 34-year period). Figure 9.1 shows changes in marriage and divorce since 1950. The number of marriages has declined by around 41% since 1972, while divorces increased by 50% but now may be slightly declining (Social Trends 2007, Fig. 2.9). Cohabiting now normally precedes marriage and many couples cohabit but never marry. In 1986, when the first data were produced, only 12% were cohabiting; now the rate has doubled to 24% in just 20 years.

Along with changes in the structure of the family, fertility rates have also declined. Table 9.1 shows a big decline in these rates since 1971, with a record low of 1.63 in 2001. The rate recovered a little to 1.79 by 2005 (partly, it is thought, due to more births to immigrants, especially from the new EU countries), but the overall drop means twenty less live births for every 1000 women since 1971. What is interesting is that in 2005 the

135

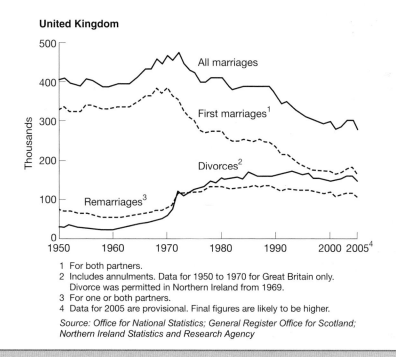

United Kingdom

1 For both partners.
2 Includes annulments. Data for 1950 to 1970 for Great Britain only.
  Divorce was permitted in Northern Ireland from 1969.
3 For one or both partners.
4 Data for 2005 are provisional. Final figures are likely to be higher.

Source: Office for National Statistics; General Register Office for Scotland; Northern Ireland Statistics and Research Agency

Fig. 9.1 Marriages and divorces in the UK (Social Trends 2007, Fig. 2.9, page 18).

TABLE 9.1	Fertility rates by age of mother at childbirth (Social Trends 2007, Table 2.16, page 21)				
	Live births per 1000 women				
United Kingdom	**1971**	**1981**	**1991**	**2001**	**2005**
Age					
under 20	50.0	28.4	32.9	27.9	26.2
20–24	154.4	106.6	88.9	68.0	70.5
25–29	154.6	130.9	119.9	91.5	98.3
30–34	79.4	69.4	86.5	88.0	100.7
35–39	34.3	22.4	32.0	41.3	50.0
40 and over	9.2	4.7	5.3	8.6	10.6
Total Fertility Rate[2]	2.41	1.82	1.82	1.63	1.79
Total births[3] (thousands)	901.6	730.7	792.3	669.1	722.5

[1] Live births per 1000 women aged 15 to 19.
[2] Number of children that would be born to a woman if current patterns of fertility persisted throughout her childbearing life. For 1981 onwards, this is based on fertility rates for each single year of age, but for 1971 it is based on the rates for each five year age group.
[3] Total live births per 1000 women aged 15 to 44.
Source: *Office for National Statistics.*

fertility rate for the 30+ age group exceeded that of the 25–29 year olds for the first time. Many more women are giving birth outside marriage, and in 2005 these women were, on average, 4 years younger than their married counterparts. The overall picture, therefore, shows that women are getting married later, having their children later in life and having fewer children. Contributing factors include increased participation in higher education and employment and better contraception (72% of women were using contraception by the end of the twentieth century). One area of particular concern is the increasing trend for women to remain childless. Only 11% of women born in 1943 remained childless at the age of 45, but this figure has risen steadily, and by 2005 of those born in 1960 18% remained childless at 45. This rise is expected to continue (Social Trends 2007).

Women and paid employment

Equality for the genders is still not obvious in the general area of paid work. Although there was an Equal Pay Act in 1970, women working full-time in 2005 earned only 83% of the average full-time male wage. This is an improvement on 1985 when the figure stood at 74%, but that is still a gender pay gap of 17% (ONS 2006a). Table 9.2 shows the percentage of males and females in various employment sectors, together with their accompanying pay gaps (ONS 2006b). The occupational sectors show big gender differences, but some things have not changed much. Nine out of ten workers in the construction industry were male in both 1972 and in 2005, while women predominated in health and education in both periods. Enormous variation was also found in pay gaps by sector, with the lowest gap of 9% in transport and communication, where only 24% of workers are female, and the highest at 41% in banking and insurance, where gender numbers are virtually equal. It is significant that women are twice as likely to work in the public sector (they make up 65% of the workforce as opposed to the 35% who are male), where pay

Industry sectors	% Women	% Men	% Pay gap
TABLE 9.2 — Percentage of men and women employed in industry sectors with pay gap percentages for each sector			
Health and social work	79	21	32
Education	73	27	12
Hotels and restaurants	56	44	17
Other community, social and personal	52	48	25
Banking, insurance and pension provision	51	49	41
Public administration and defence	51	49	20
Wholesale, retail and motor trade	50	50	22
Real estate, renting and business activities	42	58	24
Manufacturing	25	75	19
Transport, storage and communication	24	76	9
Construction	10	90	12
All Sectors	47	53	17
PRIVATE SECTOR	41	59	22.5
PUBLIC SECTOR	65	35	13.3

(Source: ONS 2006b, Social Trends 2007.) Data from: ONS (2005), Labour force survey Spring 2005 dataset; ONS (2005), Annual survey of hours and earnings 2005.

levels do not match the private sector despite the gender pay gap being only half as great (Economic and Market Review, May, 2007). Perhaps the Gender Equality Duty may have at least a little impact here. Three quarters of self-employed workers are male, and only a third of managers are women. This drops to only 17% when considering directors and chief executives of major organisations and it is at the higher levels that other benefits kick in. Apart from pay differentials, women are less likely to get access to company cars, private health insurance paid by the company, health screening and other forms of welfare, including access to sports clubs. They also have less access to subsidized canteens and company shares, and are less likely to get bonuses and overtime pay.

The patriarchal structure of paid employment is therefore heavily implicated in what has undoubtedly been the 'feminization of poverty'. Women's contribution to paid work has been significantly curtailed by their unpaid work in the household, and only 70% of all working age women are in work compared to 79% of all working age men, although since 1971 female rates have generally risen while male rates have been falling (ONS 2006a). The patriarchal structure is even more evident within the ethnic minorities, however, with only 50% of women employed, but there is wide variation, with less than 25% of Pakistani and Bangladeshi women working, while Indian and Black Caribbean women have rates close to white women. Part-time working is also a very important factor for women. In Britain, part-time working for married women and mothers became the norm after the Second World War when, unlike France (where women were called into the workforce and provided with comprehensive child-care facilities), recruitment of full-time workers was extended to the Commonwealth and women were used as cheap, part-time employees on a lower hourly pay than full-time workers and largely without benefits such as sick pay, holiday pay, redundancy pay and so on. The pattern for women became, and still is, fragmented because of reproduction. In 2005 42% of female workers were still part-time compared with only 9% of males, and females comprised 82% of the part-time workforce. Pay for part-time work averages at £5.40 less per hour than the average full-time male wage, giving a part-time gender pay gap of 38.4%. Part-time working is most common for employed mothers with dependent children, with the percentage working part-time decreasing as the children grow older. Two-thirds of employed mothers with children under five are in part-time employment, while about the same proportion of employed women without dependent children work full-time (ONS 2006b). More recently both male employees (23%) and female employees (57%) are using flexible arrangements at work to fit in with caring responsibilities, but women are much heavier users across a wider range of options (i.e. part-time work, term-time working only, flexitime, homeworking) (ONS 2006a).

Women's lifetime earnings are substantially lower than men's and both gender and motherhood independently affect the income. In 2000 a 'gender earnings gap' – the difference between equivalently skilled and childless males and females, and a 'mother gap' – the difference between equivalently educated females with and without children, were found. The average loss for each lifetime gap was £170 000 per woman (Davies et al 2000). Data like these might well push the fertility rate even lower than it is already. These findings give weight to the feminization of poverty thesis as lowered lifetime earnings are reflected in substantially reduced or absent work pension funds. Pension contributions are smaller and more erratic for women because of gendered roles and lower earnings. Women's weekly retirement income is 47% less than men, who get nearly half their incomes from non-state pensions, while women get only a quarter (ONS 2006b). It is predicted that large numbers of females will become increasingly poor as the pension system continues to be privatized and individuals become personally responsible for their maintenance in retirement. Women are also disproportionately dependent on social security benefits to raise their income to the basic level (18% of women as opposed to only 7% of men). As already indicated, women are more likely to be single parents, and this social group receives 29% of its income from benefits (ONS 2006b). The sum total of all this information is that for many women, especially those at the bottom of the class structure, life can be one long slog characterized by demands on time, energy and income which cannot be met satisfactorily. The effects on women's health are examined throughout the chapter.

Two gender issues of some importance in relation to work are the ways that occupational health research and practice have sidelined women's health issues, and the effects of sexual harassment on female health. Doyal highlighted the male gender bias in occupational health research, showing that most research in relation to chemical risk assessment has been applied to the metabolic processes of males rather than females, and that the size and shape of protective clothing also follows a male gender model, either excluding women from certain work spheres altogether, or giving them inadequate protection (Doyal 1995). Recent publications by Messing and Stellman (2006) and WHO (2006) show that the problem is one of international importance. Male biology is still being used as the focus for toxicology studies in the work place, and the research tools to measure employment risks have been designed in relation to predominantly male employment sectors. Gender differences in the patterning of these risk factors have thus been ignored, although gender-neutral terms such as 'employee' or 'worker' are frequently used, sending out false information on the risks to females.

Harassment at work is also a health risk and source of much distress to women. Common symptoms of distress include anxiety, depression, guilt and fear. Walby (1990) and Crompton (1997) both suggest that sexual harassment is a deliberate strategy used by men to exclude women from certain work contexts, while Pilcher (1999) points out that this is particularly common where women have encroached on traditional male areas. In October 2005 what constitutes 'sexual harassment' was defined in law for the first time in the UK. The Employment Equality (Sex Discrimination) regulation was created to comply with EU directives. No longer can sexual harassment be seen as a 'bit of fun', but is now 'unwanted conduct of a sexual nature', and can be verbal or physical. The regulation includes conventional sexual harassment, discrimination in workplace facilities, and rules, such as rotas, that might exclude work/home life balance, potentially discriminating against female workers. Needless to say it is still very difficult to prove harassment at the personal level, but the problem is now much more open to public scrutiny. Again the Gender Equality Duty may have a role here.

▮ The public and private spheres

Society can be visualized as two distinct and gendered spheres, the public and the private. The public world of paid work is deemed to have higher status than the private, and is constituted as the 'real world', containing the institutions and personnel necessary to create a functioning society. It has also been seen as the natural social sphere for men. Conversely, the domestic sphere is gendered female and is conceptualized as the domain of unpaid work that is performed 'for love', where the next generation is reproduced and the nurturing of families takes place. It is also seen as a place of leisure and a refuge from paid work, especially for men.

This ideology, although changing, still has a significant effect on male and female roles and subsequent access to material and social resources, despite the fact that households find it very difficult to exist on one income. Women's work in the home continues to be valued lower than paid work, and the status of 'home-worker' remains a negative one. Indeed, the current benefit structure focuses on the 'welfare to work' ideology, which clearly implies that society has little tolerance for women with dependent children who themselves depend, not on a partner's income, but on welfare. A minimal benefit level, together with strict surveillance of welfare recipients and continual public pressure to seek 'proper' work outside the home, are not deemed to be risk factors for the well-being of such women. The expectation is that they should be able to cope both with paid work and with unpaid childcare work, despite a lack of facilities or adequate income.

The low status placed on a 'woman's work' is highlighted when its lack of monetary value within the economy is addressed. In 1997 the Office of Statistics estimated the economic value of work done around the household. At equivalent value to paid employment, this would have amounted to £739 billion per annum; more than double the gross domestic produce (GDP) at that time. Women performed nearly twice as much of this work as men. Significantly, work in the home is often rendered invisible by being ignored altogether, or recognized only when child neglect or poor housekeeping emerges as a problem. Women in these circumstances might be seen as lacking in social skills (not a proper woman) and subject to public surveillance, or they could even be classified as suffering from mental illness.

The home is not necessarily a refuge for women, and there is now a wealth of information on domestic violence and its health effects. Domestic violence includes physical, emotional, psychological and sexual violence, and it ranges from slaps to murder, harassment to mental abuse. It is mainly directed towards females by males. Although domestic violence is a significant problem in Britain, it is also a global issue and in 2002 a world report on violence, including domestic violence, was published to instigate worldwide prevention policies (WHO 2002). Three years later a multicultural study showed that the prevalence for domestic violence (physical, sexual or both) ranged from 15% (Japan) to 71% (rural

Ethiopia), with rural areas showing consistently higher rates than urban areas. Sufferers were significantly more likely to report poor or very poor health than non-sufferers, and long term effects included mental distress, fatigue and thoughts of suicide. Younger, poorer or pregnant women were all at higher risk (WHO 2005).

A recent British study also shows that women are three times more likely than men to be victims, and that the majority of these are in heterosexual relationships. Only 21% of women had reported the incident to the police, while a mere 7% of men did so. One fifth of attacks required medical attention, and those most at risk were young women between 16 and 34, women in low-income households and pregnant women. These findings mirror those presented in the multicultural study above. Additionally, over one third of female homicides in England and Wales are committed by a partner or ex-partner (McVeigh et al 2005). British studies list a range of health effects of the violence including bruising, broken bones, damage to the genitalia and facial injuries, emotional distress including depression and loss of self-esteem, sleep problems and increased risk of suicide. Domestic violence is yet another indication that women have very different health profiles to men and that much still needs to be done on this aspect of the health agenda. In Britain we have already established domestic violence forums and publicity campaigns and a range of other support systems, and the WHO have recently put new global initiatives, such as screening, in place (WHO 2007), but the problem is deeply entrenched and will be slow to remove.

Dual roles and role conflict

Gender divisions still remain firmly entrenched around reproduction despite recent changes and women are finding it difficult to make significant inroads in the public sphere. The strain of dual roles has been a key issue in women's health research, and, although working patterns of younger women are changing, with the average age for childbirth now standing at 29, and many middle-class women delaying their children to the mid- or even late thirties to qualify and stabilize their careers, recent research suggests that working practice has not altered in line with these developments. There is a trend for women who have gone back to work full-time after having their first babies to give up their jobs altogether or to go part-time if they are able to. Inflexible hours of work leads to a health toll on women as they soak up the stress from trying to juggle work and home commitments. One study in Quebec in 1999 looking at the stresses of working mothers with degrees found that women who juggle difficult jobs with raising a family face greater risk of stress-related illness than their husbands: 'While tension raises the blood pressure of both sexes during the day, working mothers remain stressed for longer into the evening and may increase the danger of heart disease and strokes' (Brisson 1999).

The long hours and competitive culture in Britain (which has one of the longest working days in Europe) also disadvantages women with home responsibilities who are unable to stay late in the evenings or get into work early, or take work home. Women have reported feeling watched and valued less in their jobs than when they were childless, and let down by the system. More and more women, in the middle classes especially, are choosing to remain childless for longer periods and are assimilating into the male long-hours work culture with its heavier drinking patterns and smoking and a movement away from domesticity. Additionally, it has been noticed that young women in business are not always overtly supportive of female colleagues who are trying to juggle home and family. Many see working mothers as a drain on their own career progress as they see themselves 'carrying' them during periods of childhood illness or other domestic crises.

What is not happening at the moment is a change in the culture of work to accommodate changing expectations of young women to their life chances.

Childbirth, therefore, still remains a barrier to the progress of women throughout society, and ironically, paid work culture also now increasingly acts as a barrier to childbirth. There has been recent concern that a whole cohort of younger women are in danger of forfeiting the opportunity to bear children because they are waiting until the middle to late thirties when the dangers of genetic abnormality and lowered fertility combine to render conception difficult and childbirth risky.

LIFE EXPECTANCY

■ Gendered life expectancy in the global context

Life expectancy rates differ globally, but in almost every country women outlive men. Part of this difference can be accounted for by an innate biological advantage, which is still not fully understood, but manifests itself in, among other things, higher male deaths in utero and in the early postnatal period. Recent research focuses on the immune system and suggests that the extra T cells that women possess might give them more protection against disease over the life course. However, the social construction of gender identity and related gender roles also has a significant effect. Globally, a woman's life expectancy tends to increase as the social standing of women in her specific society improves. Only those societies which fundamentally subordinate women have equal gender life expectancy, and in a very few there is a male excess (see Arber & Thomas 2001, for data and a full discussion).

■ Gendered life expectancy in Britain

Life expectancy in Europe has not always favoured women. In Europe in the sixteenth and seventeenth centuries there was a big male advantage (Shorter 1982), and in the industrialized early nineteenth century male and female longevity was more or less the same. The female advantage began to appear in the second half of the nineteenth century, with the widest gender gap occurring in the twentieth century from the 1960s to 1980s. Since 1901 there have been large improvements in life expectancy for both males and females in the UK. In 1901 life expectancy was 45 for UK born males, and 49 for UK born females. By 2005 the rates had almost doubled with the male figure reaching 77, while the female had risen to 81 (Social Trends 2007). The projection to 2021 gives males just over 80 years and females just under 84. The gender gap has been closing since the 1980s, having peaked at 6.3 in 1969, and now stands at only four years. This trend is expected to continue until 2014 when it is expected to stabilize at 3.7 years (Social Trends 2007). Information on 'healthy life expectancy' includes a much-needed dimension on the quality of life expected and has been published since 1981 in GB. This is defined as expected years of life in good or fairly good self-assessed general health. A gender gap still appears with this measure, but is somewhat less than the general life expectancy gap. Table 9.3 (Social Trends 2007, Table 7.2) compares the gender gaps for life expectancy, healthy life expectancy and disability-free life expectancy between 1981 and the most recent figures available for 2002. The male healthy life expectancy increased by 2.8 years, while the female increased by 3.2 years. So women are still living longer lives than men, and these measures indicate that they are also spending more years in a healthy condition than men are. However, for both genders the number of years spent with disability or poor health has also increased, especially for men, narrowing that gender gap.

TABLE 9.3	Life expectancy, healthy life expectancy and disability-free life expectancy[1] at birth: by sex (Social Trends 2007, Table 7.2, page 88)			
	Years			
	Males		Females	
Great Britain	1981	2002	1981	2002
Life expectancy	70.9	76.0	76.8	80.5
Healthy life expectancy	64.4	67.2	66.7	69.9
Years spent in poor health	6.4	8.8	10.1	10.6
Disability-free life expectancy	58.1	60.9	60.8	63.0
Years spent with disability	12.8	15.0	16.0	17.5

[1] See Appendix, Part 7: Expectation of life. Healthy life expectancy and disability-free life expectancy.
Source: *Government Actuary's Department: Office for National Statistics. Social Trends 37:2000 Edition*

MORTALITY

As with the data for length of life, there are clear differences in mortality rates between the genders. The focus will be on western society and this section will examine these differences, look at the main causes of death and offer some explanations for the differences.

■ Main causes of death by gender

At the beginning of the twentieth century the major categories of causes of death for both males and females were infections and respiratory diseases (Social Trends 2001) (see Chapter 1). With the progression of the twentieth century, infections declined and for both males and females were replaced by circulatory diseases (including heart disease and stroke), then cancers, with respiratory diseases (including pneumonia) dropping to third place as the population lived longer and standards of living and health care improved. These three are still the leading causes of death today, and there have been consistent downward trends for both genders since 1971. Figure 9.2 shows these trends for the decade up to 2006 (Health Statistics Quarterly, Summer, 2007). The figures have consistently shown lower rates for females in all three major causes of death, and continue to do so. With circulatory diseases there has been a sharp downward trend for both genders since 1971, but the much greater male decline has rapidly closed the gender gap (Social Trends 2007). Table 9.4, using the most recent data for 2006, gives a breakdown of diseases in each category, and shows that death from ischaemic heart disease is the leading cause of death in both genders, followed by cerebrovascular disease (stroke). However, while ischaemic disease is higher in men, death from stroke is higher in females (Health Statistics Quarterly, Summer, 2007). Cancers have been the second major cause of death in both sexes over the last thirty years for both genders, but during that time have displayed different trends. The higher male rate peaked in the mid eighties, while the typically lower female rate did not do so until the late eighties. These differences relate both to types of cancer and to risk factors which we will deal with later. However, while the 2006 data show that the decline in the female cancer rate has been very

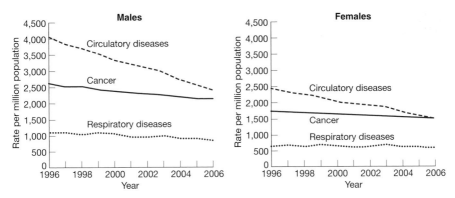

1 These rates are standardised to the European Standard Population, expressed per million population; they allow comparisons between populations with different age structures, including between males and females and over time.

2 These categories correspond to the three chapters of ICD-10 with the largest number of deaths in England and Wales.

Note: The Tenth Revision of the *International Classification of Diseases and Related Health Problems* (ICD-10) came into operation in 2001. Comparability ratios have been applied to data for 1994 to 2000. See the explanatory notes.

Fig. 9.2 Age-standardized, all age mortality rates for the three categories of cause of death (per million population), 1996–2006 (Health Statistics Quarterly 34, web supplement, Summer 2007).

gradual compared to that of the female circulatory disease rate, the most recent figures indicate that the female cancer rate has just taken over from circulatory disease as the leading cause of death in females. Males have not yet reached this point, but circulatory diseases are now closely followed by cancers as the leading cause of death in males. The male rate for respiratory diseases again exceeds the female rate, but repeats the pattern of circulatory disease by declining at a greater rate. Between 1996 and 2006 the male rate dropped by 19.6%, while over the same period the female decline was only 6.6% (Health Statistics Quarterly 2007).

Gender differences in type and risk of cancer

While cancer, therefore, is an important cause of death in both genders, the age specific incidence of all cancers by sex over the life course is significantly different. From around 30 incidence rates begin to rise, but far more rapidly in females until about 45 when the male rate accelerates and overtakes the female rate towards the late fifties, when a permanent and widening gender gap appears. The earlier rise in incidence in females (70% higher than males in the 30–34 age group) is largely due to breast (and much less so to cervical) cancer which starts to develop at lower ages than most cancers, while the excess in the male incidence at older ages (40% excess age 65–69 and 70% excess at ages 80–84) is heavily related to the onset of prostate and lung cancer which tend to manifest themselves later. Lung cancer reflects gender differences in smoking patterns (discussed later), while prostate cancer has been rising rapidly since the early 1990s to become the major form of cancer in men. For women breast cancer far exceeds other cancers and the incidence continues to rise.

Breast cancer

In England breast cancer is now the most common form of cancer overall, and represents 32% of all female cancers. It is also the most common cause of cancer death in women.

TABLE 9.4	Leading causes of mortality: by sex, 2006 (Health Statistics Quarterly 34, web supplement, Summer 2007)			
England and Wales				**Numbers**

Underlying cause of death[1]	Number of deaths	Percentage of all deaths	Age-standardized all age mortality rate per 100 000 population
Males			
Rank			
1 Ischaemic heart diseases (I20–I25)	46 316	19.2	135.0
2 Cerebrovascular diseases (I60–I69)	18 744	7.8	52.0
3 Malignant neoplasm of trachea, bronchus and lung (C33, C34)	16 964	7.0	50.7
4 Chronic lower respiratory diseases (J40–J47)	13 007	5.4	36.3
5 Influenza and pneumonla (J10–J18)	11 511	4.8	32.1
6 Malignant neoplasm of prostate (C61)	9 061	3.8	24.9
7 Malignant neoplasm of colon, sigmoid, rectum and anus (C18–C21)	7 467	3.1	22.1
8 Malignant neoplasms of lymphoid, haematopoietic and related tissue (C81–C96)	5 777	2.4	17.5
9 Dementia and Alzheimer's disease (F01, F03, G30)	5 282	2.2	14.0
10 Aortic aneurysm and dissection (I71)	4 774	2.0	13.4
All deaths	**240 889**	**100.0**	
Females			
Rank			
1 Ischaemic heart diseases (I20–I25)	36 272	13.9	63.0
2 Cerebrovascular diseases (I60–I69)	29 650	11.3	48.0
3 Influenza and pneumonia (J10–J18)	17 212	6.6	26.3
4 Dementia and Alzheimer's disease (F01, F03, G30)	12 912	4.9	18.5
5 Malignant neoplasm of trachea, bronchus and lung (C33, C34)	12 350	4.7	29.9
6 Chronic lower respiratory diseases (J40–J47)	12 281	4.7	23.9
7 Malignant neoplasms of female breast (C50)	10 942	4.2	27.7
8 Heart failure and complications and ill-defined heart disease (I50–I51)	6 567	2.5	9.9
9 Malignant neoplasm of colon, sigmoid, rectum and anus (C18–C21)	6 547	2.5	13.9
10 Diseases of the urinary system (N00–N39)	6 181	2.4	10.0
All deaths	**261 710**	**100.0**	

[1] The cause of death groups used here are based on a list provided developed by the WHO, modified for use in England and Wales. For more information see Grilfiths C, Rooney C and Brock A. Leading causes of death in England and Wales – how should we group causes? *Health Statistics Quarterly* 28, 6–17.

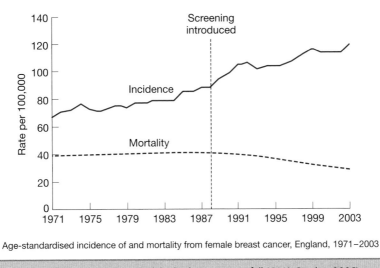

Age-standardised incidence of and mortality from female breast cancer, England, 1971–2003

Fig. 9.3 Breast cancer: incidence rises while deaths continue to fall (ONS October 2005).

There has been a rise in incidence from 78 per 100 000 women in 1981 to 120 per 100 000 women in 2003 (Social Trends 2007). In that year 36 500 new cases were diagnosed. Now 80% of new cases occur in women aged 50 or over, with a peak in the 50–64 age range. One in nine females is expected to develop breast cancer at some time in the life course. The incidence has also been rising in many EU countries and it is suspected that better screening contributes to the increase. In Britain the increase is deemed to be partly due to the NHS screening programme first introduced in 1988, resulting in earlier diagnosis in large numbers of cases. In 2003–4 75% of all those aged 50–64 who were invited to attend screening did so, and now a total of 1.4 million women aged 50 and above are screened each year. Earlier detection and more effective forms of treatment have both contributed to improvements in survival rates, with the 5-year survival rate now standing at 80%. This is higher than for cervical cancer, and much higher than the other major female cancers. Death rates began to fall around the time screening began, and it is estimated that the rate was 20% lower by 1998 than it would have been without the screening. Figure 9.3 show the trends of incidence and mortality rates before and after the introduction of breast screening (ONS October 2005). The major risk factors for breast cancer are age, with two-thirds of cases in women over 50, having a close relative with the disease, early menarche, late menopause, childlessness and late first full-term pregnancy. Other factors such as obesity, higher alcohol consumption, HRT and oral contraceptives also increase the risk.

Gender and suicide rates

In every country worldwide, except for one, men commit more suicides each year than women do. The exception is China, where young women have the highest rate. One might speculate that this relates to their already very low status, exacerbated by the incursion of capitalist upheaval. In Britain suicide follows the global trend and is starkly gendered with a long-established excess for males over females. In 1973 the suicide rate for males aged 15 and over was one-and-a-half times the female rate in that age group, but since then the gap has widened and by 2005 the male rate stood at three times the female rate. For females, the rate for those under 45 has been the lowest and has remained largely stable since the 1980s. The highest female rates have been in those aged 45–74 but their rates have more than halved in the same period. For men the picture is very different, with the much higher 15+ rate which peaked in 1998. However, the male rate has since begun to fall and by 2005 was at its lowest since 1991. Over the last decade, in contrast to the female trends, the highest male rates have occurred in the 15–44 age group with that group largely responsible for the overall male peak in the late 1990s, while the 45–74 age group has remained relatively stable at a lower level. The trend is now downward in the younger age group. In both sexes suicides in the 75+ age group have steadily declined (ONS 2007, Social Trends 2007).

EXPLAINING GENDER DIFFERENCES IN LIFE EXPECTANCY AND MORTALITY

Biological and social factors are both used to explain life expectancy and mortality. Employment is a key factor involved in the excess male mortality rate as more occupations typically followed by men involve direct risk to life, through individual accidents, dangerous machinery or machine failure, weather and environmental hazards. Underground and surface mining, oil rig work, fishing, construction and heavy industry are typical. Men are also deemed to be at higher long-term risk of danger from exposure to toxic chemicals, radiation and so on, which are implicated in a range of cancers, respiratory diseases and other conditions. What also should be noted is that it is largely lower-class males who are most at risk.

Although occupations are still heavily gendered worldwide, so too is risk-taking behaviour. Masculinity, it seems, still needs to be affirmed and continually renegotiated by men's participation in activities such as dangerous sports like hang-gliding, car and motorbike racing, rock-climbing and so on. Men also generally drive more than women and faster or under the influence of alcohol (hence the preferential insurance rates for women). Men are more at risk from death or injury in road traffic accidents than women; in 2005 men made up 60% of the annual casualty rate (ONS 2006a). Overall, males have more accidents than females and this is especially reflected in excess mortality for young men in the age group 15–25. This excess starts early in childhood in the generally more physical behaviour of young boys, implicating both biology and gender socialization. Boys engage in more dangerous pastimes in sport and in peer groups and take more risks than girls, and males from boyhood also engage in criminal activity which puts them at risk of injury, death and mental ill health. Around 90% of offenders found guilty of burglary, robbery, drug offences, criminal damage or violence are male and males from all age groups, but especially young men, also engage in more physical aggression towards one another, so excess male deaths from violence and murder can be added to the equation. The British Crime Survey for 2005/6 found that men are three times more likely than women to be attacked by a stranger (overwhelmingly male), and 'doing masculinity' for young black men in Britain is especially lethal at present, involving gang violence and gun crime. However, recent evidence suggests that violence has marginally increased among young women as they take on more behaviour patterns of young men. Recent cases of mugging, murder and assisted rape by young women might indicate a trend here. Young men are also one third more likely to take illicit drugs than young women (ONS 2006a).

Another gendered form of risky behaviour is smoking. Men have always smoked more than women, but overall trends are still downwards and the gender gap has narrowed. In 1974, 51% of males and 41% of females smoked, while in 2005 the gap had narrowed to 2% with only 25% of men and 23% of women smoking. Since the early 1990s smoking has been highest in the 20–24 age group, with 34% of men and 30% of women in this group smoking (GHS 2005). More worrying is that girls up to the age of 15 are now more likely than boys to be regular or occasional smokers (Drever et al 2000). If this cohort trend continues, smoking-related diseases will continue to rise for women. Heavy smoking (twenty plus per day) has also declined in both genders, but continues to be higher in both genders in the lower classes (Social Trends 2007). Single people also smoke more (Rainford et al 2000), and single women working in previously male strongholds, for example City finance occupations, are significantly increasing their smoking levels. Hopefully the ban on smoking in public places, which has now fully taken effect in Britain, will put the brakes on smoking in the younger age groups, especially.

Male excess mortality is also linked to higher alcohol intake via high blood pressure, cirrhosis of the liver and cancer. Table 9.5 from the General Household Survey, 2005 (Social Trends 2007), shows gender differences in excess alcohol intake. One third of males and one fifth of females exceeded the recommended daily amount on at least one day in the last week, while men drink significantly more than women in all age groups. Although young people drink less frequently than older people, when they do drink they are more likely to drink to excess, with 43% of males and 36% of females aged from 16–24 doing so. Binge drinking is also at its greatest in this group, with 30% of males and 22% of women drinking at least twice the recommended daily level. Women in this age group began increasing their intake in the 1990s and have maintained the habit. However, as the women in the youngest cohort have moved into the 25–44 age group, excess drinking has declined to only 26%, with binge drinking halved to 11%, while the equivalent male group declined only very slightly. After the age of 25 in women, and 44 in men, drinking in each gender steadily declines. While for men, higher levels of drinking show little difference across the social classes, for women, alcohol intake is higher in the professional and managerial classes (Social Trends 2007).

The masculine persona has also been implicated in the effect of differential health behaviour on risk of mortality. Men are said to shrug off the symptoms of illness in the early stages and consult later when the damage is greater, as illness is defined as

TABLE 9.5	Adults exceeding specified levels of alcohol:[1] by sex and age, 2005[2] (Social Trends 2007, Table 7.10, page 93)				
	Percentages				
Great Britain	16–24	25–44	45–64	65 and over	All aged 16 and over
Men					
More than 4 units and up to 8 units	13	17	19	12	16
More than 8 units	30	25	16	4	19
More than 4 units	43	42	35	16	35
Women					
More than 3 units and up to 6 units	14	15	14	3	12
More than 6 units	22	11	4	1	8
More than 3 units	36	26	18	4	20

[1] On at least one day in the previous week. See Appendix, Part 7: Alcohol consumption.
[2] Data for 2005 include last quarter of 2004/05 due to survey change from financial year to calendar year. See Appendix, Part 2: General Household Survey.
Source: General Household Survey (Longitudinal), Office for National Statistics.

weakness and not consistent with being a 'real' man. However, an alternative view might suggest that women's closeness with their bodies through menstruation and childbirth and the long tradition of women as carers, has rendered females more aware of bodily symptoms and more socialized into the potential illness/patient role.

MORBIDITY: GENDER DIFFERENCES AND EXPLANATIONS

Although the explanations for gender differences in mortality are rarely disputed, morbidity differentials invite more controversy. First, there is dispute about whether, indeed, the higher morbidity traditionally attributed to women actually exists or whether it is mere artefact. Second, recent interest in men's health suggests that real changes in gendered morbidity have occurred and that men are suffering more illness and are increasing their use of the health services.

For a long time it has been an accepted truism that 'women are sicker but men die quicker'. A major focus in morbidity has been self-reported data relating to gender differences in general health, long-standing illness and limiting long-standing illness. In the mid-1990s surveys were showing consistent but small female excesses in morbidity, with more females self-reporting their general health as poor or fairly poor. By 2001 male and female responses had become very similar, with 7.8% of males rating their health as 'not good' and only 8.1% of females doing so (ONS 2004). However, researchers did find a class difference, with females in the highest class 25% more likely to rate their health as poor. Women were also more likely to do so in the lower classes. The intermediate classes, interestingly, showed a small male excess (Drever et al 2004). For both measures of long-standing illness, longitudinal data from the 1970s–1990s had been showing small excesses of around 2–4% for females (OPCS 1995, Rainford et al 1998) and by 2005, as shown by Table 9.6, little had changed, with female excesses of just under 2% for long-standing illness, and around 4% for limiting long-standing illness. However, the data also show gender differences across the age groups (Social Trends 2007, Table 7.3).

Other data show that women are more likely than men to consult a professional in relation to their health. In 2004/5 females were more likely than males to see a GP in the 14 days before interview (16% of females as opposed to only 11% of males), and to take more prescribed drugs. Women also consult more than men for most conditions, although men consult more for serious illnesses relating to the circulatory system and the digestive system, while women do so more for serious musculo-skeletal conditions (ONS 2005b). Women also average five consultations per year, while males average just three (GHS 2004, 2005). Additionally, women are more likely to consult for preventive care, even after controlling for reproductive issues, while men are less likely to carry out self-examinations or to take health supplements (GHS 2004). Having said that, there has been an upsurge in health magazines for men, and more interest is being shown by men in prevention through good diet and exercise.

Studies also tend to show that women report more symptoms, overall, but that while symptoms of malaise and stress showed a clear excess, the difference in physical symptom reporting was not significant. Table 9.7, produced by the Women's Unit (2002), shows self-reported health problems by gender and age, and Arber & Thomas (2001) also report that older women are more likely to suffer from chronic but non-fatal conditions and functional impairments that affect their daily quality of life. Arthritis and rheumatism are more common in women at all ages, and rise in both sexes with age. Significantly, the gender gap increases from age 44 so that the female prevalence is double that of males in the 65–74 age group. Women also suffer markedly more than men from migraine at all ages, but especially from 16–54. The prevalence rate is three to four times

TABLE 9.6	Self-reported illness:[1] by sex and age (Social Trends 2007, Table 7.3, page 89.)	
	Rates per 1000 population	
Great Britain	**Long-standing Illness**	**Limiting long-standing Illness**
Males		
0–4	140	46
5–14	181	72
15–44	175	90
45–64	401	233
65–74	554	342
75 and over	583	402
All ages	273	150
Females		
0–4	93	28
5–14	160	67
15–44	209	114
45–64	407	245
65–74	589	370
75 and over	545	401
All ages	282	163

[1] See Appendix, Part 7: Self-reported illness.
[2] Data for 2005 include last quarter of 2004/05 due to survey change from financial year to calendar year. See Appendix, Part 2: General Household Survey.
[3] Data have been age-standardized using the European standard population. See Appendix, Part 7: Standardised rates, and European standard population.
Source: *General Household Survey (Longitudinal), Office for National Statistics.*

higher than in men, and fluctuating hormones relating to the menstrual cycle may be somewhat implicated. Irritable Bowel Syndrome (IBS) is another condition suffered more by women. IBS affects about 40% of the total population, but is between two and four times as common in women. It is associated with poor mental health, especially stress and depression (ONS 2006c, Payne 2006).

THE MASCULINE NORM AND THE CONSTRUCTION OF WOMANHOOD

Western definitions of women's mental status have concerned the women's movement since the 1970s. Concepts of normality in society are seen as constructions from a male perspective, creating the man as mentally robust and the woman as mentally fragile. This model subordinates women to a masculine construction of reality which places the male at the centre of humanity with women on the periphery. The biological, social and psychological male forms the template against which all other forms of life are compared. The male identity is superior whereas the female identity is flawed. This long-standing male/female dichotomy was strengthened when Enlightenment thinking in Europe decreed that women, bound as they were by their reproductive ties to nature, were not inherently logical or rational, or able to match the cognitive skills of men. The essential character of womanhood was said to be constructed from common sense and intuitive

TABLE 9.7	Self-reported health problems by gender (%) (ONS 2002)				
		Age range			
Problem	16–44	45–64	65–74	75 and over	All aged 16 and over
Males					
Pain or discomfort	18	39	52	56	32
Mobility	6	22	36	50	18
Anxiety or depression	12	19	20	19	15
Problems performing usual activities	5	16	21	27	12
Problems with self-care	1	6	8	14	5
Females					
Pain or discomfort	20	40	51	65	34
Mobility	6	21	37	60	19
Anxiety or depression	18	24	25	30	22
Problems performing usual activities	7	17	23	40	15
Problems with self-care	2	5	9	21	6

From OPCS (2002) General Household Survey, Office for National Statistics; Continuous Household Survey, Northern Ireland Statistics and Research Agency.

understanding. With these ideas deeply embedded in social norms, social philosophers marginalized womanhood as 'biologically ill-equipped to exercise pure uncontaminated reason' and therefore as incapable of exercising the full rights of public citizenship. The 'normal' woman was entrenched as a semi-citizen, better suited to the private sphere of the home than the rough and tumble of the public domain, and under the 'natural authority of the male head of household' (Scambler 1998).

Connell's model (1987, 1995), shown in Figure 9.4, describes the gender order in terms of three major social structures: how labour is organized, where power is held, and through sexual and emotional relations. These three interlinking structures interact constantly to create a gender hierarchy, fundamental to which is the dominance of men over women. At the top is 'hegemonic' masculinity, focused on authority and the culturally dominant ideals of paid work, physical strength and heterosexuality. Below is 'complicit' masculinity, where most men live their lives, falling short of the hegemonic ideal

Masculinities	Hegemonic masculinity
	Complicit masculinity
	Subordinated masculinity
Femininities	Emphasized femininity (compliant)
	Resistant femininity (e.g. feminist)

Fig. 9.4 Connell's model.

but gaining significant social advantages from their association with it. Further down are the 'subordinated' masculinities, spearheaded by homosexuality, where men are seen as somewhat diminished. Significantly, even the lowest masculine category exceeds the feminine in the gender order, but the whole is open to internal contestation or even crisis.

Such social constructions of masculinity and femininity, and the power relations they engender, are profoundly difficult to dislodge and structure individual and social actions deep below the surface of everyday life. Since the 1960s, theorists have been exploring how patriarchy functions at all its levels, and one of the most problematic relates to the construction of woman herself. The categories of male and female have been broken down to expose the underlying patriarchal discourse. Clearly the social gendering of the two sexes has not just empowered men at the expense of women, but was constructed by them as well. Theorists from within the post-modern perspective suggest that the source of women's oppression lies in the symbolism created by masculine power structures. Irigaray cites what she calls the 'male imaginary', asserting that men have used 'phallocentric logic' to create a symbolic order that imposes gender opposites comprising a range of dualities (rational/irrational, logical/illogical) defining women as 'other' and 'lacking', or as object in relation to the male subject (Irigaray 1985). Many feminists have additionally pointed to the fact that the traits attributed to the male are those socially valued, especially in the public domain. The female psyche, conversely, is deemed suitably placed in the devalued domestic arena.

GENDER AND ISSUES OF MENTAL HEALTH

The gendered discourse of psychiatry

The mysogynistic control of women by the emerging (male) psychiatric profession in the 19th and 20th centuries has been extensively studied. Ehrenreich & English (1979) documented the ways in which women were firstly defined as mentally fragile (they were diagnosed as suffering from hysteria, the vapours, were too overtly sexual or were insubordinate to their husbands), and the problem was then located firmly within women's reproductive systems. Remedies were then applied. One such, which would now be condemned as sensory deprivation, confined the woman to a darkened room where she was forbidden to read or exercise her mind in the interests of a cure. For cases of hysteria, slapping with wet towels was one of the techniques used to bring the woman to her senses, and for sexual proclivity the clitoris was sometimes removed. Continuing research suggests that patriarchal definitions of female mental health persisted throughout the twentieth century and are still apparent in the twenty-first. Women found themselves in a 'catch 22' situation where they were defined as mentally unstable if they conformed to the female norm, or conversely, deviated from it. The dominant discourse of psychiatry, it is contended, incorporated the gendered dualisms outlined above, rendering tenets of masculinity such as rationality, competitiveness and creativity fundamental to the notion of the mentally healthy adult, while the psychologically unhealthy female exhibited characteristics such as passivity, conformity and lower motivation for achievement. In the twentieth century unhappiness, anxiety, depression and so on were regarded as a normal part of the female condition and routine treatment with drugs such as Librium, Valium and Prozac was widespread. Prescription drug dependence also became a problem as long-term prescribing became commonplace as part of what came to be seen as the 'medicalization of female unhappiness'.

What, then, of the mental health of men? How was their unhappiness or debility defined and treated? From the perspective of social constructionism one could decree that the dominant masculine identity did not condone mental disorders deemed to be indicative of a 'weak character', such as neuroses, anxiety states and depression. These were clearly female states, or might, perhaps, emerge in males of a more artistic temperament. Thus, it has been contended, much male mental ill-health has lacked an acceptable social category and was thus rendered invisible. Doctors operating within the discourse would not define male distress as mental illness unless it appeared associated with a socially appropriate masculine form of deviance for men. Not permitted to express their mental debility in the same ways as females, men could, however, do so via aggressive behaviour, criminal behaviour, the use of drugs and alcohol, or in the more 'heroic' medically defined expressions of mental derangement such as psychotic behaviour.

This view of the gendering of mental illness suggests that men suffered alongside women but that their problems were not recognized, were redefined or the unhappiness was either suppressed or channelled into alternative forms. Within the constructionist view, an increase in male mental illness statistics must mean 'that the conceptualisation of mental disorder has changed so that men are now more likely to be diagnosed as having psychiatric problems' (Prior 1999). Indeed, in the late 1980s and into the 1990s studies in the USA indicated that if alcohol and drug dependence and personality disorders were included as psychiatric categories, a very large number of men would be pulled into the statistics on mental disorder, rather than boosting those on criminal justice. In positive terms this could mean a more sympathetic treatment of male unhappiness, but in negative terms it could simply imply greater medicalization of men. Prior contrasts the constructionist view with the 'social causation' perspective. From the latter standpoint it is contended that the actual incidence of mental problems for men is greater because their exposure to stressful life experiences has burgeoned. What becomes increasingly clear is that it is not possible to treat the issue as an either/or.

▧ Gender differences in mental illness incidence and symptom reporting

Mental illness categories are contentious and it is accepted that statistics relating to both prevalence and medical treatment have been affected by patriarchal definitions and by under-reporting of symptoms due to problems of stigma. Busfield, however, presented a clear three-fold typology of psychiatric disorders, below, which she related to gender, using data from the 1990s (Busfield 2002).

● Disorders of thought: comprising more severe conditions such as functional psychoses, including schizophrenia (gender neutral).

● Disorders of emotion: including depression, anxiety states, phobias and neuroses (female excess).

● Disorders of behaviour: including behaviour and personality disorders such as alcohol and drug dependence (male excess).

The categories used in the 2000 Psychiatric Morbidity Survey (ONS 2002) relate closely to Busfield's typology but alcohol and drug problems are dealt with separately. This study surveyed a large sample of adults aged 16–74, living in private households in Britain. Before we consider these data, however, it should be noted that childhood mental illness bucks most of the trends by exposing a male excess in all key mental health categories, and also showing that while 11% of boys between the ages of 5 and 16 suffer from mental health problems, only 7.7% of girls do so (Social Trends 2007).

In the 2000 data the category for psychotic disorders (disorders of thought), was gender neutral (as in the Busfield analysis) with prevalence rates of just 5 per 1000 for females and 6 per 1000 for males. Within this category, however, men have poorer prognosis after diagnosis. The other two categories were clearly gendered, again mirroring the direction of Busfield's findings. Neurotic disorders (disorders of emotion) including categories such as fatigue, irritability, sleep problems, anxiety and depression (frequently called symptoms of minor psychiatric morbidity) showed an overall prevalence for females of around 185 per 1000, with males at around 135 per 1000. Despite recent changes in male mental health behaviour the consistent evidence from the 1990s of a female excess for reporting psychological distress across the lifespan still persists (MacIntyre et al 1996), but the gap is beginning to close (ONS 2002). Personality disorders (disorders of behaviour) include the obsessive-compulsive, paranoid, antisocial, dependent and narcissistic, and clearly show a male bias with 54 per 1000 males and only 34 per 1000 females, and if we added in the male rates for excessive alcohol use and drug abuse, as Busfield does, the gender difference would grow considerably (ONS 2002). In the 2000 sample, those having a neurotic disorder were substantially more likely to report one or more physical complaints, 38% of those with no neuroses, 57% of those with one condition, and 67% of those with more than one. Although the data are not gender segregated this finding fits well with gendered conditions such as IBS which has already been related to poorer mental health and to stress.

Consulting and treatment for mental health problems

Besides being significantly more likely to admit to neurotic disorders such as anxiety and depression, women are also more likely to consult for such conditions, and in the 1990s women in England and Wales were two and a half times more likely to be treated for depression than men (Social Trends 2001). However, in line with the increases in male reporting of neurotic symptoms in the 2000 study, the treatment gap is now closing, and younger women, in particular, are now only twice as likely to be treated for depression as men and to be prescribed antidepressants. Older women are more likely than younger women or men to be treated for anxiety states (ONS 2005b). There is also an abundance of evidence, globally, to indicate that women are much more likely than men to be prescribed psychoactive drugs (Payne 2006).

In Britain, women make up the majority of those who receive treatment for mental health problems within primary care and they also form the majority of those referred to outpatient departments (ONS 2005a). Furthermore, they also form the majority of those being admitted to psychiatric inpatient care, and have done so since the middle of the nineteenth century. Men, however, are twice as likely to be sectioned as women. What the data do show is that, although women take more mental ill health to the GP and get more treatment overall, there is a gender imbalance in specialist care. Both Payne (2001) and Prior (1999) suggest that men pass more easily through the primary care filter, and into the specialist care sector, whereas women are more likely to be treated by their GPs. Within specialist care, women are more likely to be filtered into outpatients, while men are more likely to be referred for inpatient treatment (ONS 2005a). Payne suggests that this reflects the gender hierarchy, with men able to command access to more resources than women. However, she sees the picture as much more complicated. The changes in mental health care enacted over the past few decades, with big reductions in psychiatric beds, the placing of psychiatric care in district hospitals and the improvement in drug treatments that reduce inpatient stay or can be offered to outpatients, might have resulted in rationing of inpatient care, which has left men more at risk of incarceration than women. But why should men between 20 and 34 be so prominent in the statistics at present? Payne considers the relationship between criminal behaviour and mental ill health. Men are much more likely to be imprisoned than women (less than 5% of the prison population is female). Young men are four times less likely to be admitted to psychiatric hospital than to be imprisoned, while the reverse is true for young women (Payne 2001).

153

Recent changes do suggest that problematic young men are increasingly being seen as targets for the 'medical gaze' rather than just that of the criminal justice system. While young men have had a worryingly high suicide rate, it is beginning to decline, and men, generally, are admitting to suffering from and are also consulting more than ever before, for depressive illness. This new level of consulting may be reducing the suicide rate as young men seek help. One underlying cause might be that norms of the acceptability of males expressing unhappiness as mental illness are changing, as was discussed earlier; another might be the result of what Payne called the 'redundant male'. Men are now more likely to be unemployed than women, with young men especially vulnerable. Young women are more independent, have better careers and young people are in looser relationships for longer and having children later. One theory is that young men have lost a structure to their lives, resulting in a surge of unhappiness and mental illness. However, the dominant perception is that young men's unhappiness results in aggressive and problematic behaviour, and Payne implies that the new psychiatric interest in this group of patients mirrors the custodial response of the criminal justice system and promotes inpatient care. The same reasoning could explain the sectioning figures; simply that men under stress are seen as much more of a public threat than women and need to be closely controlled (Payne 2001).

▩ Body hatred and eating disorders

Finally one must include the effect of embodiment on female mental health. The well-being of women is often affected by negative body image resulting in loss of self-esteem. Frost (2001) contends that damaging sets of emotions focused on the body are common in females, beginning at an early age and resulting in the alienation of young women from their bodies. The range of conditions connected with what she calls 'body hatred' affects the mental and physical well-being of a large number of females. Eating disorders such as anorexia and bulimia are good examples. Central to these conditions are disturbance in perception of body weight and shape with fear of weight gain and refusal to maintain normal weight. Both anorexia and bulimia are female conditions, around 90% of all cases, although there is some evidence that male incidence may be increasing. They are largely absent outside western societies. Anorexia is characterized by inability to eat sustainable amounts of food, while bulimia, which can occur independently of anorexia, is characterized by binge eating, alternating with compensatory behaviour such as use of laxatives and self-induced vomiting. Anorexia, which seems to be increasing in prevalence, affects between 1% and 4% of women, overwhelmingly adolescent or young, and peaks between ages 15 and 19. All ethnic groups are somewhat affected, but referrals are mainly white, middle-class women (Frost 2001).

From the foregoing discussion it would seem conclusive that a woman's mental well-being is gendered in a complex range of ways that combine to make her especially vulnerable to lowered self-esteem, anxiety, tension and depression. Her whole being is rendered suspect from her femininity to her sexual competence, to her intellectual competence, to her capacity for paid work and physical activity and for mothering. She is unable to match social expectations in relation to her body and in Connell's hierarchy she is not just valued below hegemonic masculinity, she is valued lower than the masculine underclass.

CHILDBIRTH AND MEDICALIZATION

Childbirth is an issue of central importance to women and has been the subject of much debate around contentions that women have lost control of their own bodies as medicalization has progressed. Campaigns to reclaim childbirth have been prominent since the 1970s. In Britain, Oakley (1984) spearheaded some key discussions, considering especially the way childbirth seemed to have progressed from being a normal biological and family event to becoming defined as pathological and ordered by medical professionals. In this scenario the GP confirms the impending birth, defines the woman as 'patient', endows on her a status of 'risk' and despatches her to the obstetric unit for a programme of screenings. Under obstetric surveillance the woman's pregnancy culminates in a controlled birth within the maternity unit. The whole process became known as 'technological childbirth', with a fully 'managed' pregnancy and birth. The plethora of tests often resulted in what came to be known as the 'cascade of intervention'. A scan might suggest a baby not growing to expectations or a potentially small pelvic canal, for example, and early induction might ensue, culminating in an increased need for analgesics (with enhanced danger to the baby), a caesarean section or even fetal surgery. Once the train of events was set in motion it was difficult to get back to a low-tech birth. In the mid-1990s, research showed many women did not realize that antenatal screening is optional, such are the subtle pressures on women to conform (Jackson 2001), and a recent survey in 2006 showed that over 99% of English pregnant women now have at least one prenatal scan (NPEU 2007), suggesting that pressures to conform are as strong as ever.

Between 1927 and 2006 the change from home to hospital birth has been dramatic, as Table 9.8 (adapted from Lloyd & Woroch 2000 and NPEU 2007) indicates, but the percentage of home deliveries has now remained static at around 3% for the last decade (NPEU 2007). Moves to promote 100% hospitalization of births, such as the Government's Peel Report of 1970, made spurious connections between the ongoing reduction in perinatal mortality rates and the increased hospitalization of births. Tew (1990) and others, later pinpointed more significant factors, such as better nutrition and standards of living of mothers, better contraception and fewer pregnancies. Meanwhile, the average rate of caesarean sections had escalated from under 10% in the 1970s to 17% by 1997, and had reached 23.5% by 2006. The trend is still upwards, and in some London hospitals, where birth rates are soaring and services are stretched, rates are much higher. Queen Charlotte's stands at 33.8%, Chelsea and Westminster at 32% and St Mary's at 31%. This rise has been variously attributed to the heroic maintenance of borderline viable fetuses, medical fashion, the desire for pain-free or planned childbirth, and increased litigation threats. Other interventions are also on the increase. Inductions are now at 20.2% (up nearly one percent in a year), epidurals are at 22% (up 2% in a year), while 'normal' births (defined as those without the use of surgical or instrumental intervention, general anaesthetic, inductions or epidurals) are down to 46.7% from 48% a year earlier,

155

TABLE 9.8	Changes in place of birth 1927–2006										
	1927	1937	1946	1957	1968	1973	1984	1990	1993	1997	2006
Hospital	15	25	54	64.6	80.7	91.4	99	99	98	97	97
Home/ elsewhere	85	75	46	35.4	19.3	8.6	1	1	2	3	3

From Audit Commision (1997; figures for 1993 and 1997); Lewis (1980; figures for 1927, 1937 and 1946); Oakley (1984; figures for 1957,1968 and 1973); OPCS (1992; figures for 1984 and 1990); NPEU (2007; figure for 2006). Figures are percentages of live births.
Figures for hospitals include hospitals, maternity homes and poor-law institutions.

and only 62% of mothers had a midwife delivery (NHS Maternity Statistics 2006, NPEU 2007).

From the 1970s organizations – the Association for Radical Midwives (ARM), the National Childbirth Trust and the Maternity Alliance – began to respond to medicalization, and maternity care gradually came under public scrutiny. Women began to ask for women-focused birth, and to critique the notion that childbirth was a 'double medical emergency' for mother and baby. Some saw this as a confrontation between the lay sector and the experts and evidence of the use of professional power by doctors to shroud the process of childbirth in medical mystique. ARM began to ask for more independence from the obstetrical profession and middle-class women for rights to choose the type of birth and level of technology they wanted, especially for forms of 'natural childbirth', midwife-assisted births and more recognition of the experience of childbirth as a personal and family event. Interest group action from the 1980s saw the emergence of 'domino' births – hospital birth with a midwife and discharge into domiciliary midwife care after as little as 6 hours – and choices relating to pain relief and sometimes water births and other forms of birthing techniques. By the 1990s it was recognized that offering choice was politically advantageous, and the 1993 government report, 'Changing Childbirth' focused on choice for women and was proactive towards the idea of 'home birth', an issue that had suffered much negative battering from previous governments of both persuasions (DoH 1993). Birth Plans were instigated. However, recent statistics suggest that the changes these and more recent approaches have introduced are largely cosmetic and that the underlying trends are for more medicalization, with recent NICE guidelines (2003) recommending earlier antenatal attendance in order for women to benefit from all the screening available.

CONCLUSION: WHY WE STILL NEED TO FOCUS ON WOMEN'S HEALTH

It would be premature to abandon a focus on women's health issues in favour of a more 'neutral' gender approach, although there is evidence that the health of males is changing and that they might be taking on some of the health profiles usually attributed to women, especially in the area of mental health. Other evidence also seems to suggest that men are more interested than they used to be in health matters (they are subscribing to magazines on men's health and are increasingly, especially younger men, including fitness workouts and body-building in their daily routines). However, changes in women's behaviour have also tended to move them closer to masculine norms and values, and there is evidence of younger women undertaking fitness regimes, while also taking on 'male' patterns of behaviour such as heavier drinking and smoking, more participation in contact sports and in related 'laddish' behaviour. The effect on the health of females of these changes could well be mixed. Current evidence, however, does little to suggest that there are fundamental changes taking place in the power base of society or the gender order that underpins gender health profiles.

References

Arber S, Thomas H 2001 From women's health to a gender analysis of health. In Cockerman W (ed) The Blackwell companion to medical sociology. Blackwell, Oxford
Brisson C 1999 Study on work and stress. Lavel University, Quebec
Busfield J 2002 The archaeology of psychiatric disorder: gender and disorders of thought, emotion and behaviour. In Bendelow G, et al (eds). Gender, health and healing: the public/private divide. Routledge, London
Connell R 1987 Gender and power. Polity Press, Cambridge

Connell R 1995 Masculinities. Polity Press, Cambridge

Crompton R 1997 Women and work in modern Britain. Oxford University Press, Oxford

Davies H, Joshi H, Rake K, Alami R 2000 Women's incomes over the lifetime: a report to the Women's Unit, Cabinet Office. The Stationery Office, London

Department of Health (DoH) 1993 Changing childbirth: report of the expert maternity group. HMSO, London

Doyal L 1995 What makes women sick: gender and the political economy of health. Macmillan, London

Drever F et al 2000 Social inequalities. Office for National Statistics, London

Drever F, Doran T et al 2004 Exploring the relationship between class, gender and self-rated general health using the new socio-economic classification: a study using data from the 2001 census. Journal of Epidemiology and Community Health 58:590–596

Economic and Market Labour Review May, 2007 Two-thirds of public sector workers are women, London, National Statistics

Ehrenreich B, English D 1979 For her own good, 150 years of the experts' advice to women. Pluto Press, London

Equal Opportunities Commission 2006 Sex and Power: who runs Britain, EOC

Frost L 2001 Young women and the body, a feminist sociology. Palgrave, Basingstoke, UK

General Household Survey 2004 Stationery Office, London

General Household Survey 2005 Stationery Office, London

Health Statistics Quarterly, Web supplement Summer, 2007 Office for National Statistics, London

Irigaray L 1985 This sex which is not one. Cornell University Press, Ithaca, NY

Jackson E 2001 Regulating reproduction. Hart Publishing, Oxford

Lloyd C, Woroch K 2000 Visions and values in health: a case-study of childbirth. Unit 5 in Visions and values in health, which forms block one of the course Working for health. Open University, Milton Keynes, UK

MacIntyre S, Hunt K, Sweeting H 1996 Gender differences in health: are things really as simple as they seem? Social Science and Medicine 42(4):617–624

McVeigh et al 2005 Violent Britain: people, prevention and health, a report by the Centre for Public Health, Liverpool, John Moores University

Messing K, Stellman J 2006 Sex, gender and women's occupational health: the importance of considering mechanism. Environmental Research 101:149–162

National Health Service 2006 Maternity ONS Statistics, London

NPEU 2007 Recorded Delivery: a national survey of women's experience of maternity care, 2006 Redshaw M et al National Perinatal Epidemiology Unit, Oxford University

Oakley A 1984 The captured womb. Blackwell, Oxford

Office for National Statistics (ONS) 2002 2000 Psychiatric Morbidity Survey. ONS, London

Office for National Statistics (ONS) 2004 Focus on Health: health status. ONS, London

Office for National Statistics (ONS), October 2005a Breast cancer incidence rises while deaths continue to fall. National Statistics Online, London

Office for National Statistics (ONS) 2005b General Practice Research Database. ONS, London

Office for National Statistics (ONS) October 2006a Focus on gender. ONS, London

Office for National Statistics (ONS) 2006b Facts about men and women in Great Britain. ONS, London

Office for National Statistics (ONS), January, 2006c Focus on health, arthritis and migraine. National Statistics Online

Office for National Statistics (ONS) February 2007 Suicides: rates in UK men continue to fall. National Statistics Online, London

Office of Population Censuses and Surveys (OPCS) 1995 Living in Britain: results from the 1994 General Household Survey. HMSO, London

Office of Population Censuses and Surveys (OPCS) 2002 Living in Britain. General household survey. HMSO, London

Payne S 2001 Masculinity and the redundant male: explaining the increasing incarceration of young men. In Heller T, Muston R, Sidell M, Lloyd C (eds) Working for health. Sage Publications, London

Payne S 2006 The health of men and women, Polity Press, Cambridge

Pilcher J 1999 Women in contemporary Britain. Routledge, London

Prior P 1999 Gender and mental health. Macmillan, London

Rainford R, Mason V, Hickman M, Morgan A 2000 Health in England 1998: investigating the links between social inequalities and health. Health Education Monitoring Survey, Office for National Statistics/Health Education Authority. HMSO, London

Scambler A 1998 Gender, health and the feminist debate on postmodernism. In: Scambler G, Higgs P (eds) Modernity, medicine and health. Routledge, London

Shorter E 1982 A history of women's bodies. Penguin, London

Social Trends 2001 Office for National Statistics. HMSO, London

Social Trends 2007 Office for National Statistics. HMSO, London

Tew M 1990 Safer childbirth? A critical history of maternity care. Chapman and Hall, London

The Women's Unit 2002 Women and men in the UK: facts and figures 2000. Cabinet Office. HMSO, London

Walby S 1990 Theorizing patriarchy. Blackwell, Oxford

Women and Equality Unit 2006 Women in public life: key facts. HMSO, London

World Health Organization (WHO) 2002 World report on violence and health. WHO, Geneva

World Health Organization (WHO) 2005 Multicultural study on women's health and domestic violence. WHO, Geneva

World Health Organization (WHO) 2006 Gender equality, Work and health: a review of the evidence. WHO, Geneva

World Health Organization (WHO) 2007 World report on violence and health, follow up. WHO, Geneva

CHAPTER

10

Ethnicity and health

Moira Kelly
James Nazroo

INTRODUCTION

Ethnic minorities on the whole have the same health needs as the rest of society. However, there are significant variations in some disease rates and health disadvantage is clearly seen to exist. The relationship between ethnicity and health is understandably complex and efforts to understand this relationship have involved considerable discussion about the concepts of ethnicity, race and culture, and how they should be defined and measured. There has also been debate about competing explanations for ethnic health differences and, importantly, what our healthcare goals should be regarding ethnic variations in health. At the same time health professionals are increasingly concerned about how best to provide 'culturally competent' care for their patients.

Health researchers, policy makers and service providers need to be responsive to the changing ethnic make-up of societies such as the UK. A number of factors have contributed to this: post-colonial migration; the speed of globalization and related movement of people in recent years; the identification of risk factors associated with ethnicity through epidemiological research; evidence of the importance of social inequality as a factor in ethnic health difference; evidence of individual and institutional racism in health care; and improved understanding of differences in the experience of illness in ethnic minority populations gained through qualitative research. The challenge is how to address the issue of ethnicity without reifying cultural difference, or applying stereotypes.

This chapter aims to explore the relationship between ethnicity and health by covering four main areas. First of all we will discuss definitions of race, ethnicity and culture. We will go on to describe the demographic structure of the UK in relation to ethnicity. This will include a brief review of the history of inward migration, family structure, education and employment patterns. The third section will incorporate an outline of the main differences in disease rates between ethnic minorities compared with the UK in general, and a discussion of how these differences can be explained. Examples will be used in order to illustrate the way in which particular conceptions of ethnicity and health can influence how the relationship may be understood (or misunderstood as the case may be). Finally we will consider the different ways in which ethnicity is relevant to the practice of medicine. This will include a review of the nature and role of cultural competence in health care.

WHAT ARE RACE, ETHNICITY AND CULTURE?

Underlying discussions of 'ethnicity and health' is an interest in the way we view and respond to diversity and change in the societies in which we live. We can consider diversity in relation to the concepts of race, ethnicity and culture. These concepts provide us with different, and at times contentious, ways of understanding the relationship between ethnicity and health.

Race is a concept that is used to differentiate groups of people biologically on the basis of supposed differences in their genetic make-up. Differentiation between people on the basis of race generally reflects relatively superficial characteristics, such as skin colour and facial features. For example, early racial theory identified three main types of people: Negroid, Caucasian and Mongoloid. Race has no legal definition in the UK and is justifiably a controversial concept due to the way it has been used to support racist views of different ethnic groups. Indeed, an essential core to the concept is that some 'races' are better than others, so justifying negative discrimination. For example, it has been used to justify segregationist policies, as in the southern states of the USA until the 1960s and in South Africa until the 1990s, to explain differences in intelligence across 'racial' groups (Herrnstein & Murray 1994), and, of course, racist violence.

As with race, ethnicity reflects our social identities, or how we and others view us and how we relate to each other. For example, people from seemingly similar ethnic backgrounds may describe themselves as 'British, 'British Asian', 'Pakistani', or 'Mixed race', depending upon how they view their identity and who they are interacting with. The UK Commission for Racial Equality (2006), while acknowledging the difficulty in defining 'ethnic group', has used the following definition which was initially provided by the House of Lords:

'A group that regards itself, or is regarded by others, as a distinct community by virtue of certain characteristics that will help to distinguish the group from the surrounding community. Two of these characteristics are essential:

A long shared history, of which the group is conscious as distinguishing it from other groups, and the memory of which it keeps alive; and

A cultural tradition of its own, including family and social customs and manners, often but not necessarily associated with religious observance.'

Ethnicity is tied to culture. Culture and ethnicity are often used interchangeably, but are not the same thing. For example, the term 'multi-cultural society' is frequently referred to in the press, with 'culture' taken to mean ethnicity. Culture can be defined as: 'complexes of shared usages that distinguish a community, a setting or a situation' (Gubrium & Holstein 1997, page 14). It consists of shared experiences, beliefs and values. As we may have multiple ethnic identities, so we may be part of a number of cultural groupings. For example, we may be first or second generation Jamaican, be male or female, a teenager, a medical student, a nurse, a parent, a pensioner, or a combination of these things. These may all constitute different cultural groups with particular experiences, beliefs and attitudes. In this way, ethnicity may be an important aspect of culture, but does not necessarily define us culturally. This has implications for our understandings of ethnicity and health, because it highlights the need to be sensitive to difference within ethnic 'groups', and to change in the meaning and significance of being part of a particular ethnic or cultural group.

As we have seen, the concepts of race, ethnicity and culture are not straightforward and definition is difficult. The ethnic make-up of developed societies, such as the UK, is increasingly diverse and dynamic. Global migration patterns and mixing between different ethnic groups also mean that our cultural experience is dynamic and subject to change. Care therefore needs to be taken in defining ethnicity and culture and using them as concepts uncritically. Such 'inflexible assessments of ethnicity that treat ethnic categories as undifferentiated groups' (Karlsen & Nazroo 2002: 2) may lead to stereotyping and contribute to racism.

We have indicated that ethnicity is an important component of social identities, that is, it influences how we relate to and interact with each other. A central element of this is how groups are racialized – that is how racism operates in peoples lives. The Macpherson Report (1999), following the Stephen Lawrence Inquiry, defined racism in the following way:

'Racism in general terms consists of conduct or words or practices which disadvantage or advantage people because of their colour, culture, or ethnic origin. In its more subtle form it is as damaging as in its overt form.'

Incidences of racism are taken seriously and are often covered by the press, such as in highlighting institutional racism in public bodies and the provision of services, or cases where racism is a barrier to equal opportunities for promotion. Racism, as with sexism and ageism, can be both overt and covert. Covert racism often occurs when people are unaware that their actions are undermining the position of people from ethnic minorities. It may be inherent in the structures of institutions, such as workplaces and hospitals, and is often referred to as 'institutional racism', which can be defined in the following way:

'those established laws, customs, and practices which systematically reflect and produce racial inequalities in society. If racist consequences accrue to institutional laws, customs or practices, the institution is racist whether or not the individuals maintaining those practices have racial intentions.' (CRE submission to the Stephen Lawrence Inquiry, section 6.30. Macpherson Report)

Institutional racism may be hard to identify unless the systems through which it operates are scrutinized closely, as happened in the Stephen Lawrence Inquiry. People who experience racism may not be aware that it is operating and how it is affecting their health care. For example, ethnic minority patients may not be aware if they are being treated differently from other patients.

WHO ARE THE UK'S ETHNIC GROUPS?

Patterns of immigration

The UK has a long history of immigration, with the early inhabitants of the British Isles believed to have come from mainland Europe. The first millennium saw invasions by the

Romans, Angles, Saxons, Vikings and Danes, ending in the Norman Conquests in 1066. In the early part of the second millennium there were small but significant waves of immigration, including Jews from mainland Europe in the 13th century, Lascar seamen from South Asia and China recruited to work in Britain's increasing trading empire in the 17th century, and French Huguenots fleeing religious persecution in the late 17th century. The Irish potato famine and the UK industrial revolution led to significant numbers of Irish economic migrants settling in Britain in the 19th century, as well as smaller numbers of Chinese people settling in London and Liverpool. However, immigration to the UK occurred in relatively small numbers until the middle of the 20th century when the pattern changed dramatically.

After the Second World War the UK's expanding economy led to the proactive recruitment of workers from the Caribbean, South Asia and Ireland in the 1950s and 1960s. Immigration from India, Pakistan and Bangladesh continued through the 1960s and 1970s. The next significant wave of immigration came in the 1970s when political unrest in Uganda and Kenya led to the expulsion of South Asian people, some of whom came to the UK. Towards the end of the 20th century immigration became more diverse with immigrants from countries such as Ghana, Somalia, Sri Lanka and Turkey coming to the UK for economic reasons, or as refugees. By the 2001 Census 7.9% of the UK population identified themselves as members of an ethnic minority group (see Table 10.1). Since that census there has been a significant increase in economic immigration from Eastern Europe, following the expansion of the European Economic Union.

Social circumstances of ethnic minorities

As indicated above, there have been waves of immigration from different countries at particular times for different social reasons. Most ethnic minorities have settled in urban areas, with 45% of the non-White population living in London in 2001, and only 4 to

TABLE 10.1 Population of the United Kingdom by ethnic group, 2001 Census

	Total population		Percentage of non-white population
	Number	Percentage	
White	54153898	92.1	n/a
Mixed	677117	1.2	14.6
Asian or Asian British/Scottish	2331423	4.0	50.3
Indian	1053411	1.8	22.7
Pakistani	747285	1.3	16.1
Bangladeshi	283063	0.5	6.1
Other Asian	247664	0.4	5.3
Black or Black British/Scottish	1148738	2.0	24.8
Black Caribbean	565876	1.0	12.2
Black African	485277	0.8	10.5
Black Other	97585	0.2	2.1
Chinese	247403	0.4	5.3
Other	230615	0.4	5.0
All minority ethnic population	4635296	7.9	100.0
All population	58789194	100	

5% living in the South West and North East of England (ONS 2005). The social reasons for immigration are reflected in the varying pattern of socioeconomic circumstances across different ethnic minority groups, including family structure, educational achievement, employment and economic well-being.

Family structure tends to vary between different ethnic groups. Immigrant populations on the whole tend to be younger and have higher rates of fertility than the majority population. For example, 74% of Bangladeshi households contain at least one dependent child compared with 28% of White British households (ONS 2005). There is considerable variation between ethnic groups in fertility, which is also influenced by migration patterns. This can be seen in statistics on family size. South Asian households are larger than those for other ethnic groups, though there is variation between different South Asian groups, with the average Bangladeshi household size being 4.5 people, the average Pakistani size being 4.1, and for Indian households it is 3.3. The smallest households are in the White Irish (2.1), Black Caribbean (2.3) and White British (2.3) groups (ONS 2005).

There is considerable variation in education, employment and economic well-being between and within ethnic groups. For example, regarding education, Chinese and Indian pupils do better at school than White pupils. However, Black Caribbean, Pakistani and Bangladeshi pupils do less well on average than White pupils. It should be noted that there are significant gender differences in educational achievement, with girls doing better than boys across all ethnic groups. In terms of economic position, while on the whole higher proportions of ethnic minorities tend to be in lower socioeconomic groups and live in deprived areas, there is great variation between groups. If we consider household income, which works well as a summary marker, after housing costs are taken into consideration, 21% of White families were on low incomes in 2001 compared with 30% of Indian, 68% of Bangladeshi/Pakistani, 31% of Black Caribbean and 49% of Black Other households (ONS 2005). This pattern is repeated across a variety of indicators of economic well-being (class, employment, housing, etc.); Pakistani and, particularly, Bangladeshi people are worst off, while Indian and, particularly, Chinese people are closest to White people.

163

THE HEALTH OF ETHNIC MINORITY GROUPS

▓ Ethnic differences (inequalities) in health: patterns and explanations

Differences in health across ethnic groups, in terms of both morbidity and mortality, have been repeatedly documented in the UK (Erens et al 2001, Harding & Maxwell 1997, Nazroo 2001), as they have in other developed countries. They seem to be a consistent feature of the social distribution of health. Here we will first describe the ethnic patterning of health and then go on to discuss possible explanations for this patterning.

In the UK mortality data are not available by ethnic group, because ethnicity is not recorded on death certificates. However, country of birth is recorded and mortality rates have been published by country of birth using population data drawn from the Census. Some of these analyses are summarized in Table 10.2, which shows variation in mortality rates by country of birth and gender (using the 'standardized mortality rate' statistic, which adjusts for differences in age profiles of different groups and where the value '100' is the average population rate, and rates higher than this indicate higher death rates). The table reproduces some repeatedly documented findings:

● Men born in the Caribbean have low mortality rates overall, and particularly low mortality rates for coronary heart disease, but high rates of mortality from stroke. Women born in the Caribbean have similarly high rates of mortality from stroke.

164

TABLE 10.2 Standardized Mortality Ratio by country of birth for those aged 20–64 years, England and Wales 1991–1993

	All causes		CHD		Stroke		Respiratory disease		Lung cancer	
	Men	Women	Men	Women	Men	Women	Men	Women	Men	Women
Caribbean	89*	104	60*	100	169*	178*	80*	75	59*	32*
Indian subcontinent	107*	99	150*	175*	163*	132*	90	94	48*	34*
India	106*	-	140*	-	140*	-	93	-	43*	-
Pakistan	102	-	163*	-	148*	-	82	-	45*	-
Bangladesh	137*	-	184*	-	324*	-	104	-	92	-
East Africa	123*	127*	160*	130	113	110	154*	195*	35*	110
West/South Africa	126*	142*	83	69	315*	215*	138	101	71	69
Ireland	135*	115*	121*	129*	130*	118*	162*	134*	157*	143*

Source: Office for National Statistics.
* P < 0.05.

- This high mortality rate from stroke and low mortality rate from coronary heart disease is also found among those born in West/South Africa, who also have a high overall mortality rate.

- Men and women born in the Indian subcontinent and East Africa (presumed to be South Asian migrants) have high rates of death from coronary heart disease, with the highest rates found among those born in Bangladesh.

- Those born in the Indian subcontinent also have high mortality rates from stroke.

- Those born in Ireland have high mortality rates for all of the diseases covered in the table.

- On the whole, the non-White migrant groups have lower mortality rates from respiratory disease and lung cancer.

- Not shown in the table are the very high mortality rates in non-White migrants for conditions relating to diabetes (Marmot et al 1984).

Although these findings are statistically robust, applying them to ethnic categories comes with important problems, including, most obviously, that they do not include ethnic minority people born in the UK. However, such data have been supplemented by the growth in data on ethnic differences in morbidity. These, perhaps not surprisingly, contain some contradictions with the immigrant mortality data (Nazroo 2001), but are basically similar. Figure 10.1, drawn from the 1999 Health Survey for England (Erens et al 2001), shows differences in self-reported general health across ethnic groups. It charts the odds ratio and 95% confidence intervals, in comparison with a White English group (who consequently are indicated by the value of '1'), for a broad measure of health – reporting your health as fair, bad or very bad rather than good or very good. So a value greater than '1' indicates a greater risk of fair, bad or very bad health than White English people (and a value less than '1' indicates a smaller risk). Immediately obvious is the heterogeneity in experience across ethnic groups. Most notable is the wide variation for the three South Asian groups – Indian, Pakistani and Bangladeshi – who are typically treated as one group in epidemiological data and health policy.

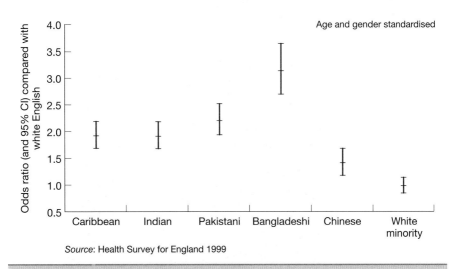

Source: Health Survey for England 1999

Fig. 10.1 Ethnic differences in reported fair or bad general health in England.
Source: Health Survey for England 1999.

But how do we make sense of the data showing differences in health across ethnic groups? The typical list of explanations is a simple extension of the categories used in the Black Report to explain class inequalities in health (Townsend & Davidson 1982), such as:

● They are a statistical artefact (an explanation that the growing body of data suggests is not the case and which will not be further discussed);

● They are a consequence of the migration process;

● Genetic/biological differences between ethnic groups lead to the health differences;

● Differences in culture and consequent health behaviours;

● They are a consequence of socioeconomic disadvantages between ethnic groups;

● Experiences of racism and racial harassment result in health differences.

This list can, of course, be adapted and extended. But the following discussion will identify and illustrate the key arguments and underlying evidence.

Perhaps not surprisingly, explanations for the ethnic patterning of health are commonly reduced to claims of genetic or cultural difference. This is a direct result of the temptation to read meaning directly into the categories the statistical data provide. So, for example, when attempting to understand the poorer overall health of Bangladeshi people we seek an explanation in the nature of what it is to be 'Bangladeshi', and resort to explanations based on our understandings of a stereotyped category. The high rates of coronary heart disease found in South Asian populations provide a good example of how this explanatory approach operates.

A *British Medical Journal* editorial (Gupta et al 1995) attributed the high rate of coronary heart disease among South Asian people to a combination of genetic and cultural factors that are apparently associated with being 'South Asian'. Concerning genetic factors, the suggestion was that 'South Asians' have a shared evolutionary history that involved adaptation 'to survive under conditions of periodic famine and low energy intake'. Here it is postulated that the evolutionary development of a 'thrifty' gene in South Asian populations, to deal with inconsistent food supplies, has led to a greater likelihood for people in these ethnic groups to develop non-insulin dependent diabetes in the form of 'insulin resistance syndrome', which apparently underlies a 'South Asian's' greater risk of coronary heart disease (McKeigue et al 1989). Of course this perspective requires crude 'race' thinking, allowing 'South Asians' to be viewed as a genetically distinct group with a *unique* evolutionary history. In terms of cultural factors, the use of ghee in cooking, a lack of physical exercise and a reluctance to use health services were all mentioned in the editorial – even though ghee is not used by all of the ethnic groups that comprise 'South Asians', and evidence suggests that 'South Asians' do understand the importance of exercise (Beishon & Nazroo 1997) and do use medical services (Nazroo 1997, Rudat 1994). This example is by no means unique, but the key point made here is that the relationship between ethnicity and illness is necessarily complex and cannot be explained by simple models.

An alternative approach is to examine how far explanatory factors that correlate with ethnic categories actually statistically explain ethnic differences in health. Important here is to consider how the ethnic patterning of health relates to wider social and economic inequalities. It is worth noting that the ethnic patterning of health shown in Figure 10.1 mirrors the broad patterning of socioeconomic inequality across ethnic groups described earlier. Although initial studies suggested that differential death rates by country of birth (the immigrant mortality rates shown in Table 10.2) could not be explained by occupational class (Harding and Maxwell 1997), it is now reasonably clear that socioeconomic factors make a major contribution to ethnic differences in health and are the most likely explanation for these differences (Nazroo and Williams 2005). Figure 10.2 shows rates of reporting fair or bad general health by house-hold income for a range of ethnic groups (Nazroo 2003). There is a clear relationship between reported general health and income for each ethnic group.

It is worth noting that the graph points to heterogeneity within broad ethnic groupings. It is misleading to consider, for example, Caribbean people to be uniformly disadvantaged in terms of their health; those in better socioeconomic positions have better health. There is nothing inevitable, or inherent, in the link between being Caribbean, Bangladeshi, Irish, etc. and a greater risk of mortality and morbidity. This points to the need to move beyond explanations that appeal to fixed ethnic (cultural) or race (genetic) effects. In addition, once statistical adjustments are made for socioeconomic indicators, ethnic differences in health diminish greatly (Nazroo 2003). For example, analysis of US data showed that crudely adjusting for household income reduced the relative risk for all-cause mortality of Black compared with White men from 1.47 to 1.19, so 'explaining' about two thirds of the ele-vated mortality risk (Davey Smith et al 1998). Adjusting for a number of medical risk fac-tors (diastolic blood pressure, serum cholesterol, cigarette smoking, existing diabetes, and prior hospitalization for coronary heart disease) only decreased the relative risk from 1.47 to 1.40. This demonstrates that socioeconomic position is a considerably more important determinant of Black–White differentials in mortality among men in the US than the typical markers of risk that are used for explanation and targeted in health promotion activities.

An additional explanation that needs to be considered as part of the social and eco-nomic inequalities faced by ethnic minority groups in developed countries is the possibil-ity that stress resulting from racial harassment and discrimination is related to poorer health. In the few but growing number of studies that have been conducted in this area, experiences of racial harassment and discrimination appear to be related to health. US studies have shown a relationship between self-reported experiences of racial harass-ment and a range of health outcomes, including hypertension, psychological distress, poorer self-rated health and days spent unwell in bed (Krieger 2000, Krieger & Sidney 1996, Williams et al 2003). In the UK, analyses have shown that reporting experiences

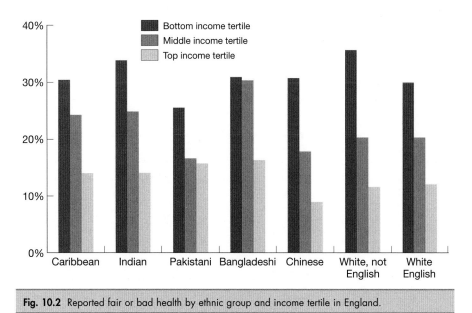

Fig. 10.2 Reported fair or bad health by ethnic group and income tertile in England.

of racial harassment and perceiving employers to discriminate against ethnic minority people are independently related to likelihood of reporting fair or poor health (Karlsen & Nazroo 2002), that reporting being fearful of racism is also related to poor health (Karlsen & Nazroo 2004), and more recent data have shown the relationship between experiences of racism and discrimination and mental health outcomes for a wider range of ethnic groups (Karlsen et al 2005).

So, there is a growing body of evidence showing the importance of social and economic disadvantage for explaining ethnic inequalities in health. However, the data available on such inequalities do not reflect how disadvantages are experienced over the life-course. The limited evidence that does exist suggests that inequalities increase with age (Nazroo & Williams 2005), perhaps reflecting both the accumulation of risks over the life-course ('weathering') and the long-term consequences of exposure to hazards at crucial develop-ment stages in early life. The cross-sectional pattern of increasing differences in risk over age could also reflect differences between first and second generation migrants, as older peo-ple are more likely to be migrants and younger people are more likely to be born in the UK. Such a life-course perspective alerts us to a number of issues relating to migration:

- Selection into a migrant group will be related to both health and human capital, potentially leading to the migration of a healthy sub-set of the population (Marmot et al 1984).

- The childhood experiences of migrants will be very different from those of the second generation, so insofar as these lead to long-term adverse health outcomes, or onto pathways that lead to an accumulation of social and health disadvantage, differences in health across generations might be expected.

- The experience of migration itself will occur alongside social and economic uphea-vals, which might have a direct impact on health.

- The contemporary social and economic experiences of a migrant and non-migrant gen-eration might be quite different, with the non-migrant generation more likely to do well economically and to have less traditional ethnic identities (Nazroo & Karlsen 2003).

- And such generational differences may well also be driven by the varying influences of events particular to specific periods (for example, the civil rights movement), and the con-sequent changes in the nature of ethnic relations, and ethnic inequalities, over time.

Inequalities in access to and quality of health care

Although the discussion above has concentrated on the causes of ethnic differences in health, it is also worth considering the role of health services in ameliorating, or aggravating, ethnic inequalities in health. In the USA a large body of research has repeat-edly documented ethnic/racial inequalities in access to and quality of health care, inequal-ities that are consistent across a range of outcomes and types of providers. A recent Institute of Medicine (IOM) study, requested by Congress, identified ethnic/racial differences in healthcare insurance status as a key determinant of these inequalities (Smedley et al 2003). In the UK there is, of course, (almost) free universal access to its publicly funded National Health Service (NHS), so one might expect ethnic inequalities in access to health care and quality of health care to be minimal, or at least smaller than those in the USA.

Evidence from the UK indicates that while there are not inequalities in access to health care, there are inequalities in the quality of care received, supportive of an institutional rac-ism hypothesis. UK studies have shown that ethnic minority people on the whole make greater use of primary healthcare services than White people (with Chinese people being the exception) (Balarajan et al 1989, Erens et al 2001, Nazroo 1997), even when adjustments are made for self-reported morbidity (Nazroo 1997). However, this does not appear to be reflected in greater use of secondary care services (Nazroo 1997), and there are suggestions that the quality of services received by ethnic minorities are poorer. For example, in primary care ethnic minority people are more likely to be dissatisfied with various aspects of the care received (Raleigh et al 2004), to wait longer for an appointment (Raleigh et al 2004) and to face language barriers during the consultation (Nazroo 1997). Other evidence suggests that South Asian people with coronary heart disease wait longer for referral to specialist care than Whites (Shaukat et al 1993), are less likely to receive revascularization procedures (Feder et al 2002, Mindell et al 2005), and among those who have suffered an acute heart attack one study has suggested that Indian patients are less likely to be treated with thrombolysis, or to be referred for exercise stress tests (Lear et al 1994a, b). Nevertheless, research in the UK is limited, with only a few studies to date covering a limited range of diseases and often local rather than nationally representative populations.

Mental health – the case of Black Caribbean people in the UK and psychotic illness

The evidence presented in the section on inequalities in access to and quality of care indicates that health services cannot operate outside of the context of broader processes of racialisation and institutional racism. This is perhaps most acutely seen when considering the evidence on ethnic differences in mental health. One of the most striking findings in the literature on ethnic inequalities in health – perhaps *the* most striking finding – is that Black Caribbean people are three to five times more likely to be admitted to a psychiatric hospital with a diagnosis of first episode of psychosis than White people (Harrison et al 1988, Van Os et al 1996). This difference is larger than that for any other condition or ethnic group except diabetes, where differences between White and most ethnic minority groups are of a similar order of magnitude (Erens et al 2001). However, the increased rates are even higher for young Caribbean men (Cochrane & Bal 1989), and especially British-born young men – 18 times higher in one widely cited study (Harrison et al 1988).

As you might imagine, these findings have been used in a number of ways by commentators. On the one hand they are interpreted as reflecting real differences in the incidence of psychotic illnesses – the methods used in studies are considered robust and, importantly, it is assumed that psychotic illness is sufficiently severe for all cases to appear in treatment data, so there is no clinical iceberg. Such an interpretation inevitably leads to a questioning of the causes of these high rates of illness. Not surprisingly, the full range of explanations associated with ethnic categories has been examined, including the possibility that the high rates are a consequence of genetic factors. However, differences in the risk of psychotic illness across Black Caribbean people in different contexts raise doubts about such explanations. For example, low rates of psychotic illness in Jamaica and Trinidad (Bhugra et al 1996, Hickling & Rodgers-Johnson 1995) and the large differences in risk between those who migrated to the UK and those who were born in the UK (noted above), suggest that there is not a straightforward ethnic difference in genetic risk. So, commentators have instead expressed concern that the social circumstances of Black Caribbean people in the UK, such as socioeconomic inequalities and racism, might result in such consequences (Harrison et al 1988, King et al 1994) and empirical work has supported this possibility (Karlsen et al 2005).

An alternative interpretation is that these high treatment rates are a consequence of the adverse interactions between ethnic minority people and social structures as represented, in this case, by the social institution of psychiatry (Fernando 2003, Sashidharan & Francis

1993). It is argued that psychiatry is not only institutionally racist, but part of a broader oppressive system that reinforces ethnic disadvantage. For example, evidence suggests that there are differences in the routes of admission into treatment for psychosis, with Black Caribbean people over-represented among patients compulsorily detained, despite them being both less likely than White people to display evidence of self-harm and no more likely to be aggressive to others prior to admission (Davies et al 1996, McKenzie et al 1995). In addition, studies of the prevalence of illness in the wider community (rather than studies of rates of treatment) suggest that the prevalence of psychotic illness among Black Caribbean men, young men, and men born in the UK is no greater than that for White men (King et al 2005, Nazroo 2001).

Taken together, the evidence suggests that there are a variety of potential problems with straightforward interpretations of existing data and, consequently, that the higher rates of psychosis reported among Black Caribbean people need to be examined critically. This position is understandably contentious (see Singh & Burns 2006). However, the limited investigations of institutional racism that have been conducted in psychiatric services have indicated that it is present (Sainsbury's Centre for Mental Health 1998, King's Fund 1998). Further research is required to understand how it operates and connects with wider social processes and to identify ways in which it can be addressed.

■ Placing ethnic differences in health in context

Ethnic differences in health in the developed world have been clearly documented, across countries, across groups and over time. On the whole, ethnic minority groups have poorer health than the ethnic majority, but there are variations in the nature of this across ethnic groups and across specific types of disease. The detail of the variation in morbidity, and emphasis on specific diseases, can lead to a focus on presumed fixed characteristics of ethnic groups when seeking explanation. An example is the focus on genetic differences and culturally-rooted health behaviours when attempting to explain the higher rates of heart disease among South Asian populations. Such an approach, however, neglects the social character of ethnicity and ethnic identities and it detaches health experiences from social context. Instead, accumulating evidence suggests that variations in health across ethnic groups in developed countries can best be understood as inequalities in health – that is, they are rooted in the wider social inequalities faced by ethnic minority groups.

Socioeconomic inequalities across ethnic groups statistically explain a large proportion of ethnic differences in health and this is the case across groups and national contexts and for measures of general health and specific diseases. Other elements of social disadvantage faced by ethnic minority groups, such as experiences of discrimination and racism, are also strongly related to health. Inevitably, there are exceptions – complex phenomena can never be so easily explained – with, for example, lower rates of respiratory symptoms among some ethnic minority groups in the UK explained by differences in the prevalence of smoking (Nazroo 2001). But this is the general pattern. The implication of this is, of course, that there are not inevitable links between ethnic/racial categories and health experiences, because the social inequalities associated with these categories vary over time and place. This is exemplified in differences between the health experiences of Black Caribbean people in England and the US, with those in the US doing much better in terms of their health, and their socioeconomic position (Nazroo et al 2007).

IMPROVING THE HEALTH OF ETHNIC MINORITIES

As discussed above, social and economic inequalities are the most significant explanation for differences in health across ethnic groups. In this section these explanations will be incorporated into a diagrammatically represented conceptual model that enables identification of the various ways in which ethnicity may be related to health. The model draws on the work of Dahlgren and Whitehead (1991) who developed a similar conceptual approach to understanding socioeconomic inequalities in health. See Figure 10.3.

The health of an individual is influenced by a wide range of different factors that operate in various ways. The influences on the health of ethnic minorities, as described above, add to this complexity. These factors are identified in research studies and in policy aimed at improving outcomes. This model aims to both demonstrate the potential intricacy of the relationship between ethnicity and health, and to simplify it so that we can see how different factors may inter-relate. The factors that may influence health have been grouped into three different layers surrounding 'the individual' at the centre. Four key over-arching influences on the health of ethnic minorities sit at the corners of the model. At the micro level, there are individual characteristics that are generally fixed, namely, gender, age and genetic make-up. The meso layer contains social networks that an individual may be part of, relating to their involvement with community, friends, family and religion. These may of course overlap but can also be viewed as distinct influences on health. The macro layer incorporates the wider determinants of health including employment, education, housing, which have all been consistently linked to health (Acheson 1998, Department of Health 2003), as well as health care (treatment and preventive services) and institutional racism. Ethnic minority health is also influenced both directly and indirectly by social

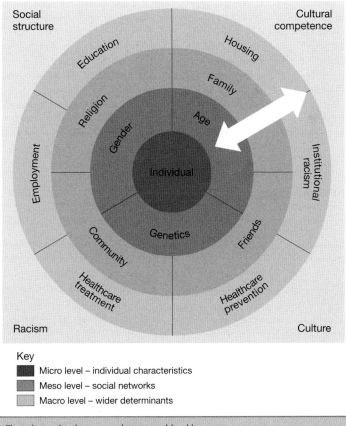

Key

■ Micro level – individual characteristics

■ Meso level – social networks

□ Macro level – wider determinants

Fig. 10.3 The relationship between ethnicity and health.

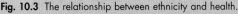

structure, racism, culture and the cultural competence of healthcare staff, which can be considered to impact on all other dimensions in the model.

There are infinite ways in which the different factors included in the model may interact. Let us take an example that looks at two hypothetical individuals from the same ethnic background and consider a number of possible ways in which the categories included in the model may influence an individual's health experience. One individual is a young single man who came to the UK three years ago from China to work in the financial services industry. The other individual also comes from China and has lived in the UK for 3 years. She is a young married woman with a baby, and her husband works long hours as a cook. The health of both individuals may be influenced in a variety of ways by their ethnicity. The young woman has poor English and finds it difficult to communicate with her GP about her symptoms. There is no interpreter or health advocate available when she attends. Her husband finds it difficult to get time off work to go to her GP with her. Her GP wonders about her attitudes towards western medicine, but he is unable to explore this with her due to communication difficulties. The young woman may also have limited social support in the form of family members and other people to share information about life in general, including health and health services, and to help with childcare. These circumstances depend upon the social networks she has in the UK. Her health may also be influenced by her living conditions, such as her housing and limited finances resulting from her husband's low wages. The young man, on the other hand, speaks fluent English and is able to communicate his health problems to his GP without much difficulty. He attends a gym, which is subsidised through work. He has a good social network through his firm, but finds the pressure to consume large quantities of alcohol with colleagues after work difficult. He finds it strange that his GP asks him about his attitudes towards traditional Chinese medicine, which he has never used.

The factors included in the different layers in the model are not fixed, that is, they are not to be seen in simple terms as cause and effect. Movement can take place between the layers in either direction, as indicated by the arrow. For example, social networks have been found to be a source of support and to be protective against illness (Stansfeld, 2006; Berkman and Syme, 1979). However, they may also be associated with particular life-styles that can be viewed as healthy or unhealthy, such as those related to eating, smoking and drinking patterns. Providing social support through caring for a sick relative or friend may mean that the carer cannot work, thereby influencing his/her financial circumstances. The number and type of social networks an individual is part of may also influence their access to the wider influences on health, such as work and housing.

In relation to health care, the recognition of institutional racism has contributed to the development of the notion of 'cultural competence', which can be defined as:

> '... the capacity to provide effective healthcare taking into consideration people's cultural beliefs, behaviours and needs ... cultural competence is the synthesis of a lot of knowledge and skills which we acquire during our personal and professional lives and to which we are constantly adding ... transcultural health is the study of cultural diversities and similarities in health and illness as well as their underpinning societal and organisational structures in order to understand current healthcare and to contribute to its future development in a culturally responsive way.' (Papadopolous 2003: page 5; cf. Papdopolous et al 2004: page 109).

The need for guidance on cultural competence is a concern for doctors and other health professionals who feel that they do not have the skills necessary to provide the level of care they would like to ethnic minority patients. A model of cultural competence has been developed by Papadopolous, Tilki and Lees (Papadopolous 2006, Papadopolous et al 2004), which involves the synthesis and application of awareness of one's own culture, cultural knowledge and cultural sensitivity. The first step is to increase self-awareness of cultural identity so that individuals can see how it is constructed and how it may shape values, beliefs and practices. Cultural knowledge can be gained in a variety of ways, including having meaningful contact with people from different ethnic backgrounds. This leads to increased understanding of similarities and differences in health beliefs and practices between and within ethnic minority groups, such as gender and generational differences, as well as experiences of social inequality. Cultural sensitivity refers to how health professionals relate to the people they are caring for. A foundation of trust, empathy and respect is needed in order to have constructive facilitation, negotiation and advocacy. Synthesis of these three stages into 'cultural competence' includes the ability to recognize and challenge forms of discriminatory practice such as essentialism, ethnocentricity and racism.

Cultural competence needs to be considered in relation to healthcare services that focus on the treatment and management of illness and those that focus on prevention of disease. As discussed above, ethnic minority groups have been found to have good access to primary care services, but the quality of the services they receive may not be as good. There is consequently a growing body of research into ethnic minority people's experiences of illness and health services (including doctor–patient consultations) in order to improve what we know about how ethnicity relates to health care, including the effects of social inequality and racism. For example, how and why might a doctor treat the Chinese patients discussed above differently from White patients? How does this relate to the (un)conscious use of cultural stereotypes (for example around diet or family structure), or institutional structures that cannot equitably accommodate ethnic diversity? Also important is the possibility that the doctor will treat the two Chinese patients differently from each other, leading to the need to consider how ethnicity and socioeconomic characteristics might interact with each other.

CONCLUSION

There is considerable evidence that ethnic differences in health exist and that they are complex. In part this arises from the complex nature of ethnicity in modern societies, which requires rigorous and critical examination, and sensitivity to the contextual nature of the significance of ethnic categories and the forms that ethnic relations take. Considering the issue sociologically, it can be seen that ethnic differences in health are related to social and economic inequalities, of which racism is a fundamental part. There is a need for a greater understanding of the processes involved in the enactment of institutional racism in social institutions in general, and in health services. Related to this is a need for institutions and practitioners to develop and practise culturally competent care.

References

Acheson D 1998 Independent inquiry into inequalities in health report. The Stationery Office, London
Balarajan R, Yuen P, Raleigh V 1989 Ethnic differences in general practitioner consultations. British Medical Journal 289:958–960
Beishon S, Nazroo JY 1997 Coronary heart disease: contrasting the health beliefs and behaviours of South Asian communities in the UK. Health Education Authority, London
Berkman L, Syme SL 1979 Social networks, host resistance, and mortality: nine year follow-up study of Alameda County residents. American Journal of Epidemiology 109(2):186–204
Bhugra D, Hilwig M, Hossein B et al 1996 First-contact incidence rates of schizophrenia in Trinidad and one-year follow-up. British Journal of Psychiatry 169:587–592
Cochrane R, Bal S 1989 Mental hospital admission rates of immigrants to England: a comparison of 1971 and 1981. Social Psychiatry and Psychiatric Epidemiology 24:2–11

Commission for Racial Equality 2006 Race, ethnicity and national origin. http://www.cre.gov.uk/diversity/wordsandmeanings/essay2.html (Accessed 12 July 2007)

Dahlgren G, Whitehead M 1991 Policies and strategies to promote social equity in health. Institute of Futures Studies, Stockholm

Davey Smith G, Neaton JD, Wentworth D et al 1998 Mortality differences between black and white men in the USA: contribution of income and other risk factors among men screened for the MRFIT. Lancet 351:934–939

Davies S, Thornicroft G, Leese M et al 1996 Ethnic differences in risk of compulsory psychiatric admission among representative cases of psychosis in London. British Medical Journal 312:533–537

Department of Health 2003 Tackling health inequalities: a programme for action. Department of Health, London

Erens B, Primatesta P, Prior G 2001 Health Survey for England 1999: The health of minority ethnic groups. Stationery Office, London

Feder G, Crook AM, Magee P et al 2002 Ethnic differences in invasive management of coronary disease: prospective cohort study of patients undergoing angiography. British Medical Journal 324:511–516

Fernando S 2003 Cultural diversity, mental health and psychiatry: the struggle against racism. Brunner-Routledge, East Sussex

Gubrium JF, Holstein JA 1997 The new language of qualitative method. Oxford University Press, New York

Gupta S, de Belder A, O'Hughes L 1995 Avoiding premature coronary deaths in Asians in Britain: Spend now on prevention or pay later for treatment. British Medical Journal 311:1035–1036

Harding S, Maxwell R 1997 Differences in the mortality of migrants. In: Drever F, Whitehead M (eds) Health inequalities: decennial supplement Series DS no 15. Stationery Office, London

Harrison G, Owens D, Holton A et al 1988 A prospective study of severe mental disorder in Afro-Caribbean patients. Psychological Medicine 18:643–657

Herrnstein R, Murray C 1994 The bell curve. Free Press, New York

Hickling FW, Rodgers-Johnson P 1995 The incidence of first contact schizophrenia in Jamaica. British Journal of Psychiatry 167:193–196

Karlsen S, Nazroo JY 2002 The relationship between racial discrimination, social class and health among ethnic minority groups. American Journal of Public Health 92:624–631

Karlsen S, Nazroo JY 2004 Fear of racism and health. Journal of Epidemiology and Community Health 58:1017–1018

Karlsen S, Nazroo JY, McKenzie K et al 2005 Racism, psychosis and common mental disorder among ethnic minority groups in England. Psychological Medicine 35(12):1795–1803

King M, Coker E, Leavey G et al 1994 Incidence of psychotic illness in London: comparison of ethnic groups. British Medical Journal 309:1115–1119

King M, Nazroo J, Weich S et al 2005 Psychotic symptoms in the general population of England: A comparison of ethnic groups (The EMPIRIC study). Social Psychiatry and Psychiatric Epidemiology 40(5):375–381

King's Fund 1998 London's mental health. The Report to the King's Fund London Commission, King's Fund Publishing, London

Krieger N 2000 Discrimination and health. In: Berkman L, Kawachi I (eds) Social epidemiology. Oxford University Press, New York

Krieger N, Sidney S 1996 Racial discrimination and blood pressure: the CARDIA study of young black and white adults. American Journal of Public Health 86:1370–1378

Lear JT, Lawrence IG, Burden AC, Pohl JE 1994a A comparison of stress test referral rates and outcome between Asians and Europeans. Journal of the Royal Society of Medicine 87:661–662

Lear JT, Lawrence IG, Pohl JE, Burden AC 1994b Myocardial infarction and thrombolysis: a comparison of the Indian and European populations in a coronary care unit. Journal of the Royal College of Physicians 28:143–147

Macpherson Report 1999 The Stephen Lawrence Inquiry. London: The Stationery Office. http://www.archive.official-documents.co.uk/document/cm42/4262/4262.htm

Marmot MG, Adelstein AM, Bulusu L & OPCS 1984 Immigrant mortality in England and Wales 1970–78: causes of death by country of birth. HMSO, London

McKeigue P, Marmot M, Syndercombe Court Y et al 11988[9] Diabetes, hyperinsulinaemia, and coronary risk factors in Bangladeshis in East London. British Heart Journal 60: 390–396

174

McKenzie K, van Os J, Fahy T et al 1995 Psychosis with good prognosis in Afro-Caribbean people now living in the United Kingdom. British Medical Journal 311:1325–1328

Mindell J, Klodawski E, Fitzpatrick J 2005 Using routine data to measure ethnic differentials in access to revascularization in London. London Health Observatory, London

Nazroo JY 1997 The health of Britain's ethnic minorities: findings from a national survey. Policy Studies Institute, London

Nazroo JY 2001 Ethnicity, class and health. Policy Studies Institute, London

Nazroo J 2003 The structuring of ethnic inequalities in health: economic position, racial discrimination and racism. American Journal of Public Health 93(2):277–284

Nazroo JY, Karlsen S 2003 Patterns of identity among ethnic minority people: diversity and commonality. Ethnic and Racial Studies 26(5):902–930

Nazroo JY, Williams DR 2005 The social determination of ethnic/racial inequalities in health. In: Marmot M, Wilkinson RG (eds) Social determinants of health, 2nd edn. Oxford University Press, Oxford, p 238–266

Nazroo J, Jackson J, Karlsen S, Torres M 2007 The black diaspora and health inequalities in the US and England: does where you go and how you get there make a difference? Sociology of Health and Illness (in press)

Office for National Statistics 2005 Focus on ethnicity and identity. Office for National Statistics, London

Papadopolous I 2003 The Papadopolous, Tilki and Taylor model for the development of cultural competence in nursing. Journal of Health, Social and Environmental Care 4:1 http://www.mdx.ac.uk/www/rctsh/modelc.htm

Papadopolous I, Tilki M, Lees S 2004 Promoting cultural competence in healthcare through a research-based intervention in the UK. Diversity in Health and Social Care 1:107–115

Papadopolous I (ed) 2006 Transcultural health and social care : development of culturally competent practitioners. Churchill Livingstone Elsevier, Edinburgh

Raleigh VS, Scobie S, Cook A et al 2004 Unpacking the patients' perspective: variations in NHS patient experience in England. Commission for Health Improvement, London

Rudat K 1994 Black and minority ethnic groups in England: health and lifestyles. Health Education Authority, London

Sainsbury's Centre for Mental Health 1998 Keys to engagement: review of care for people with severe mental illness who are hard to engage with services. Sainsbury's Centre for Mental Health, London

Sashidharan S, Francis E 1993 Epidemiology, ethnicity and schizophrenia. In: Ahmad WIU (ed) Race and health in contemporary Britain. Open University Press, Buckingham

Shaukat N, Cruickshank J 1993 Coronary artery disease: impact upon black and ethnic minority people. In: Hopkins A, Bahl V (eds) Access to health care for people from black and ethnic minorities. Royal College of Physicians, London

Singh SP, Burns T 2006 Race and mental health: there is more to race than racism. British Medical Journal 333:648–651

Smedley BD, Stith AY, Nelson AR (eds) 2003 Unequal treatment: confronting racial and ethnic disparities in health care. Institute of Medicine of the National Academies, Washington

Stansfeld S 2006 Social support and social cohesion. In: Marmot M, Wilkinson RG (eds) Social determinants of health. Oxford University Press, Oxford

Townsend P, Davidson N 1982 Inequalities in health (the Black Report). Penguin, Middlesex

Van Os J, Castle DJ, Takei N et al 1996 Psychotic illness in ethnic minorities: clarification from the 1991 Census. Psychological Medicine 26:203–208

Williams DR, Neighbors HW, Jackson JS 2003 Racial/ethnic discrimination and health: findings from community studies. American Journal of Public Health 93(2):200–208

Further/recommended reading

Commission for Racial Equality http://83.137.212.42/sitearchive/cre/diversity/wordsandmeanings/index.html

Sproston K, Mindell J (eds) 2006 Health survey for England 2004: the health of minority ethnic groups. The Information Centre, London http://www.ic.nhs.uk/statistics-and-data-collections/health-and-lifestyles/health-survey-for-england/health-survey-for-england-2004:-health-of-ethnic-minorities–full-report

175

Later life, health and society

Paul Higgs

DEMOGRAPHIC TRANSITIONS

The existence of large numbers of older people in countries such as Britain is a relatively recent feature, characteristic only of the last century and a half. This is not to say that there were no old people in the past; many individuals survived until their 70s and 80s, but there were not enough for them to constitute a significant part of the population. Surviving into old age was an achievement – not an expectation – for the majority of the population. By contrast, in modern Britain the vast majority of the population can expect to live beyond the age of retirement; indeed, many will live beyond the age of 80. In 2005, life expectancy at birth in Britain was 77 years for men and 81 years for women (ONS 2007); in 1841 the figures were 41 years for men and 43 years for women and, according to Victor (1994), it had taken 400 years for these figures to increase by 8 years. As can be seen, the increase in life expectancy that accompanied industrialization is not surprising. The advent of public health measures that substantially controlled the impact of infectious diseases had the effect of lowering the infant and maternal mortality rates and ensuring that a greater proportion of the population survived at each age (see Chapter 1). Consequently, the majority of deaths in England and Wales occur in those aged over 65, with the rate increasing with age. This process has been described as 'rectangularization of the survival curve' (see Fig. 11.1) and describes a move to an idealized situation where there is little or no infant mortality and little attrition in the proportions of the population living until they reach their natural lifespan.

Not only has life expectancy increased but the nature of the population has also changed. In 2014 it is projected that the number of people aged 65 and over is expected to exceed those aged under 16 for the first time. This projected increase is caused in part by the relative balance between the birthrates of different generations. As those born during the post-war 'baby boom' grow older they affect the composition of the population, because relatively fewer people were born in the decade that followed. Since the 1970s the younger population has declined as both a proportion of the population and in absolute terms. In 1971 25% of the population were aged under 16 compared with 13% aged over 65. By 2005 these proportions were 19 and 16% respectively, an increase in the older population of 2.2 million. In 2005 the population of people aged 85 or over reached 1.2 million, to make up almost 2% of the UK population (ONS 2007).

These changes are not unique to Britain. In 1990, just under 20% of the total population of the European Union was aged 60 or over (Walker & Maltby 1997). In numerical terms, this was about 60 million people. By the year 2020, the corresponding percentage of the population is calculated to be a quarter of all EC citizens. As in Britain, the number of over-80s is also set to increase; by the year 2025 they are projected to rise by up to 115% in Portugal and by nearly an extra million in both Italy and Germany.

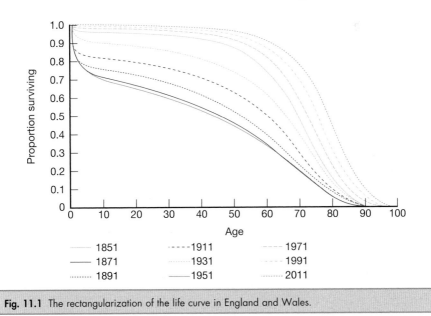

Fig. 11.1 The rectangularization of the life curve in England and Wales.

Life expectancy has also been increasing throughout Europe over the past 30 years, and has increased by up to 10 years in some countries. However, it is important to note that 16 out of the 25 European Union nations had larger populations of those aged under 15 than aged over 65 and that Ireland has the lowest proportion of older people in its population of any nation in the EU (ONS 2007).

The composition of the older population of the UK reflects the fact that the country has historically consisted of people from a White British ethnic background. The pattern of migration to the UK since the 1950s has favoured younger age groups and has meant that most ethnic minority groups in Britain have a younger age structure than the White British population, with only 11% of Black Caribbeans and 3–7% of South Asians being 65 or over compared with a figure of 17% for White British. Conversely, the migration patterns of the early 20th century have meant that the White Irish group have an older age profile than that of the White British category with over 25% being aged 65 or over (ONS 2007).

HEALTH AND ILLNESS

Although, as has been noted throughout history, there is a strong connection between old age and physical disability, the extent of this is not as profound or pervasive as popular image would have it. Acute health problems such as colds or accidental injuries increase with age, but even among the very oldest age groups these only affect 20% of males and 25% of females. On average, people over 75 lost 77 days over a year because of acute sickness. This compares with an average of 21 days for those aged 16–44 (HMSO 2000). Chronic health problems do increase with age and according to the 2002 General Household Survey, 72% of the over-75 age group reported a long-standing illness (HMSO 2004). In Table 11.1 we can see how both long-standing and limiting long-standing illnesses increase with age with the latter including arthritis, back pain, heart disease and mental disorders (ONS 2007). It is important to note that both of these are self reported measures of health and may reflect people's increased expectations about health and the fact that individuals vary in how much they are troubled by the same symptoms (HMSO 2004). In order to integrate the fact that age is associated with illness and disability researchers have constructed tables based on life expectancy, healthy life expectancy and disability-free life expectancy (See Table 11.2). This shows that while life expectancy has been increasing, healthy life expectancy measured as years lived in self-reported 'good' or 'fairly good' health have not increased as quickly. Disability-free life expectancy is calculated as the number of years lived free from a limiting long-standing illness. People can expect to live more years experiencing disability than they will in poor health. Again, because this measure is based on self-reported data, whether people are living longer and sicker is the subject of a fierce debate with considerable evidence to suggest that there has been a decline in disability of about 2% per year during the 1990s and that this is a global trend (Fries 2003).

ACTIVITIES OF DAILY LIVING

Many researchers have looked at the health status of older people from the perspective of their ability to undertake what are called 'activities of daily living' (ADL). There are many different ways of measuring these abilities but most concentrate on a few distinct activities, such as bathing, climbing stairs and cutting toenails (Table 11.3). Again, it should be noted that the majority of older people can undertake these activities. Using data from the 1985 General Household Survey, Johnson & Falkingham (1992) point out that even

TABLE 11.1 Self-reported illness: by sex and age, 2005

Great Britain	Rates per 1000 population[3]	
	Long-standing illness	Limiting long-standing illness
Males		
0–4	140	46
5–14	181	72
15–44	175	90
45–64	401	233
65–74	554	342
75 and over	583	402
All ages	273	150
Females		
0–4	93	28
5–14	160	67
15–44	209	114
45–64	407	245
85–74	589	370
75 and over	545	401
All ages	282	163

Source: Social Trends 37, Office for National Statistics.

TABLE 11.2 Life expectancy, healthy life expectancy and disability-free life expectancy at birth: by sex

Great Britain	Years			
	Males		Females	
	1981	2002	1981	2002
Life expectancy	70.3	76.0	76.8	80.5
Healthy life expectancy	64.4	67.2	66.7	69.9
Years spent in poor health	6.4	8.8	10.1	10.6
Disability-free life expectancy	58.1	60.9	60.8	63.0
Years spent with disability	12.8	15.0	16.0	17.5

Source: Social Trends 37 Office for National Statistics.

among those aged over 85, 14% of males and 11% of females are described as having no functional disability. However, nearly half of all women in this age group are deemed to have severe disability. In a recent study of older Europeans it was found that disability and need for help in self-care activities was less common than in mobility abilities and that successive cohorts of older people had better physical functioning when measured against a range of ADL items (Äijänseppa et al 2005).

TABLE 11.3	Help needed by elderly people with various tasks: by age (1996–7)					
	65–69	**70–74**	**75–79**	**80–84**	**85 and over**	**All aged 65 and over**
Climbing stairs	5	7	11	15	30	10
Bathing/showering	5	6	8	15	24	9
Dressing/undressing	3	2	4	5	8	4
Getting in and out of bed	2	2	1	3	4	2
Getting around the house	1	1	0	1	4	1
Going to the toilet	1	1	1	1	3	1
Eating	0	0	1	1	1	0

From General Household Survey, Office for National Statistics. HMSO (2004)

MULTIPLE PATHOLOGY

One important conclusion acknowledged explicitly by those who construct and use ADL scales is the importance of what is known as 'multiple pathology' among older people. This refers to the fact that an older person is likely to have more than one medical condition, and these will often be of a disabling nature. But, again, although the average number of multiple pathologies increases with age, it should be remembered that nearly two-fifths of older people are not subject to any disabling conditions.

One common belief about old age is that it is inextricably linked with mental decline, so much so that senile, which is the Latin word for old, has become a pejorative term for mental incapacity. The idea of mental decline as an accompaniment of the ageing process is not supported by the evidence. Alzheimer's disease is probably the most well known organic disorder of the brain to affect old people. Its most common symptoms include memory loss and behavioural disturbances, but the prevalence of dementing conditions is in fact less than 10% for older people living in the community. There were 700 000 people with dementia in the UK at the time of writing. The incidence of dementia does increase with age with the proportion doubling with every 5 years of life and one-third of those aged over 95 are affected (PSSRU 2007). More hidden is the fact that affective disorders such as depression do feature highly among the older population, with around one-quarter reporting either a mild or severe clinical affective disorder. Suicide rates seem to increase with age, with people over 65 accounting for 27% of male and 32% of female successful suicides in England and Wales (Victor 1994).

RESIDENTIAL AND INSTITUTIONAL CARE

Another common image of older people is that many of them are residents in some form of institution. This could be an old people's home, a residential or nursing home or a long-stay ward in a geriatric hospital. It is true that nearly 500 000 older people were in some kind of institutional setting by 1990, and that this had grown from 250 000 in 1970 (Henwood 1992). However, such absolute numbers should not be allowed to disguise the fact that these only represent a small fraction of the older population. Even among those aged over 90, nearly three-fifths lived in private households (Bury & Holme 1991). Moreover, while 64% of residents of care homes have some degree of dementia, two-thirds of people with dementia live in the community. Although the numbers of places in institutions nearly doubled between 1970 and 1990, the real growth occurred within the private sector. Places in private residential homes increased from 24 000 in 1970 to 156 000 in 1990, and places in private nursing homes grew from 20 000 in 1970 to 123 000 in 1990. Over the latter part of the past decade the provision of residential and care homes for older people has been dominated by financial uncertainty due to changes in the funding of places and the rise in property values. In certain areas such as London and the south of England, the provision of nursing homes has become very disparate because many have gone out of business. It has been estimated that there was a fall of 5% in the numbers of places between 1992 and 1999 (HMSO 2001). Some estimates suggest that this situation is untenable in the long term and that there will be a 63% rise in the numbers of people with cognitive impairment between 1998 and 2031, leading to a need for another 140 000 places in residential care (PSSRU 2003).

USE OF HEALTHCARE SERVICES

Older patients comprise the largest single group of users of hospital services. This is not just confined to those specialisms with an interest in the conditions of old age such as geriatric medicine, but applies throughout most of the major specialities. The admission rate increases with age, with the 1998 General Household Survey (HMSO 2000) showing 21% of men aged over 75 and 15% of women in the same age group reporting an inpatient stay in the previous year. The same survey reported that 17% of those aged over 75 had been inpatients compared with only 12% of those aged 65–74. It is also the case that inpatient length of stay increases with age. Those aged over 75 spend three times as long in hospital as those aged between 16 and 44, with the average length of stay being 12 and 4 days, respectively.

Consulting the general practitioner (GP) also increases with age, as does the average number of consultations made. In 1998, 21% of those aged over 75 had visited a GP in the previous fortnight (HMSO 2000). Women tend to consult the GP more often than men, and they are more likely to receive a home visit. However, Victor (1994) notes that less than 10% of older people in Canada accounted for 35% of all visits to the GP.

Older people are major users of prescribed medicines, having on average more than two-and-a-half times more items than the rest of the population. When non-prescribed drugs are taken into account, only a small proportion of older people are not on medication of any sort. Consequently, one of the notable features of older patients is the existence of what is known as polypharmacy – the taking by one patient of many different medicines. This is a particular problem often associated with the fact that many items are prescribed on repeat prescriptions, leading to a build-up over time. This can lead to problems in acute hospital care, where doctors might not be sure what medication older patients are on when they are admitted.

GENERATIONS, AGEING POPULATIONS AND HEALTH POLICY

Infirmity and illness are often seen to define later life and policy makers often assume that a population with a high proportion of older people is also one that leads to greater expenditure on health care. In Britain, the government calculates what is known as a 'dependency ratio' based on the proportion of the population aged under 16 and over 65 to those of working age. It is assumed that the young and the old represent a drain on expenditure that those of working age will have to pay for. As the percentage of older people in the population increases, so does the burden on the working population. This is not just a British phenomenon. A study by the International Labour Organization suggests that, throughout

Europe, medical expenditure on health care for the over 65s will increase from 37% of all healthcare spending in 1985 to 58% by the year 2015. Individual countries such as Switzerland could find their expenditure rising to 70% (Walker & Maltby 1997).

Important dimensions of these issues are the similarities or differences that exist between different succeeding generations. Evandrou & Falkingham (2000) have attempted to model the impact on British society of the retirement of different birth cohorts. Most of our experience of old age is derived from cohorts who were born in the 1910s. Their experiences will be very different from those born in the 'baby boom' that occurred between the late 1940s and early 1960s. It is this latter group who will be retiring in the first few decades of the twenty-first century. Evandrou & Falkingham (2000) focus on three areas – living arrangements, health and access to resources. They point out that the proportion living alone is likely to increase because of social factors such as divorce, childlessness and low birth rates. In terms of health, as we have already seen, more recent generations report more long-standing illness than their predecessors at similar ages. However, offsetting this, younger cohorts are less likely to smoke but tend to work more hours. In terms of access to resources, later generations have greater work participation rates for women than earlier ones, and women are much more likely to work full time. This means that both men and women are more likely to have private pensions and to have benefited from the rise in home ownership. Evandrou & Falkingham conclude that the baby boomers are likely to be 'better off in retirement than today's older people' (Evandrou & Falkingham 2000, p 34). Taken together, the evidence suggests a mixed set of implications for social and health policy.

The questions that policy makers ask are whether expenditure on the coming cohorts of older people will continue to rise or will it stabilize as each succeeding generation brings its own experiences into the equation and sets the balance between the responsibilities of the individual and the state. In Britain the Wanless Report (Wanless 2001) sought to answer these questions and concluded that the issues that faced the NHS were not mainly about an ageing population but were about the levels of disability people experienced in later life and the extent to which the 'compression of morbidity' was occurring. The key issue, as we have seen, is whether the level of disability and chronic illness is diminishing, stabilizing or increasing as people live longer? As we have seen above, the evidence is mixed. One argument is that there has been a decrease in morbidity among higher socioeconomic classes in later life. This is seen to relate to the prevention or delayed onset of many non-fatal conditions that increase the age of onset of disability without affecting age of death. If this compression of morbidity could be extended to the rest of the population, then the nature of later life would be transformed as would the demands created by an ageing population. The Wanless Report gave some credence to the position of declining disability rates in later life by pointing out that most health care costs occurred in people's last year of life irrespective of their age, suggesting that age in itself was not responsible for greater costs. The report did, however, carry an important caveat, namely that people's expectations of services were increasing all the time and this may be the cause of increases in spending. While the compression of morbidity may represent a model of 'successful ageing' at minimal extra cost, in practice all European healthcare systems are preparing for a significant rise in demand. This has led Harry Moody (1995) to argue that modern societies face four possible scenarios (Box 11.1). Although each of these scenarios can be assessed separately in terms of their implications, what is probably more likely to happen is that they are all going to happen simultaneously. No single approach to the future of ageing is likely to be dominant. Even Moody's preferred solution of the voluntary acceptance of limits assumes that there

BOX 11.1   Moody's (1995) four scenarios for the future of old age

1. **Prolongation of morbidity:** the state whereby an increase in years is not accompanied by an equal increase in quality of life. This prompts demands for the 'right to die' and rationing based on quality-of-life measures
2. **Compression of morbidity:** a situation where the majority of the population experiences good health almost up to the end of their lives and are then subject to a 'terminal drop' just before they die. This strategy advocates health promotion and individual responsibility as the way forward in health care
3. **Lifespan extension:** the abilities and successes of modern medicine are such that the natural lifespan can be extended upwards, leading to the delaying or abolition of many of the features of 'normal ageing'. The emphasis is put on basic medical research into the ageing process. Problems of who gets access to discoveries and treatments would emerge
4. **Voluntary acceptance of limits:** recognizes the problems inherent in the other three positions and argues for a shared 'meaning of old age' that maintains the common good by stressing limits beneficial to coming generations. It is accepted that there must be a point where interventons should be appropriate rather than life extending

183

can be general agreement on the desirability of such an approach. What Moody directs us to is the uncertainty and contradictions facing the future of ageing.

OLDER PEOPLE AND SOCIETY

The only characteristic shared by all older people is chronological age, and even this is not consistent between societies. In Britain, the state retirement age is often used to designate the onset of old age. This has meant that until recently men became old on their 65th birthday whereas women did so on the occasion of their 60th birthday. In many countries such as Kenya, employees of the State often retire at 40 and live on their pensions, so that younger people can be employed. The arbitrariness of when retirement occurs means that all we can safely say about it is that it marks the end of participation in the formal economy. Even this has been eroded with the widespread phenomenon of people taking early retirement in their 50s, but others not fully leaving the labour market until much later than the state retirement age. When old age is deemed to begin is therefore increasingly difficult to ascertain.

It is not the case that older people are either richer than the rest of the population or poorer. There are considerable numbers of relatively well-off older people, but it is also the case that some of the poorest people in Britain are old. However, it is a situation that is changing over time. In 1979, 47% of pensioners were in the bottom 20% of the distribution of the income distribution for the whole population. By 2005/6 this figure had fallen to less than 25%. During the same period, there were increases in the proportion of pensioners falling into the other four-fifths. In 2005/6, pensioners were most commonly found in the second fifth (Fig. 11.2). One reason for this change is that pensioners' income has grown at a faster rate than other sectors of the population. It has been estimated that pensioners' income has grown by over 60% in real terms between 1979 and 1997 and by 26% between then and 2005/6 (Department for Work and Pensions (DWP) 2007). By way of comparison, average earnings grew by 36% and 16% in the same period.

Obviously, such averages hide considerable differences between different groups of retired people. The major source of income for older people was the State Retirement Pension; however, that has begun to have less significance as the determining factor in most older people's income and state benefits represent an average of 45% of pensioners'

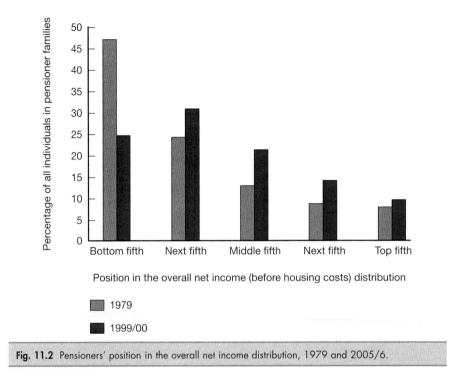

Fig. 11.2 Pensioners' position in the overall net income distribution, 1979 and 2005/6.

income allowing for a greater variation in older people's incomes to occur. Among recently retired pensioner couples, the proportion of total income received from benefits amounts to only 32% of their income, as opposed to 54% for pensioner couples over 75. For single pensioners aged over 75 this figure is 67% (DWP 2007).

Income from occupational pensions rose by 162% in real terms between 1979 and 1997 whereas that from state benefits rose by 41% (DWP 2000). Since 1997 the growth of occupational and state benefit has been equalized at around 25% however, 23% of pensioner households were in receipt of disability benefits. Household structure also has an important effect. 59% of pensioners have income from occupational pensions but pensioner couples receive twice the level of occupational pensions and investments as single pensioners. Younger pensioner couples have higher incomes than older ones, as do male pensioners and those living in London or the South East of England for those over that age. Among retired households, the poorest seem to be ones comprising older single women (DWP 2007). This is sometimes described as the 'feminization of poverty'and is in part a result of the fact that widowhood and now divorce particularly affect women's income because they are less likely to have occupational pensions and more likely to be reliant on state benefits (Arber & Ginn 2004).

It would be a mistake, therefore, to assume that poverty is a natural state for all older people. The poverty of many old people is because many of them rely upon state benefits as their main source of income. Because these entitlements were set low relative to the rising standard of living of the rest of the population and have not yet caught up, it is not surprising that large numbers are poor. It should also be noted that households with children but only one adult are also disproportionately likely to be in poverty. Both of these groups are the subject of targeted policy interventions whose success is yet to be established.

DOMESTIC CIRCUMSTANCES

The social circumstances of older people also vary greatly. Family structures are dominated by the cultural norm of the nuclear family, where only two generations of a family live under the same roof. This is different from the extended family, where many different generations live together, which is prevalent in some other cultures. Older people who have been married have tended to live in forms of nuclear family when their children have left home. As older people have aged so the chances of them still living with their spouses decreases. This, combined with the relatively high number of women who have never married, means that a substantial number of older people live alone. Social networks therefore become crucial. Although the vast majority of older people do not live with their children, this does not mean that they have little contact. The majority of older people have children and/or a sibling living close to them and contact is frequent. The family does not provide the only source of social contact. Surveys report, unsurprisingly, that friends and neighbours play an important part in maintaining the older person's place in social networks. Age does affect the nature of these contacts: 'younger' old people tend to visit friends whereas 'older' old people tend to be visited. The percentage of reported contact with both family and friends tends to diminish with age. Victor & Scharf (2005) using the ONS Omnibus Survey found that 5% of their sample had a high score for social isolation and that only 2% reported that they always felt lonely.

Most care for physically frail and mentally confused older people is provided by members of such social networks. There are 6 million carers in Britain and 75% are looking after an elderly person. Family relationships are of extreme importance to this process of informal care, with 80% of carers looking after a relative (Henwood 1992). Women, and especially daughters, are the main carers. However, a third of all carers are men, although they often do different things. Sometimes the caring relationship can continue for so many years that the carers themselves become elderly people. The effect of caring on carers can be immense, both in physical and financial terms. The majority receive no help from formal agencies and what help is offered is often designed to stop the informal caring relationship breaking down rather than alleviating stresses. Community care policy depends on informal care 'by the community' to keep costs down.

SOCIOLOGY AND OLDER PEOPLE

The existence of a state of retirement for large numbers of the population is a feature of most industrialized societies. As such, it has prompted the interest of many different sociologists who have constructed a number of different theories to account for the position of older people.

Disengagement theory

One of the first generalized accounts to look seriously at old age was an American approach centred on the theme of 'disengagement' (Cumming & Henry 1961). This was a process whereby older people in industrial societies disengaged themselves from the roles that they occupied in the wider society. This was so younger generations would have opportunities to develop and society could continue. Such disengagement not only occurred in relation to work roles but also in relation to families, when retired generations became much less central to the lives of their children. Seen from this perspective, old age presented the individual with many difficulties. In preindustrial societies, the inheritance of skills and property accorded older people a social function. In industrial societies, the lack of property or skills that could be handed on meant that older people did not have 'scripts' with which to negotiate their new roles. This led many researchers to stress the importance of finding ways to facilitate 'successful ageing' with the priority being psychological adjustment.

Research was undertaken in the USA during the 1950s and 1960s to provide evidence for this theory. A longitudinal study in Kansas City (Neugarten et al 1964) showed that older people did indeed disengage, although women started this process at widowhood whereas men began on retirement. Again, the processes were seen as involving difficulties in the roles being played by older people and the answers in psychological adaptation. This approach, which for a long time was the dominant paradigm in social gerontology, saw the way in which old age occurred in modern societies as an inevitable and natural process. Questions about whether older people wanted to 'disengage' or were forced to do so by society were not asked. The emphasis on psychological adjustment also avoided looking at the very real social processes that structured old age.

▒ Structured dependency theory

If the disengagement approach centred on the perspective of the individual older person, then the analysis put forward by the predominantly British 'structured dependency' school (Townsend 1981) stressed the importance of social policy. For the structured dependency writers the most important fact about the ageing process is the existence of the notion of retirement. In most industrial societies the age at which this occurs has been set by the State, and it is from this point that people are entitled to the State retirement pension. Retirement not only marks the withdrawal from the formal labour market but also the shift from making a living to being dependent on the State. In fact, until the 1990s it was a requirement that, to receive a State pension, the recipient was not allowed to undertake paid work, at the risk of having the money deducted from his or her pension. In this way the State pensioner was treated in the same 'punitive' way as the unemployed person seeking benefit.

Consequently, decisions made by the government have a dramatic effect on how older individuals live their lives. A good example is the decision by the post-war government to set different retirement ages for men and women. Women were to retire at 60 because it was estimated that the average age difference between a husband and wife was 5 years. If men retired at 65 it would therefore be intolerable that their wives would still be working and have access to independent income. After all, this might challenge the moral authority of the male head of the household. For similar reasons, many governments allowed married women to opt out of paying a full national insurance contribution on the grounds that they could share their husband's pension rather than having one in their own right.

We know that a significant section of older people experience poverty. For the structured dependency school this is not a coincidence. State retirement pensions are kept at a deliberately low level, even falling in relation to average living standards. One study concluded that they were worth only 20% of average earnings and that their value will drop by half by 2020 (Evandrou & Falkingham 1993). It is suggested, therefore, that the 'disengaged' nature of many old people is the result of low pensions, and not any process brought on by the ageing process. That this can be seen as a continuing feature of modern Britain can be seen by the abolition of the State Earnings Related Pension Scheme (SERPS). This pension scheme had been set up in the 1970s to create a more generous pension for those not covered by private or occupational schemes. It was effectively abolished by the Conservative government in the 1990s after a long period of atrophy.

The post-1997 Labour governments have chosen not to reintroduce the scheme, preferring instead to rely on the private sector and 'stakeholder' pensions.

Structured dependency is not just limited to the economic sphere but rather pervades the whole of society as an effect of this inferior status. The association of age with infirmity might not be factually true but it does 'represent' the position of older people, as does the exclusion of older people from various forms of social involvement. Often, lack of resources is the main reason for what are taken to be the characteristics of older people. The cultural emphasis on 'youth' is one that sees ageing in negative terms. This can lead to 'ageism', where it becomes culturally acceptable to discriminate against older people. This can manifest itself in policies seeking to limit medical or healthcare resources to older people, in discriminatory employment practices and in the treatment of physically frail or mentally confused older people.

If, as the structured dependency school argues, the dependency of older people is structured by society then the obvious response to it is to change those policies that most reinforce the inferior position of older people. Increasing the value of State pensions is one obvious answer. This is controversial, given that the general move in policy circles is towards seeing post-retirement income as an individual responsibility. However, structured dependency theorists remain committed to an egalitarian approach to later life and would argue that it is the State's responsibility to provide a good standard of income for all. Otherwise, what is being perpetuated is class inequality, with prosperity in earlier life ensuring prosperity after retirement. Taking this class inequality as their cues the 'political economy' school has linked the position of older people to more neo-Marxist themes around the role of the older person within the capitalist economy (Phillipson 1982, Walker 1981). In more recent works the mixed fortunes of older people in the globalized economy have been a focus for theorising (Estes et al 2003).

◼ Theory of the third age

The whole approach of the structured dependency school has been challenged by writers such as Peter Laslett (1996), who saw that modern societies created opportunities for a fulfilling 'third age' of relative good health and affluence as well as for dependency. He argued that the portion of most people's lives spent in retirement is increasing. The idea of a fixed retirement age is being challenged by the many individuals who have chosen early retirement. For many, Laslett argued, this provides possibilities for undertaking the self-enriching activities that there was not enough time for when they were preoccupied with the tasks of working or bringing up children. Laslett identifies education as one of the key areas for a successful third age and to this end he has been a proponent of the University of the Third Age.

This theme meshes well with the work of sociologists of culture such as Featherstone & Hepworth (1991), who argue that there has been a blurring of the distinction between 'middle' and 'old' age. This has occurred because of the increasing influence of life-style and consumerism on significant numbers of people outside of the younger age groups who have been typically associated with these developments. An important aspect of these processes is that old age becomes seen as a 'mask' detracting from the person beneath. Older people feel that they are just the same as they were when they were younger. The 'mask of ageing' is accentuated in modern societies where the collapse of clear age-appropriate distinctions of clothing has meant that clothing such as jeans can be worn by people of very different ages. This contributes to what has been described as the 'postmodernization of the life course' where the idea of a linear life course, with clearly defined stages, has become more and more problematic. The distinction between adolescence and adulthood has become blurred as teenagers become more adult in their pursuits and adults become used to an extended period of pleasure-seeking non-responsibility, often waiting until their 30s or 40s to have children. Similarly, with the popularity of early retirement among the more affluent (and male) members of society, the idea of a simple work and child-rearing trajectory to life suggests an ideal that is no longer the case.

Cultures of ageing

Gilleard & Higgs (2000) have argued that these changes to the nature of old age suggest that we need to see later life in the context of what they call the 'cultures of ageing'. It is not just the individualized 'mask' of ageing that needs to be understood but the whole social terrain on which ageing occurs. They argue that the issues of individual ageing are caught up in a number of cultural processes such as not wanting to be identified as 'old' or being seen in terms of a category of 'loss'. This leads to growing opportunities for the anti-ageing industry's products. These products reach back across all age groups so that the impact of cultures of ageing is felt at earlier and earlier ages. Wrinkles and greying hair are only small examples of the concerns of such 'nutraceuticals'. It is equally important to establish that there are no activities outside the ambition of older people, whether it is running a marathon or indeed, as the astronaut John Glenn has done (aged 77), going back into space. As examples of this it is possible to point to the growing involvement of older people in entertainment and tourist markets, where they are able to enjoy pleasures previously deemed inappropriate for their age group. The importance of consumerism and consumer culture for third-age lifestyles is central to this approach. As the cultural distinctions previously dominated by social class are replaced by individually focused lifestyles, the consequences of ageing become one of the principal arenas where identity is played out. It is not surprising that at the core of many of these changes to later life is the impact of the post-war 'baby boom' cohorts who in the circumstances of expanding choice and economic prosperity created a 'generational schism' between themselves and those who had grown up in less prosperous times. This schism manifested itself in music and clothes but most significantly in life-styles where there have been cumulative changes to the nature of families, relationships and sexuality. An important part of this 'generational habitus' (Gilleard & Higgs 2005) is that it has not been discarded as the teenagers of the sixties became the middle-aged of the 1990s. It is this generationally located set of dispositions that Gilleard and Higgs see as transforming the experience of later life.

Gilleard & Higgs (2000) accept that a lot of the transformation of later life depends on older people having the resources to be able to participate in the various cultural activities now open to them. This brings in themes associated with the structured dependency approach. The association of age with poverty has been a historical reality for the last two centuries at least. However, is this connection about the nature of poverty rather than of age? The ability to participate in social life has always been dependent on having sufficient resources, and may not necessarily be a consequence of reaching retirement age. Industrialization created a class of wage labourers who spent most of their lives in poverty. Only in the latter part of the 20th century did the standard of living of the mass of workers start to approach a degree of affluence. As these cohorts of relatively affluent workers reached retirement they brought with them some of the benefits they had accrued during their working lives which they could use to pursue the life-styles that they had developed earlier in life.

Gilleard & Higgs (2000, 2005) argue that a major difficulty that many studies of later life suffer from is that they assume that old age is a stable phenomenon, rather than being one that is changing constantly. Present cohorts of retired people, as we have seen, are better off than the ones that preceded them and have their own dispositions This transformation of later life might not continue indefinitely as some of the unique factors associated with the 'baby boomer' generation disappear. Equally, it is difficult to imagine that later life will return to the circumstances that marked out the problem of 'old age' in earlier decades of the twentieth century. Each cohort of people entering retirement needs to be studied separately to fully understand the circumstances and experiences that have fashioned them and upon which they will draw.

CONCLUSION

If the 20th century was the first century to see large numbers of people survive into old age, then it is likely that the 21st century will be one where the implications of this transformation will become apparent. Not only will the assumptions of social and health policy be challenged, but so also will the whole of our understanding of the 'stages of life'. If it is now possible for post-menopausal women to give birth to babies through assisted conception then it is likely that other fundamental features of the ageing process will be turned on their head. How, or whether, these changes will be addressed is unclear, but it is an inescapable fact that they will become a more and more pressing context for all of us.

References

Äijänseppa S et al 2005 Physical functioning in elderly Europeans: 10 year changes in the north and south: the HALE project. Journal of Epidemiology and Public Health 59:413–419

Arber S, Ginn J 2004 Ageing and gender: diversity and change. Social Trends 34:1–14. Stationery Office, London

Brocklehurst A, Tallis R, Fillet H 1992 Textbook of geriatric medicine and gerontology. Churchill Livingstone, Edinburgh

Bury M, Holme A 1991 Life after ninety. Routledge, London

Cumming E, Henry W 1961 Growing old: the process of disengagement. Basic Books, New York

Department for Work and Pensions (DWP) 2000 The pensioners' income series 1999/2000. National statistics. HMSO, London

Department for Work and Pensions (DWP) 2007 The pensioners' income series 2005/2006. National statistics. HMSO, London

Estes C, Biggs S and Phillipson C 2003 Social theory, social policy and ageing. Open University Press, Maidenhead

Evandrou M, Falkingham J 1993 Social security and the life course: developing sensitive policy alternative. In: Arber S, Evandrou M (eds) Ageing, independence and the life course. Jessica Kingsley, London

Evandrou M, Falkingham J 2000 Looking back to look forward: lessons from four birth cohorts for ageing in the 21st century. Population Trends 99:21–30

Featherstone M, Hepworth M 1991 The mask of ageing and the post-modern lifecourse. In: Featherstone M, Hepworth, Turner B (eds) The body: social process and cultural theory. Sage, London

Fries J 1983 The compression of morbidity. Milbank Quarterly 397–419

Gilleard C, Higgs P 2000 Cultures of ageing: self, citizen and the body. Prentice Hall, Harlow

Gilleard C, Higgs P 2005 Contexts of ageing: class, cohort and community. Polity, Cambridge

Henwood M 1992 Through a glass darkly: community care and older people. The King's Fund, London

HMSO 2000 Living in Britain 1998. General household survey. HMSO, London

HMSO 2001 Social trends 31. HMSO, London

HMSO 2004 Living in Britain 2002. General household survey. HMSO, London

Johnson P, Falkingham J 1992 Ageing and economic welfare. Sage, London

Laslett P 1996 A fresh map of life, 2nd edn. Weidenfeld and Nicholson, London

Moody H 1995 Ageing, meaning and the allocation of resources. Ageing and Society 15:163–245

Neugarten B et al 1964 Personality in middle and late life. Atherton, New York

Office of National Statistics 2007 Social trends 37. Palgrave Macmillan, London

PSSRU 2003 Cognitive impairment in older people: Its implications for future demand for services Discussion paper 1728. PSSRU, London

PSSRU 2007 Dementia UK. Alzheimer's Society, London

Phillipson C 1982 Capitalism and the construction of old age. Methuen, London

Townsend P 1981 The structured dependency of the elderly. Ageing and Society 1:5–28

Victor C 1994 Old age in modern society. Chapman and Hall, London

Victor C, Scharf T 2005 Social isolation and loneliness. In: Walker A (ed) Understanding quality of life in old age. Open University Press, Maidenhead

Walker A 1981 Towards a political economy of old age. Ageing and Society 1:73–94

Walker A, Maltby T 1997 Ageing Europe. Open University Press, Buckingham

Wanless D 2001 Securing our future health: taking a long term view, an interim report. HM Treasury, London

The social process of defining disease

CHAPTER

12 The limits and boundaries to medical knowledge

Paul Higgs

WESTERN MEDICINE

In the contemporary world, the existence of infective agents as a cause of ill health is seen as such as an obvious truth that it hardly needs stating. In a similar fashion, most people are aware that they risk infection if they don't try to keep wounds clean. Two hundred years ago such precautions were not so obvious. The threat to health posed by microorganisms was not part of everyday understanding because such organisms had not yet been identified by science. This did not mean that until the introduction of the theory of sepsis people did not know about the dangers of leaving a wound open to the air. However, an individual's understanding of what was happening was often very different from one centring on the idea of infective agents.

All societies have had ways of dealing with the problems of illness and disease and these ideas made (and in many cases still do make) perfect sense to the people involved. From our vantage point at the beginning of the 21st century, the dominant views of earlier centuries or other cultures might seem strange, if not irrational. Modern medicine can seem to be qualitatively different from these other approaches because it is based on the obviously superior rationality of modern science. The evidence to support this view is compelling, given that medical science can diagnose, treat and cure many of the afflictions that have affected human beings for thousands of years. The difficulty with this approach is that it tells only part of the story. Both medicine and science exist in social contexts that can place limits as well as challenges to their activities. This chapter looks at some of the issues involved.

As an example, we can return to germ theory. The discovery of germs is only part of the picture, especially when this particular theory of illness causation can be overextended to account for many other 'social' processes. This can happen because an idea like that of the 'germ' can catch the public imagination and become part of popular mythology (Lupton 1994). It has been used both to label certain individuals or groups as potentially dangerous, and as a metaphor for social persecution where the undesired group are seen as 'germs' infecting the wider society (Bauman 1995).

To understand fully the workings of medicine in the modern world we must look at the circumstances in which medical knowledge comes about. We must also examine how people understand and are influenced by medical knowledge. Our starting point must be the inextricable link between modern medicine and the world of science. Again, this might seem an unnecessary point to make but the history of medicine need not have culminated in the dominance of what has been described as 'western scientific medicine'. Other highly complex systems of medicine have flourished in other cultures, often for thousands of years (Porter 1998).

Conventional accounts of the development of western science stress its emergence out of irrationalism and magic. Applauding prescientific thinkers for their energy in trying to understand and change the natural world, science and the work of scientists starts to come into existence when the metaphysics is replaced by approaches based on observation and experiment. Seeking-out the regularities of phenomena and explaining why they should be so allows science to be both rational and neutral. Such understanding is seen to form the basis for technological innovation.

Normal science and paradigm shifts

However, as some historians and philosophers of science have pointed out, the idea of a simple distinction between irrational prescience and rational science is not always convincing. In his work 'The structure of scientific revolutions', Thomas Kuhn (1970) pointed out that the way in which science operates is often very far from a rigorous objective assessment of evidence. Instead, Kuhn argues, scientific ideas are organized into definable paradigms of ideas that create a state of what he describes as 'normal science'. Such paradigms define the areas of acceptable knowledge and most scientists work within the framework of ideas provided by such approaches. This means that theories that work in accordance with the paradigm are regarded as the common sense of scientific investigation. Where problems concerning evidence occur they are treated as anomalies to the paradigmatic understanding. New phenomena can provide the basis for a new theory only when the conceptual understanding necessary for the new theory has been established. When scientific change does occur it is often the result of a crisis in the existing theory that brings about a radical change in ideas. This change is what Kuhn calls a 'paradigm shift'. This, rather than the empirical 'falsification' of theories, is what happens in the development of science.

Jewson and the disappearance of the patient from medical cosmologies

Bedside medicine

The idea that scientific knowledge can be understood as a series of successive paradigms, each one replacing the last, has been applied to the development of western medicine.

Jewson (1976) noted that there has been a progressive displacement of the patient from the centre of medical interest. He argues that prescientific medicine can be characterized as 'bedside medicine' because the doctor or physician had to have a very close relationship with the paying patient who provided his income. This ensured a concern with the particular complaints, symptoms and circumstances of individual patients.

The nature of the medical knowledge at the time was based on the notion of imbalances in the four basic humours of the sanguine (blood), the choleric (yellow bile), the melancholic (black bile) and the phlegmatic (phlegm). Diagnosis and treatment were in terms of restoring the appropriate balance between the humours whose disequilibrium had brought about the illness. In this system of medicine, illness was the same thing as the symptoms reported and not the outward sign of something else. Hence, the focus of medical activity had to be individual patients and their concerns.

This system of medicine had its origins in the works of ancient Greeks and Romans and was still the basis of medical knowledge well into the 17th century. However, according to the work of the American sociologist Robert Merton (1970), the impact of the Protestant Reformation in 16th century Europe provided the impetus for a more experimentally-based theory of how the body worked. Crucially, it allowed the anatomical dissection of corpses, which had been suppressed under conventional Catholicism. This was of tremendous importance because up until this point the knowledge that most physicians had about anatomy was gleaned from Galen's treatise 'On the conduct of anatomy', which was written in the second century AD and was based on the dissection of monkeys rather than humans. Consequently, the publication of works using direct observation to illustrate a human dissection provided one of the bases for an empirical programme of comparative anatomy where the normal could be distinguished from the pathological.

Hospital medicine

The ability to look at patients in the context of what was normal allowed medicine to move away from bedside medicine and towards what Jewson described as 'hospital medicine'. The requirement to provide material for scientific investigation resulted in a need for 'cases' to study. Hospitals came to dominate the healthcare scene in the 19th century, where the poor would often be allowed access to medical diagnosis if they would offer themselves up for study. Patients' reports of their symptoms became less important than the physical signs their bodies manifested, and both were merely indications of underlying pathological lesions that were the real problem.

Under hospital medicine, the patient's physical body became crucially important in aiding the understanding of illness. The way in which medicine was practised also changed. The physical examination came to be seen by doctors as a more objective method of investigation than the personal accounts provided by the patient. As the 19th century progressed, medical science developed a number of methods for investigating the bodies of patients, such as the stethoscope and the X-ray. The invention of the stethoscope by the French physician Rene Laennec in 1816 was particularly important because it allowed the patient to be examined rather than just observed. Pathology could be localized, confirmed by autopsy and compared with the experience of other physicians. In turn, essential bodily activities such as the pulse could be quantified, leading to standardized measures of physical functioning.

Laboratory medicine

To hospital medicine Jewson adds a further development specific to the 20th century – that of 'laboratory medicine'. Here, the importance of the body and the physical examination is undermined by the molecular processes underlying normal physical functioning. By studying these, and by the patient providing specimens, medicine can diagnose difficulties that might not even give rise to symptoms or expressions of illness, and through pharmacology deal with them.

Surveillance medicine

The development of western biomedicine results in the essential 'dualism' of the body and mind in medical practice, where the individual's body is treated as separate from his or her understanding of it. That such approaches have had a negative effect on the practice of medicine is suggested by the popularity of holistic approaches to medical care. Possibly in response to this, Armstrong (1995) suggests a new development in the emergence of what he describes as 'surveillance medicine'. In this development it is not just the ill patient who is the focus of concern but the whole population. Using the results of health surveys, surveillance medicine starts from the premise that absence of disease is not the same as health. As people go about their everyday lives they exhibit, to varying degrees, many different risk factors, such as diet, weight, behaviour, and so on. Instead of localized pathology occurring at specific moments, all symptoms, signs and diseases become 'factors' of constructed 'risks'. Diets rich in saturated fats allied to obesity (measured by the body–mass index) found among people who smoke are illustrative of factors increasing the risk of coronary heart disease. Unlike the underlying pathology identified by hospital medicine, which would eventually erupt into illness or 'clinical consciousness', all that risk factors identify are propensities to future outcomes, which might in turn be transformed into new risk factors. The time frame for medicine becomes the whole lifespan. This has effects on the form of clinical intervention, which must approach health care through information campaigns and that seeks to encourage the self-monitoring of risk by individuals, as well as behavioural change. More recently Nettleton & Burrows (2003) have pointed out that if Jewson's schema depended upon a demarcation between the producers and users of biomedical knowledge, then in the circumstances of the growth of information technology such a distinction is being broken down to create what they call 'e-scaped medicine'. As they write, modern medicine is no longer exclusive to the medical school or the medical text. It is no longer contained within the institutional frameworks of medicine but has 'escaped' into wider domains where it can be 'accessed, assessed and reappropriated'. In such a scenario Nettleton and Burrows argue the sites of the production of medical knowledge are more diffuse and accompany a shift away from the expertise of the individual clinician and towards a mediation of the views of users, consumers and pressure groups as well as those of the medical profession.

SOCIAL CONSTRUCTIONISM
Michel Foucault and the clinical gaze

The French philosopher Michel Foucault has been extremely influential in developing what are known as social constructionist approaches. Foucault claims that the development of modern medicine has taken the particular route that it has because it simultaneously constructs its own object of inquiry and comes up with ideas to explain and deal with it. To the prescientific physician the evidence for the existence of humours was as compelling as the modern doctor's acceptance of the evidence provided by X-rays. The medieval anatomists using Galen's account of the body could 'see' what he had told them was there because that was what they were supposed to see. Foucault (1976) argued that with the creation of the hospital came what he describes as the 'clinical gaze', which established the idea that disease was a discrete phenomenon of the human anatomy. For Foucault, the gaze is a way of seeing and understanding that becomes identical with the thing itself.

■ Social constructionism and the sociology of the body

For Foucault, there are no fixed meanings or even the possibility of an appeal to an external reality. Such 'social constructionism'.is marked by an interest in how health and illness is created and understood by society and by social processes, rather than seeking to find a biological basis for them. The anthropologist Mary Douglas (1970) has written that in many cultures the body has often been seen as an image of society. As a result, our notions about the body will often relate to prevailing ideas about society.

Consequently, for Foucault, it is not only how medical science sees the body that is affected by discourses of knowledge, but also how people themselves view their own bodies. The shift from traditional agricultural forms of society to modern industrial ones, as Shilling (1993) points out, has also been marked by a transition from a concern with the 'fleshy' body to an interest in the 'mindful body'. What this means is that instead of the body being just an object synonymous with the person, the mind is given a central role in directing what the body does and is made responsible for it. We can see in the emphasis given to health promotion an echo of this approach.

The rise of the 'mindful body' itself also changes the nature of health and illness, as new 'problems' and new 'solutions' become commonplace in medicine. In the 19th century, Foucault (1981) argues, a concern developed regarding the nature of sexuality and the problem of the 'hysterical woman' and the 'masturbating child'. The worry arose that if these tendencies were not countered then the health of the nation would be harmed. In a different way, current worries regarding fitness and slimming are seen as ways of being desirable and attractive in a consumer society that puts great store on image.

The work of Michel Foucault has acted as a challenge to many sociologists to look at how what is taken as normal and benign is in fact the product of our own contemporary imagination. In fields as diverse as dentistry and surgery, Foucaldian analyses have been put forward to account for what is described as the 'fabrication' of discourses and to locate the operation of 'micro-power'. Ultimately, Foucault was interested in how power permeated every aspect of society to such a degree that everybody was involved in the exercise of it. In his studies of madness (Foucault 1973) and penal policy (Foucault 1977) he demonstrated that far from there having been progress to a more humane position, what resulted from psychiatry and penology was more controlling and more invasive. Ironically, one of the dilemmas that resulted from these pieces of research has been the relativization of the subject under study. It can become impossible to see the benefit in any system of knowledge and, as a consequence, impossible to believe there is any point in changing it. This has been particularly true of some feminist researchers who have been influenced by Foucault.

■ Erving Goffman and bodily idiom

The work of the American sociologist Erving Goffman provides another way in which the body plays a role in constructing our understanding of health and illness. Goffman argues that fundamental to human interaction and communication is the level of non-verbal language in which the body plays a major part. What is called 'body idiom' indicates to all those who share a culture all sorts of important knowledge. What a person says needs to be backed up with the appropriate clothes, gestures, expressions, and so on, if it is to be accepted. Body idiom allows people to classify, label and grade others. It is a continual process that is ever-present in all public interactions. It plays a crucial role in creating individuals' self-identities, as well as their social identities.

Control over the body is therefore important for people in social interactions with strangers. People with physical disabilities are at a disadvantage because if they lack control over parts of their bodies this might interfere with the process of communication. Goffman argues that this can lay the basis for the 'stained' identity that forms the basis of 'stigmatization'. It is not at all surprising, therefore, that many people with disabilities would prefer to 'mask' and 'pass' off their disablement rather than be classified in terms of their disability. However, this strategy also has its drawbacks given the continual need for the individual to be wary of 'leaking' their discredited identity to others. Epilepsy is one condition where this can occur (see Chapter 13).

Goffman's (1968) account of the social construction of disability as stigma is very useful when we look at how the interaction of people in society plays an important role in creating healthcare problems. The existence of stigma leads one part of medicine to become involved in attempting to find ways of countering the visible signs of stigmatizing conditions with techniques such as corrective surgery, whereas another part attempts to find causes and cures. As a result, medicine becomes involved with issues such as erasing face-disfiguring port-wine birthmarks, providing prosthetic limbs and providing growth hormones for children of lower than average height.

MEDICINE, MEDICALIZATION AND SOCIAL CONTROL

The fact that medicine is wrapped inextricably in social processes means that it is continually expected to move into fresh areas and deal with new problems. Part of the reason for this is the very success of medical science and technology. The capacities opened up by drug research, computerization and the new genetics mean that – potentially – most areas of life can be the focus for medical intervention. Although this is widely welcomed as providing more and more sick people with ways of being made better, it also represents problems on a number of fronts. People can feel that many of their own life experiences are being taken over by a detached biomedical elite. The experience of many women giving birth has been precisely this: that pregnancy is treated like an illness and that the procedures involved in giving birth to a child have been constructed with the doctor in mind rather than the mother. A dispute still rages as to whether hi-tech deliveries are less hazardous than ones that perhaps take place in the mother's home and at the mother's pace. However, the very fact that such a debate exists illustrates that there is some unease at the direction taken by modern medicine.

It is not only patients who are wary of the increased expectations placed upon them by both the public and pharmaceutical companies. The *British Medical Journal* (BMJ) conducted a poll on its website to identify the top ten non-diseases that healthcare workers were supposed to deal with. These included boredom, baldness, bags under eyes and ugliness (Smith 2002). Part of the problem is that biomedicine has become an integral part of what has been termed 'aspirational medicine' (Gilleard & Higgs 2000) where the individual desires of the population are transformed into biomedical priorities. Top of the BMJ list of non-diseases was, unsurprisingly, ageing. The research into avoiding the physical signs of ageing crosses over into research on overcoming ageing itself. Expectations on medicine are therefore created and these can lead to disappointment when reality does not match the ideal.

This can become even more of a problem if expectations are combined with a belief that risks to health can be avoided if people are forewarned. Anthony Giddens (1991) has described modern societies as experiencing what he calls 'manufactured uncertainty' in relation to risk. Such uncertainty is the result of too much information about risks and no real way of assessing their true impact. The controversy over the safety of eating beef against its potential for causing the devastating dementia of Creutzfeldt–Jakob disease illustrates this phenomenon. A similar fear arose about the safety of the combined measles, mumps and rubella (MMR) inoculation given to children and its potential to trigger autism. Both examples demonstrate the power of information simultaneously to make individuals aware of an issue but provide no conclusive answers to their concerns.

Iatrogenesis

Another aspect of the increasing involvement of medicine in many different aspects of social life is what the radical Latin American priest Ivan Illich (1975) calls 'iatrogenesis', or self-caused disease. He claims that there are three distinct types of iatrogenesis: clinical, cultural and social. 'Clinical iatrogenesis' is when medical treatment makes that patient worse or creates new conditions. As the old joke goes, the last place you want to be if you are ill is a hospital because that is where all the other sick people are and you'll catch whatever they have got. Although this might be a gross simplification it is not entirely without foundation. It is also possible that the medical intervention itself could be unnecessary or irrelevant. 'Social iatrogenesis' is the label Illich attaches to the way in which medicine expands into more and more areas, creating an artificial demand for its services. This in turn leads on to 'cultural iatrogenesis', whereby the ability to cope with the issues surrounding life and death is eroded progressively by medical accounts. This leads to a reliance on medicine to solve problems and a corresponding decrease in autonomy. Illich believes that, as a consequence, the scope of modern medicine should be demystified if not curtailed.

Connected to these notions is the fact that medicine can, as we have seen, create its own problems by medicalizing hitherto non-medicalized areas of life. A good example is the case of heroin addiction (Dally 1995). At first sight, this might seem an area of obvious medical action but through most of the 19th century it was regarded as a pastime and not a medical concern. This changed when it became a controlled drug in 1906. However, even up to the 1960s a small but significant number of addicts were enabled to maintain their addiction through private prescriptions provided by some GPs in private practice. What this meant was that these addicts were not criminalized and were thus enabled to live lives of relative stability. What problems these individuals had were ones of lifestyle and not necessarily the result of a medical condition. What changed this state of affairs was a number of people abusing the system and the identification of the medical category – 'drug dependency' – as a field of activity for the speciality of psychiatry. Addiction was to be cured rather than controlled. Gradually there was a change in the approach taken towards addicts; now they were to be actively treated to remove their dependency on heroin. Methadone replacement therapy was offered as an alternative. Unfortunately, it did not have a particularly high success rate and many addicts dropped out of the programmes, usually resorting to illegal 'street' heroin. This in turn brought them into conflict with the police and ensured that, to maintain supplies for their addiction, they had to adopt a criminal lifestyle.

In this manner it could be argued that medicine, by being morally pressurized to do something about a social problem, ends up adding to, rather than dealing with, the real issues of drug addiction. Part of this attitude can be seen in the dilemma about the high rates of HIV infection among intravenous drug users. Do you give out syringes and thereby condone illegal drug use, or do you refuse and let infection rates increase?

■ Mental illness

A way of understanding these issues is to utilize the concept of social control. All societies need to have some form of generally accepted value system if they are to remain relatively stable. This, by definition, creates people who refuse to, or cannot, fit in. These people become seen, and are often treated, as deviants. Various groups at different times can be seen to occupy this category. They could be members of youth subcultures, new-age travellers or criminals but they all play the same role in that they enable the majority to define themselves in terms of who they are not. Medicine can, and has, played a role in defining populations of deviants by finding medical conditions for them. This happened most notoriously in the former Soviet Union, where people opposing the nature of the State were often diagnosed as having severe psychiatric problems necessitating hospitalization. However, similar things happened in Britain up until the early decades of the 20th century, where pregnancy outside marriage was regarded as indicative of an absence of morals, which could only have a medical cause. To this end, a number of 'rebels' within the psychiatric profession, such as Szasz (1966), have argued that psychiatry's main role is to control deviant populations because of the tremendous legal and categorizing powers capable of being invoked. Often, those subject to psychiatric control lose all social and civil rights and are subject to controversial treatments such as electroconvulsive therapy. In addition, those labelled as mentally ill are completely at the mercy of those treating them and can regain their lives only if they agree with these people.

In contrast to the 'anti-psychiatrists', Hirst & Woolley (1982) argue that it would be wrong to assert that there is no real negative context to mental illness. They point out that all cultures have categories to express the idea that a person is not functioning properly. These might be seen as episodic occurrences or more long-term difficulties, but they are identified by most people as problems none the less. Psychiatry does become involved in controlling some members of society, but this is not sufficient reason to claim that this is its only function.

MEDICINE, SOCIAL STRUCTURE AND SOCIAL POLICY

The practice of medicine is not confined to the ideas that determine what is and what is not a medical problem. Modern medicine has come into being at the same time as industrialization and has become an integral feature of it. As countries have become more technologically advanced so has medicine. Since the Second World War, breakthroughs connected to groups of drugs such as antibiotics have meant that many infectious diseases can now be successfully dealt with. Previously deadly diseases such as smallpox have been officially eradicated from the planet. With this success has come a growth in demand for modern health services throughout the world. Because modern medicine is perceived as being capable of achieving great things with people's health, then more and more people want access to it. This has meant that many developing nations are put in impossible situations trying to provide costly hi-tech medicine in environments where there are few resources.

At this point it is useful to remember McKeown's argument that the improvement in the health of the British population during the 19th and early 20th centuries was a result of improvements in diet, sanitation and public health (McKeown 1979). The efforts of doctors did not make much impact until the second part of the 20th century (see Chapter 1). The impressive strides made by medical knowledge therefore depend crucially on the existence of a wider social infrastructure that can support such advances. In most societies this is formalized into some form of healthcare system. There are many different types of healthcare system (Roemer 1989) (see Chapter 19). Some organize health care on free-market principles with the State playing a minimal role except to provide a safety-net for certain underprivileged groups, whereas others are based on compulsory State insurance, as in France. Britain is quite unusual in the way it organizes its health service because it is funded out of general taxation rather than through individual contributions.

However, the differences between healthcare systems do not just reflect national characteristics but are different solutions to the problems of providing access to medical and health services and being able to pay for it. At its most simple, this accounts for the disparities in healthcare provision in some developing countries. The possession of wealth or being an expatriate of a western nation means that you have access to medical facilities as good as those in the industrialized countries. Correspondingly, if you are poor your access to services is likely to be minimal and might in fact be rudimentary.

■ Power and the politics of health

The existence of welfare states in the industrialized countries is a relatively recent phenomenon. Britain introduced old age pensions and a limited medical insurance scheme at the beginning of the 20th century, and the welfare state of which the National Health Service was a cornerstone did not come into being until 1948. Among the reasons put forward for this delay was the belief that State welfare was a victory for the working class because it shifted responsibility for paying for individual welfare away from the poorest sections of society. Marxist writers (Ferguson et al 2002, Gough 1979, Navarro 1994) argued that the provision of health care was a key battlefield in the conflict between labour and employers in all societies. The working class wants to ameliorate as many of the adverse conditions created by capitalism as it can, whereas the employers want to make as much profit as they can at as little cost. Sometimes, as in post-war Britain, the Marxist position holds, concessions regarding the provision by the State of welfare services have to be made to allow the overall profitability of the market ecnomy to continue. At other times, such as during the 1970s and 1980s, cuts will be made to this 'social wage' in order that the maximum amout of money flows to profit-making sectors. This is not to suggest that health care is only an outcome of political struggle. Marxist theorists also identified the role of the welfare state in sustaining a profitable capitalism over the medium to long term. The welfare state can be seen to carry out three roles: to ensure the health and education of the existing workforce; to produce the next generation of workers; and to justify the inequalities of capitalism. Of course, not all of these things can be done successfully all of the time, and this is why the welfare state seems in a constant state of crisis.

It is not only Marxists who have noted the close connection between the economy and the welfare state that has resulted in a crisis for the idea of a welfare state. Mishra (1984) noted that if money is to be spent on welfare the first thing that has to be established is economic prosperity. During the last few decades of the 20th century many different governments, from New Zealand to Holland, sought to reduce state expenditure and overcome what was sometimes known as the 'fiscal crisis of the state' which was seen to result from the tendency for welfare, and particularly health spending, to increase inexorably over time. This led many policy analysts to argue that a limit to public spending was essential if health care was to continue to be publicly funded and organized. Much of the impetus to reform healthcare systems in Britain and throughout the industrialized world was concentrated on finding ways of controlling costs and making the delivery of health care more effective and efficient. This was often interpreted as diminishing the range and quality of services provided by the welfare state in the interests of the wealthier sections of the population who had less need for them. From the 1980s Britain saw the introduction of what has been known as 'managed competition' or 'quasi-markets' and the widespread introduction of 'privatization' of services and function. The focus was on reducing the size of the public sector and of allowing market forces to operate wherever possible. This was politically contentious and since 1997 has been replaced by a 'third way' politics which seeks to accommodate the market within the processes of health care commissioning as well, through the introduction of public-private partnerships to build hospitals and other healthcare facilities. While the extent to which it is possible to be both financially efficient and socially equitable is still keenly debated in the context of changes to the NHS, what is also clearly evident is that the provision of health services is so intrinsically political that it cannot be reduced to a question of administration.

■ The emergence of the 'consumer citizen' and social policy

One important direction in which social policy is going is the development of what has been described as the 'consumer-citizen' which has radically transformed the relationship between the State and its citizens. The idea of mass citizenship entitlements, which was fundamental to the creation of the welfare state and of the National Health Service, has become seen as an anachronism not suitable for modern times. To many sociologists the world is no longer made up of people defining themselves in terms of class or seeing their interests represented collectively in trade unions or nationalist parties. Instead, individuals need to negotiate among the many potential identities that can form the basis of a more individualized relationship with society. These can relate to culture, sexuality, religion and generation to name a few. Such a focus on ideas of identity leads directly to the role of consumption and consumerism in transforming many facets of everyday life including notions of citizenship. Instead of thinking about how social policies are related to national political concerns, modern citizen-consumers are expected to have a very different approach to government at both local and national levels. Policies are to be viewed in much the same way that other aspects of individuals' consumer lives are judged, that is, in terms of choice and value for money. In this environment league tables, performance indicators and the provision of alternatives are seen as crucial in establishing public satisfaction (Vidler & Clarke 2005). Government on the other hand sees its role as the enabling of individuals to operate successfully in an increasingly consumerized world (Giddens 2000). In fields as diverse as pensions, education and unemployment, the onus is on the individual to take responsibility and make choices. This approach accepts that there will be differences of outcome but such differences reflect a complex world where government oversees the various markets but is loathe to intervene unless security or larger interests are affected.

The nature of medicine and the provision of health services reflect this approach. The idea of medical paternalism that has been dominant throughout earlier periods of modernity is increasingly challenged. Professional autonomy and regulation finds itself under public scrutiny. The role of the General Medical Council (GMC) in regulatng the medical profession has been seriously challenged by the impact of a number of medically related scandals, from the the Bristol Royal Infirmary Inquiry into heart surgery on children to the conviction of Harold Shipman for multiple murders. The notion that professional status is a sufficient guarantee for both ethical and effective behaviour is one that no longer chimes with wider concerns. This transformation extends further to the very shape of modern medicine itself. In a consumer society, not only has the hierachy of knowledge and power broken down but what the public has a right to expect from the providers of health care has now become subject to consumer demand and interests. The simple distinction between dealing with disease and enhancing health in its most comprehensive form can be illustrated by the public response to the prescribing of Viagra for erectile dysfunction. Not only has Viagra become a lifestyle drug promising better sex but it has also entered the public consciousness as a recognizable brand, shape and metaphor.

In return for this choice and enablement the citizen-consumer is at the centre of a process of constant monitoring and surveillance of both practitioners and patients. The new citizen is not expected to be passive or reluctant to engage with the opportunities presented to him or her. A term coined by Michel Foucault, 'governmentality', is useful to situate this process. What it refers to is the guiding of behaviour or organizing the 'conduct of conduct'. The emphasis is on ensuring that individuals choose the 'correct' way to do something. In the arena of health there have always been correct ways to act such as cleaning your teeth or not smoking. This has now extended to many other areas such as diet, exercise and sexual behaviour. The role of the healthcare system becomes increasingly one that is involved in attempting to modify individual behaviours in accordance with contemporary knowledge. This role is a double-edged sword because it can easily lead to the conclusion that individual behaviour is the source of many social problems as well as being their solution. An example of this can be found in the early 'New Labour' government's response to UK health inequalities, where recommendations of income redistribution were rejected in favour of promoting health behaviour change. While individual change can bring some benefits to some individuals, it can only be partially successful and of necessity leaves those who are unable or unwilling to change to their fate. This form of 'double jeopardy' is one that the poor and the sick have had to deal with from the inception of modern medicine. National healthcare systems were often justified in terms of ensuring that this inequity was consigned to the past. It would be a tragedy if in the name of choice and empowerment the marginalized were once again left to their fate.

203

CONCLUSION

This chapter has attempted to cover some of the boundaries to the practice of medicine that exist in the modern world. It has drawn attention to the social and cultural aspects of the construction of medical knowledge. It has also pointed out that medicine and health care can, and have, been involved in the construction and maintenance of forms of social power through the socially sanctioned authority to define what are medical or health problems. These concerns might seem incidental to the way that modern medicine is practised today with its emphasis on consumption and choice. However, to ignore these issues is to neglect in some part the way in which we have reached this point of success and the way in which this is not equally shared. A failure to integrate the practice of medicine with its social context, or to face up to some of the difficult implications of its practice, may blunt the potential of medicine to be a truly humanitarian project rather than just a set of technical skills.

References

Armstrong D 1995 The rise of surveillance medicine. Sociology, Health and Illness 17:393–404

Bauman Z 1995 Life in fragments: essays in postmodern morality. Blackwell, Oxford

Dally A 1995 Anomalies and mysteries in the war on drugs. In: Porter R, Teich M (eds) Drugs and narcotics in history. Cambridge University Press, Cambridge

Douglas M 1970 Natural symbols: explorations in cosmology. Cresset Press, London

Ferguson I, Lavallette M, Mooney G 2002 Rethinking welfare: a critical perspective. Sage, London

Foucault M 1973 Madness and civilisation. Tavistock, London

Foucault M 1976 The birth of the clinic. Tavistock, London

Foucault M 1977 Discipline and punish. Penguin, London

Foucault M 1981 History of sexuality, vol. 1. Penguin, Harmondsworth

Giddens A 1991 The consequences of modernity. Polity Press, Cambridge

Giddens A 2000 The third way and its critics. Polity Press, Cambridge

Gilleard C, Higgs P 2000 Cultures of ageing: self, citizen and the body. Prentice Hall, Harlow

Goffman E 1968 Stigma. Penguin, Harmondsworth

Gough I 1979 The political economy of the welfare state. Macmillan, London

Hirst P, Woolley P 1982 Social relations and human attributes. Tavistock, London

Illich I 1975 Medical nemesis. Calder and Boyars, London

Jewson N 1976 The disappearance of the sick man from medical cosmology. Sociology 10:225–244

Kuhn T 1970 The structure of scientific revolutions. University of Chicago Press, Chicago

Lupton D 1994 Medicine as culture. Sage, London

McKeown T 1979 The role of medicine. Oxford University Press, Oxford

Merton R 1970 Science, technology and society in seventeenth century England. Howard Fertig, New York

Mishra R 1984 The crisis of the welfare state. Harvester Wheatsheaf, Hemel Hempstead

Navarro V 1994 The politics of health policy. Blackwell, London

Nettleton S, Burrows R 2003 E-scaped medicine? Information, reflexivity and health. Critical Social Policy 23:165–185

Porter R 1998 The greatest benefit to mankind: a medical history of humanity. Harper Collins, London

Roemer M 1989 National health services as market interventions. Journal of Public Health Policy 10:62–77

Shilling C 1993 The body and social theory. Sage, London

Smith R 2002 In search of 'non-disease'. British Medical Journal 324:883–885

Szasz T 1966 The myth of mental illness. Harper, New York

Vidler E, Clarke J 2005 Creating citizen-consumers: New Labour and the remaking of public services. Public Policy and Administration 20(2):19–37

Deviance, sick role and stigma

Graham Scambler

INTRODUCTION

Social norms are definite principles or rules that people are expected to observe in a given culture or milieu. Only a tiny minority of norms is likely to be codified as laws. Deviance can be defined as non-conformity to a norm, or set of norms, which is accepted by a significant proportion of local citizens or inhabitants. Deviant behaviour is behaviour that, once it has become public knowledge, is routinely subject to sanctions – to punishment, correction or treatment. Importantly, behaviour that is acceptable in one culture might be deviant in another. For example, smoking marijuana is deviant in British culture whereas consuming alcohol is not; the reverse is the case in some Middle Eastern cultures.

ILLNESS, DEVIANCE AND THE SICK ROLE

Few analysts before the 1950s regarded illness as a form of deviance. The term 'deviance' was reserved for behaviour for which individuals could be held responsible; infractions of the law were seen as paradigmatic. A significant change of outlook dates from the work of Parsons (1951), who defined illness as a form of deviance on the grounds that it disrupts the social system by inhibiting people's performance of their customary or normal social roles. If such disruption is to be minimized then the behaviour associated with illness – which, unlike other forms of deviant behaviour cannot be prevented by the threat of sanctions – must be controlled. Control is exercised through the prescription of social roles for the sick and for physicians (see Chapter 4).

According to Parsons, the sick role consists of two rights and two obligations. The rights are that sick people are exempted: (1) from performing their normal social roles; and (2) from responsibility for their own state. Sick people are at the same time obligated: (1) to want to get well as soon as possible; and (2) to consult and cooperate with medical experts whenever the severity of their condition warrants it. Failure to meet either or both of these obligations could lead to the charge that people are responsible for the continuation of their illness and – ultimately – to sanctions, including the withdrawal of the rights of the sick role. Gerhardt (1987) describes Parsons' sick role as a social 'niche' where 'the incapacitated have a chance to recover from their weakness(es), and overcome their urge to withdraw from rather than actively tackle the vicissitudes of the capitalist labour market'. In fact, it can afford its incumbents a legitimate breathing space from a wide range of social demands, and not only from those associated with the labour market.

The sick role is a temporary role into which all people, regardless of their status or position, can be admitted. It is also 'universalistic', in that physicians are held to draw upon general and objective criteria in determining whether individuals are sick, how sick they are and what kinds of sickness they are suffering from. Its main function is to control illness and to reduce its disruptive effects on the social system by ensuring that sick people are returned to a healthy state as speedily as possible. Physicians serve as 'gatekeepers', policing access to the sick role by authoritatively determining who is sick and who is healthy. They also spur the urge to leave the sick role (Gerhardt 1987). Unlike some other commentators, Parsons is not at all critical of physicians functioning as agents of social control. Indeed, he sees the sick role, and physicians' policing of it, as important contributions to the stability and health of the social system.

Among those who are less sanguine about physicians' social control functions is Freidson (1970), who acknowledges Parsons' pioneering work in linking illness and deviance but insists that the argument must be taken a step further:

> Unlike Parsons, I do not argue merely that medicine has the power to legitimize one's acting sick by conceding that he really is sick ... I argue that by virtue of being the authority on what illness 'really' is, medicine creates the social possibilities for acting sick. In this sense, medicine's monopoly includes the right to create illness as an official social role.

Freidson adds that it is in medicine's interests – because it enhances the demand for its practitioners' skills – to pursue actively 'the proliferation of situations that create "deviant illness roles"'.

It is not necessary to adhere to a thesis of 'medical imperialism' – namely, to claim a conspiracy on the part of physicians to 'medicalize' society – to acknowledge either that a multiplicity of new deviant illness roles were created in the twentieth century (perhaps most conspicuously as a product of the growth of psychiatry) or that this has accorded physicians greater powers and responsibilities as agents of social control. Freidson's contribution is to have pointed out that these powers and responsibilities have social – not merely scientific – origins, and require careful analysis and evaluation. After all, to diagnose disease is to define its bearer as in need of correctional 'treatment' of body or mind (even if in practice this often involves little more than recognizing a disease's self-limiting natural history). Unlike Parsons, Freidson sees physicians' social control functions as extending far beyond the policing of the sick role and as possessing negative as well as positive potential for society.

THE FORCE OF A LABEL

In modern societies, professionally trained physicians are generally responsible not only for (collectively) constructing but also for (individually) selecting and applying diagnostic labels. It is now recognized, however, that the application and communication of some diagnoses can have especially serious and unwelcome consequences for patients. This occurs most conspicuously when the conditions being diagnosed are themselves regarded as deviant. Deviant conditions can be defined as conditions that set their possessors apart from 'normal' people, which mark them as socially unacceptable or inferior beings. Thus, people experiencing deafness, mental illness, severe burns, diabetes, psoriasis, acquired immunodeficiency syndrome (AIDS) and numerous other diseases or symptoms of disease have been in the past and continue to be avoided, rejected or shunned to varying degrees by others.

Another unhappy consequence of being labelled in this way is that people's conditions can come to dominate the perceptions that others have of them and how they treat them. In the vocabulary of sociology, an individual's deviant status is transmuted into a master status: whatever else he or she might be (mother or father, teacher or school governor) he or she is regarded primarily as a diabetic, cancer victim or whatever. In other words, the individual's deviant status comes to dominate and push into the background his or her other statuses. Even the past might be unsafe and subject to retrospective interpretation. Especially pertinent to this line of reasoning are the concepts of 'cultural stereotyping' and 'secondary deviation'.

▓ Cultural stereotyping

Those afflicted with a deviant condition might be expected to conform to a popular stereotype. An American study, for example, found that blind people are often attributed distinctive personality characteristics that differentiate them from sighted people: 'helplessness', 'dependency', 'melancholy', 'docility', 'gravity of inner thought' and 'aestheticism' (Scott 1969). However far-fetched or misleading such stereotyping might be, the blind person cannot ignore how others expect him or her to behave; to do so might well be to ignore key factors in his or her interaction with them. The author goes on to claim that blind people adapt to cultural stereotyping in five major ways: (1) simply concurring; (2) 'cutting themselves off' to protect their self-conceptions; (3) deliberately adopting a facade of compliance for expediency's sake; (4) making people pay something for a 'performance' (e.g. begging); or (5) actively resisting. It should be mentioned that they might also be obliged to respond to stereotypes of blindness held by physicians and other health professionals.

▓ Secondary deviation

One distinction that has gained currency among those investigating links between crime and deviance is that between 'primary' and 'secondary' deviation (Lemert 1967). Study of the former focuses on how deviant behaviour, for example stealing, originates. Study of the latter focuses on how people are assigned symbolically to deviant statuses, for example thief or criminal, and the effective consequences of such assignment for subsequent deviation on their part. The importance of studying secondary deviation has been increasingly acknowledged since the 1960s. It is now accepted, for example, that disapproving cultural and professional reactions to deviant behaviour can often foster rather than inhibit a continuing commitment to deviance.

Similarly, some have claimed that a negative, stereotyped reaction to a particular illness or handicap can confirm individuals in their deviant status, can constrain them to see themselves as others see them and to behave accordingly. For example, a blind person who is expected to be and is consistently treated as 'helpless' and 'dependent' might actually become so; he or she might find it less exacting to concur with and ultimately adopt the prescribed role than to resist it. Those in institutional or custodial care for long periods are particularly vulnerable in this respect.

Perhaps the area in which 'labelling theory' has had the most controversial impact in relation to medicine has been that of mental illness. In the mid-1960s the American sociologist Scheff claimed that labelling is the single most important cause of mental illness (Scheff 1966). He argued that a residue of odd, eccentric and unusual behaviour exists for which the culture provides no explicit labels: such forms of behaviour constitute 'residual rule-breaking' or 'residual deviance'. Most psychiatric symptoms can be categorized as instances of residual deviance. There is also a cultural stereotype of mental illness. When for some reason or other residual deviance becomes a salient or 'public' issue, the cultural stereotype of insanity becomes the guiding imagery for action. In time, contact with a physician is established, a psychiatric diagnosis made and, perhaps, procedures for hospitalization put into effect. Problems of secondary deviation follow with a degree of predictability.

Scheff's theory has been criticized by others, notably Gove (1970). Gove agreed that there is a cultural stereotype of mental illness, but not that people are treated as mentally ill because they inadvertently behave in a way that 'activates' this stereotype. If anything, he argued, 'the gross exaggeration of the degree and type of disorder in the stereotype fosters the denial of mental illness, since the disturbed person's behaviour does not usually correspond to the stereotype' (Gove 1970). Scheff is also wrong, according to Gove, in suggesting that, once publicly noticed, the person will be routinely processed as mentally ill and admitted for institutional care; public officials, he argued, 'screen out' a large proportion of those who come before them. Finally, Gove claimed that Scheff overstated the degree to which secondary deviation is associated with hospitalization for mental illness. Although the dispute between Scheff and his critics continues, it seems reasonable to conclude that he fell foul of the temptation to explain too much in terms of a single, if important, insight.

▪ Deviance and stigma

So far the term 'deviance' has been used in a general or inclusive fashion. Mankoff (1971) has made a distinction between 'ascribed' and 'achieved deviance'. The former refers to a condition, attribute or form of behaviour for which the individual is not held accountable: no blame attaches to it. The latter refers to a condition, attribute or behaviour for which the individual is in some way held to be culpable. Thus blindness can be described as ascribed deviance, and stealing as achieved deviance. In practice, of course, this analytic distinction is not always easy to apply. Consider injecting drug use for example, or alcoholism, or risk behaviours like smoking. Sometimes individuals who have lost their sight or experienced a myocardial infarct are chastised for behaviours judged irresponsible and implicated in the aetiology of their conditions.

Goffman's (1963) influential work on stigma overlaps with Mankoff's notion of ascribed deviance. He suggests that stigmatized individuals offend against specific types of social norm, namely, norms of identity or being: stigmatized individuals have 'spoiled identities'. It is a question, he says, of an individual's condition, not his or her will; 'it is a question of conformance, not compliance'. Picking up on this point, it has been proposed that relations of stigma imply an *ontological deficit*, while relations of deviance imply a *moral deficit* (Scambler 2004). Thus people to whom a stigma is imputed are regarded as 'imperfect beings', possessed of defects for which they are not responsible and which are beyond their capacity to correct. People to whom deviance is imputed, on the other hand, are said to be morally responsible, 'guilty' as opposed to 'innocent' in their norm-breaking. Stigma, in short, invokes norms of shame, and deviance norms of blame.

Stigma and deviance can be either 'enacted' of 'felt'. Whereas enacted stigma and deviance denote discrimination by others, felt stigma and deviance denote (1) an internalized sense of shame and blame respectively, and (2) a frequently distressing and disruptive fear of being discriminated against. In the following section we shall chart in particular the negative effects of enacted and felt stigma on the lives of some people with chronic conditions. To enacted and felt stigma and deviance might be added the notion of 'project' stigma and deviance. This recognizes the fact that some people with troublesome identities or statuses respond without either internalizing norms of shame or blame or becoming fearful, defensive or subdued by prospects of discrimination. Most studies of chronic or disabling illness reveal people who develop their own positive strategies that acknowledge the risks of enacted stigma and deviance while trying to avoid the pitfalls of felt stigma and deviance. These strategies can be said to constitute their projects (see Box 13.1 for a summary).

LIVING WITH A STIGMATIZING CONDITION

Stigmatizing conditions vary in terms of their visibility and obtrusiveness and of the extent to which they are recognized. Not surprisingly, there is an equivalent degree of variation in their effects on individuals' lives. People who are 'discredited', to use Goffman's (1963) terminology, are those whose stigma is immediately apparent, such as amputees, or widely known, such as someone whose fellow workers know of his suicide attempt. The discredited will often find they have to cope with situations made awkward by their stigma: their problem will be one of managing tension. Davis (1964) found that

BOX 13.1	Types of stigma and deviance
Stigma: an ontological deficit, reflecting infringements against norms of shame	**Deviance**: a moral deficit, reflecting infringements against norms of blame
Enacted: discrimination by others on grounds of 'being imperfect'	**Enacted**: discrimination by others on grounds of immoral behaviour
Felt: internalized sense of shame and immobilizing anticipation of enacted stigma	**Felt**: internalized sense of blame and immobilizing anticipation of enacted deviance
Project: strategies and tactics devised to avoid or combat enacted stigma without falling prey to felt stigma	**Project**: strategies and tactics devised to avoid or combat enacted deviance without falling prey to felt deviance

the physically handicapped typically pass through three stages when meeting with strangers: the first is one of 'fictional acceptance' – they find they are ascribed some sort of stereotypical identity and accepted on that basis; the second stage is one of 'breaking through' this fictional acceptance – they induce others to regard and interact with them normally; and the third stage is one of 'consolidation' – they have to sustain the definition of themselves as normal over time.

One major criticism of Davis' account is that it overestimates people's strength of will and psychological stamina to engage in what he calls 'deviance disavowal'. It was noted earlier that some blind people regard it as less taxing to defer to than to contest cultural stereotypes of blindness. Higgins (1980) found that deaf people sometimes actually 'avow' their deviance, and even extend it by acting mute in order to simplify and smooth their relations with the hearing: written messages can minimize misunderstandings and save time and embarrassment.

People who are 'discreditable' are those whose stigma is only occasionally apparent, such as people with epilepsy who suffer infrequent seizures, or little known, such as someone whose status as human immunodeficiency virus (HIV) positive is known only to his or her doctor. The discreditable will usually find they have to take care to manage information; to 'pass as normal' they will have to censor what others know about them. In Goffman's (1963) words, the main quandary is: 'To display or not to display; to tell or not to tell; to lie or not to lie: and in each case, to whom, how, when and where'. People with epilepsy frequently opt to pass as normal, and hence find themselves having to manage information with extreme caution. The following paragraphs illustrate this, and these and the succeeding sections on rectal cancer and HIV/AIDS afford some indication of the types of factors that affect adjustment to stigma.

■ Epilepsy

The adults with recurring seizures that Scambler & Hopkins (1986) studied clearly felt that, in an important sense, physicians had 'made them into epileptics' by selecting and communicating the diagnosis of epilepsy. It was a diagnostic label that most found unpleasant and threatening and some openly resented and contested, largely, it seems, because they saw the status of 'epileptic' as highly stigmatizing. Those who had been diagnosed in childhood often seemed to have learned to think of their epilepsy in this way as a result of their parents' behaviour: for example, well-intentioned advice never to use the word 'epilepsy', especially outside the home. Schneider & Conrad (1983), reporting the same finding in the USA, refer graphically to such parents as 'stigma coaches'. They add that careless or overprotective physicians can also function as stigma coaches.

Once applied, diagnostic labels tend to be difficult to shake off. Nevertheless, the stigma of people with epilepsy is dormant between seizures; for much of their time, therefore, they are discreditable rather than discredited. Scambler & Hopkins (1986) found that, fearing discrimination, people tended to conceal their epilepsy whenever possible. Witnessed seizures were often 'explained away' – for example, as faints – and 'stories' constructed to account for the fact that they could not drive – 'because of the law, or drink' – because of their anticonvulsant medication. Two-thirds of those experiencing epileptic seizures at the time of marriage hid the fact from their partners, at least until after the ceremony. Of those with full-time jobs outside the home, 28% had disclosed their epilepsy to their employers, and only 1 in 20 – all of whom were experiencing seizures daily at the time – had done so before taking the job.

The same authors made a distinction between felt stigma and enacted stigma. The former refers to the shame associated with 'being epileptic' and, most significantly perhaps, to the fear of being discriminated against solely on the grounds of an imputed cultural unacceptability or inferiority; and the latter refers to actual discrimination of this kind. Scambler (1989) has utilized this distinction to formulate a 'hidden distress model' in relation to epilepsy. This states that the sense of felt stigma is so strong that people with epilepsy typically do their utmost to maintain secrecy about their symptoms and the diagnostic label: they disclose only when it strikes them as prudent or necessary. Non-disclosure, in turn, reduces the likelihood of encountering enacted stigma. Thus felt stigma leads to a policy of concealment that has the effect of reducing the incidence of enacted stigma. Paradoxically, felt stigma was more disruptive of people's lives and well-being than was enacted stigma, which was in fact rarely experienced. Interestingly, Jacoby (1994) has since shown that felt stigma can remain salient even for people whose seizures are extremely infrequent or who are in remission. Both Scambler and Hopkins in Britain and Schneider and Conrad in the USA identified small groups of people who deliberately resisted the stigmatizing connotations of their epilepsy, thus coming into the category of project stigma outlined earlier.

◾ Rectal cancer

If in the 19th century tuberculosis stood out as the disease arousing the most dread and repulsion, cancer became its 20th-century equivalent. Sontag (1977) has argued that it is likely to occupy this role until its aetiology is clarified and its treatments as effective as those of tuberculosis. Rectal cancer accounts for 10% of cancer diagnoses. Two-thirds of those with rectal cancer are left with a permanent colostomy following amputation of the anus and rectum. A colostomy is an incontinent, artificial anus that, with no sphincter to control it, can release faeces and flatus unpredictably, generally into a plastic bag attached to the abdomen. MacDonald (1988) has examined patients' perceptions of what amounts to a family of stigmas: 'the shame, taboos and fears associated with mutilation of the body, with faecal incontinence, with seeing and handling faeces, and with cancer'.

MacDonald found that 49% of her sample reported 'some stigma' and 16% 'severe stigma'; these proportions rose to 54% and 26%, respectively, for those with a colostomy, most of whom said they felt as though they had been assaulted and were unclean. Like those with epilepsy, many opted for concealment as a first-choice strategy, felt stigma once more being the motivating factor. They were ashamed by noise and odours from the stoma and filled with self-disgust at the need to handle bags of faeces and to clean faeces from their bodies. They feared exposure because they thought others would be embarrassed or offended and drift away. Some practised 'withdrawal' rather than confront the potential hazards of passing as normal. Many of those in situations where they were discredited rather than discreditable adopted a strategy of 'covering': they took all possible steps to reduce the salience of their stigma for others, to render it unobtrusive (Goffman 1963). A third had never shown the colostomy to their spouses, and more than four-fifths had never shown it to anyone outside the hospital. MacDonald concludes that, although most people in her study learned to accommodate their stomas fairly well, 'a large fraction' suffered impaired quality of life because of their experiences of the stigma of cancer and colostomy'.

◾ HIV/AIDS

Since its recognition in 1981, the human immunodeficiency virus (HIV) has aroused strong responses. In the USA, where the HIV epidemic emerged among gay men and intravenous drug users, a persistently negative societal reaction has continued to play a

---

| **BOX 13.2** | HIV/AIDS disease trajectory |

1. A transient flu-like syndrome associated with seroconversion, developing within weeks or months of infection
2. An asymptomatic period of more than 4 years average duration
3. Symptomatic HIV infection of more than 5 years average duration
4. AIDS characterized by opportunistic illnesses, HIV wasting syndrome, HIV dementia, lymphomas, and other neoplasms, averaging 9–13 months for treated and untreated individuals combined, and 21 months for those receiving antiviral medical treatments

Reproduced with kind permission from Elsevier Science Ltd from Alonzo & Reynolds (1995).

---

vital role in the experiences of individuals with the virus. Alonzo & Reynolds (1995) suggest that individuals' adjustments to HIV/AIDS must be seen against the background of a 'biophysical disease trajectory'. They note that disease progression varies widely among individuals, but suggest that over a period of 12 or more years they will usually experience a number of stages. These are summarized in Box 13.2.

The authors then go on to identify four phases of an 'HIV stigma trajectory', which is linked to, but can vary independently of, the biophysical disease trajectory. These four phases are outlined in Box 13.3. They again stress individual variation, and also add that stigma can on occasions be 'expansive', pervading all corners of an individual's biography and identity, and on other occasions 'containable, limited and controllable in terms of consequences and, more importantly, personal and social identity'.

COURTESY STIGMA

It is apparent that those close to people with conditions like epilepsy, rectal cancer or HIV/ AIDS, like partners, family and friends (those Goffman (1963) calls the 'wise') are likely to

---

| **BOX 13.3** | Four phases of the HIV stigma trajectory |

1. At risk – pre-stigma and the worried well: this does not correspond to a stage of the disease trajectory, it denotes a time of uncertainty when an individual thinks behaviours might have put him at risk of HIV. He may cope through denial or disassociation. Much depends on the support available. The phase can end with testing for HIV
2. Diagnosis – confronting an altered identity: an individual can be diagnosed early or late in the disease trajectory. A typical stress response involves disbelief, numbness and denial, followed by anger, acute turmoil, disruptive anxiety and depressive symptoms. Identity and self-esteem can be threatened, stigma becomes salient, and decisions on disclosure have to be negotiated
3. Latent – living between health and illness: this is when the disease is asymptomatic and perhaps at its least disruptive. Individuals can normalize, conceal and even deny their positivity. They might choose to pass as normal, thereby avoiding enacted stigma, but felt stigma can exact a heavy price
4. Manifest – passage to social and physical death: there is often no fixed disease course because of widespread individual variation. However, there are fewer symptom-free periods and opportunistic infections accumulate. Stigma tends to be less salient as matters surrounding social and biological death become paramount. Intense felt stigma may nevertheless be associated with isolation and withdrawal as means of concealing 'abominations of the body'. Courtesy stigma may extend to carers who hesitate to reveal cause of death

Reproduced with kind permission from Elsevier Science Ltd from Alonzo & Reynolds (1995).

be deeply affected not only by the impact of the conditions themselves on everyday life but by their stigmatizing connotations. The spread of the stigma associated with the condition from the person directly affected to others close to him or her is known as courtesy stigma (Goffman 1963). A study that illustrates this is MacRae's (1999) investigation of courtesy stigma and Alzheimer's disease, a degenerative organic disorder of the brain for which there is as yet no effective treatment or cure. MacRae interviewed 47 family members of persons diagnosed with probable Alzheimer's disease: 31 of these were primary care-givers (either spouses or children). In response to a direct question, 54% of the spousal caregivers and 53% of the child caregivers said they had on occasions been embarrassed and/or ashamed; rather fewer, 37%, of those family members who were not primary care-givers responded affirmatively to this question. Embarrassment and/or shame tended to be experienced 'where it was apparent that the ill family member's behaviour was clearly in violation of social norms' (for example, rudeness to strangers or lapses of etiquette). MacRae argues that whereas for Goffman courtesy stigma is acquired simply by virtue of the individual's relationship to the person who possesses the stigma, her study suggests that this acquisition is in fact far from automatic. She commends further study into why it is that some of Goffman's wise develop strong senses of courtesy stigma whereas others reject or otherwise escape it.

STIGMA AND PHYSICIAN–PATIENT ENCOUNTERS

Whether patients have epilepsy, rectal cancer, HIV/AIDS or any other stigmatizing condi-tion, the quality of the care they receive is a major concern. The enhanced salience of medical audit will be important here. But quality of care encompasses more than biomed-ical thoroughness and numerous studies have documented patient unhappiness at physi-cians' preoccupation with diagnosis and management and apparent lack of interest in psychological and social aspects of care. Scambler (1989) has noted that the accusation that physicians, especially hospital specialists, lack the time, training or motivation to elicit and address patients' own perspectives on their epilepsy is a common one. He goes on to distinguish analytically between three dimensions to patients' perspectives: (1) 'felt stigma' – a sense of shame and apprehension at meeting with discrimination; (2) 'ratio-nalization' – a deep need to make sense of what is happening, to restore cognitive order; and (3) 'action strategy' – a need to develop modes of coping across a diversity of roles and situations. Research suggests that physicians tend to be interested in those aspects of patient rationalization that promise to facilitate diagnosis or management, but not in the process per se. Neither felt stigma nor action strategy tend to be on the medical agenda for consultations, and are typically handled inexpertly and cursorily if raised by patients.

The point has often been made that patients' perspectives need to be respected and explored in their own right. Physicians do not merely need to inform and advise, but also to listen. To do this effectively, particularly in relation to stigmatizing conditions, requires what Schneider & Conrad (1983) have termed 'co-participation in care'. Scambler (1990) has argued that physicians need to provide a competent and up-to-date technical service covering the investigation, diagnosis and management of epilepsy – at optimum cost – and to engage in health education oriented to demythologizing and destigmatiz-ing epilepsy in the community. As far as physician–patient encounters are concerned, he suggests four guiding principles, which are summarized in Box 13.4. The literature suggests that these prescriptions are pertinent to a wide range of chronic and stigmatiz-ing illnesses, and to surgical procedures such as mastectomy and colostomy, which have stigmatizing results.

> **BOX 13.4** Four criteria of good care
>
> 1. Acceptance of the principle of co-participation in care, which involves coming to terms with 'patient autonomy', or the patient as decision-maker
> 2. Acceptance of an open agenda in physician–patient encounters
> 3. A holistic rather than exclusively biomedical orientation to care, with the emphasis on informing, advising and helping 'persons in context' rather than merely managing disease
> 4. The development of counselling skills to complement technical skills, which presupposes both an awareness of the impact of epilepsy on quality of life and learned expertise in advising on coping strategies
>
> Reproduced with permission from the Royal Society of Medicine from Scambler (1990).

NEW THEMES

Political economy of stigma

In the recent literaure on stigma as applied to health and illness a new emphasis on political economy has emerged. Link & Phelan (2001), for example, have stressed that stigma is typically associated with other forms of disadvantage, like poverty and political powerlessness. Writing of HIV/AIDS, Parker & Aggleton (2003: 5–6) call for a post-individualist analysis of stigma that acknowledges its functioning 'at the point of intersection between *culture, power* and *difference*'. Relations of stigma, they maintain, are pivotal for social order, and the social order 'promotes the interests of dominant groups as well as distinctions and hierarchies of ranking between them, while legitimating that ranking by convincing the dominated to accept existing hierarchies through processes of hegemony'. Relations of stigma tend to mirror those of material well-being, status and power. Deacon & Stephney (2007) suggest that stigma follows the 'fault lines of society' and use the term 'layered stigma' in this context. Thus, for example, the poor in many regions of the world are more vulnerable to HIV/AIDS, more likely to suffer its effects publicly, whether at the household or individual level, and more likely to encounter discrimination. While there are of course exceptions – the poor can also stigmatize the wealthy – it is the affluent and powerful who are best positioned to ignore, avoid or weather cultural sanctions. At the global level, the stigma associated with HIV/AIDS has been stronger and enacted stigma more intense against marginalized groups like men who have sex with men, women, poor people, Africans, drug users, Haitians and African Americans (Deacon & Stephney 2007).

In similar vein, Scambler (2004, 2006) has argued that the study of relations of stigma and deviance cannot be conducted without reference to social structures like class, status, gender, ethnicity and age. These structures, it is suggested, influence norms of shame and blame as applied to health and illness. Parsons' sick role, discussed earlier, is an example. But who is shamed or blamed for what has varied historically and continues to vary culturally, even subculturally? Moreover, the dynamic between stigma and deviance can also vary. Scambler contends that the emphasis in British government policy on the notion of 'personal responsibility' over the last decade has meant that the stigma associated with chronic and disabling conditions has often been transmuted into deviance. Blame has been added to shame, for example for many of those who resist re-integration into the workplace. The introduction of American 'welfare-to-work' policies into Britain has meant that people may have their benefits cut off if they fail to demonstrate a willingness to find work, even if the jobs available to them are unsuitable and not well paid. In this way the onus is put on people who are 'socially excluded' to 'self-include' (Scambler 2006).

Disability politics and oppression

It is important to note the emergence in disability politics of another radical challenge to conventional, biomedical and 'common-sense' thinking in relation to chronic illness and disability. This has had an important bearing on appreciations of stigma; in particular, the understanding of chronic illness and/or disability as personal tragedy has been criticized. It has been argued, for example, that the system of knowledge based on such 'natural' dichotomies as normal/abnormal, healthy/pathological, socially acceptable/socially unacceptable, and so on, has arisen through a general cultural commitment to a discourse that dominates thinking and practice in the contemporary developed world. Many advocates of the 'disability politics movement' refuse to accept or respond to conventional notions of what is abnormal, unhealthy and unacceptable (Campbell & Oliver 1996). Moreover, their challenge to orthodox biomedical thinking is in many ways in tune with a changing culture in which identity and 'difference' are becoming key issues. As far as stigma is concerned, it is contended that there is no longer any compulsion or necessity to act out social evaluations that mark some people as imperfect, deviant or disabled, and thus as 'outsiders'. Difference should be a source of celebration rather than a rationale for rejection. What such a perspective suggests is the need for a sociological understanding of the often oppressive ways in which agents of social control, including doctors, sanction and enforce social evaluations which have their historical origins in economic and political interests (Barnes et al 1999; see Chapter 12). It is a perspective that is increasingly likely to require health workers to re-examine and re-appraise the social and moral bases of their 'scientific' programmes of treatment and care. As far as sociology is concerned, Thomas (2007) is one of a number of disability theorists to insist that its longstanding 'social deviance' paradigm be replaced by the 'social oppression' paradigm pioneered within disability studies.

STIGMA REDUCTION

It is beyond the scope of sociology to judge the appropriateness of norms of blame and shame, although it has often been pointed out that all societies have such norms and that the public definition and policing of the unacceptable has important functions for maintaining social order. It is acknowledged, however, that stigma and deviance can put people's health at risk and constitute barriers to health care and health promotion. There is a long history of public interventions to combat or allay stigmas associated with a wide range of diseases, including leprosy, tuberculosis, schizophrenia, HIV/AIDS and epilepsy. Up to the 1960s in Britain the stigma of epilepsy was in part addressed by the removal of patients from the community and their incarceration in 'epileptic colonies'. More recently, efforts have been put into initiatives in health education and promotion. Specifically, it has for example been recommended that the continuing problem of the negative impact of enacted and felt stigma on the quality of life of people with epilepsy be countered by: optimum access to medical information, treatment and care, especially in the early stages of epilepsy; legislation against prejudicial and unacceptable discrimination against people with epilepsy on the part of employers and other third parties; and programmes to foster self-advocacy (or project stigma) and to raise self-esteem (Morrell 2002).

It is not always possible to counter the stigma associated with particular conditions effectively without also confronting the relationship between cultural norms and social structures. Rhodes and colleagues (2005) underline the complexity of social contexts while discussing what they call the 'risk environment' for HIV (especially drug use). They identify a range of factors as critical in the social production of risk for HIV: cross-border trade and transport links; population movement and mixing; urban or neighbourhood deprivation and disadvantage; specific injecting environments (including shooting galleries and prisons); the role of peer groups and social networks; the relevance of social capital at the level of networks, communities and neighbourhoods; the role of major social change and political and economic transition; political, social and economic inequities in relation to ethnicity, gender and sexuality; the role of social stigma and discrimination in reproducing inequity and vulnerability; the role of policies, laws and policing; and the role of upheavals and emergencies like armed conflict and natural disasters. What is evident here is that interventions either to minimize the risk of HIV among drug injectors, *or to reduce the stigma often associated with HIV/AIDS, or indeed other chronic illnesses,* are faced with arenas in which cultural and structural factors intermingle and where political and economic factors may play a predominant role. Arguably, such interventions need to be set in a framework concerned to alleviate inequity in health, welfare and human rights (Rhodes et al 2005). This is far removed from the notion of chronic illness as personal tragedy.

References

Alonzo A, Reynolds N 1995 Stigma, HIV and AIDS: an exploration and elaboration of a stigma strategy. Social Science and Medicine 41:303–315

Barnes C, Mercer G, Shakespeare T 1999 Exploring disability: a sociological introduction. Polity Press, Cambridge

Campbell J, Oliver M 1996 Disability politics. Routledge, London

Davis F 1964 Deviance disavowal: the management of strained interaction by the visibly handicapped. In: Becker H (ed) The other side. Free Press, Glencoe, IL

Deacon H, Stephney I 2007 HIV/AIDS, stigma and children: a literature review. HSRC Press, Cape Town

Freidson E 1970 Profession of medicine. Dodds, Mead & Co, New York

Gerhardt U 1987 Parsons, role theory and health interaction. In: Scambler G (ed) Sociological theory and medical sociology. Tavistock, London

Goffman E 1963 Stigma: notes on the management of spoiled identity. Prentice-Hall, New York

Gove W 1970 Societal reaction as an explanation of mental illness: an evaluation. American Sociological Review 35:873–884

Higgins P 1980 Outsiders in a hearing world: a sociology of deafness. Sage, Beverley Hills. CA

Jacoby A 1994 Felt versus enacted stigma: a concept revisited. Social Science & Medicine 38:269–274

Lemert E 1967 Human deviance, social problems and social control. Prentice-Hall, New York

Link B, Phelan J 2001 Conceptualizing stigma. Annual Review of Sociology 27:363–385

MacDonald L 1988 The experience of stigma: living with rectal cancer. In: Anderson R, Bury M (eds) Living with chronic illness: the experience of patients and their families. Allen & Unwin, London

MacRae H 1999 Managing courtesy stigma: the case of Alzheimer's disease. Sociology of Health & Illness 21:54–70

Mankoff M 1971 Societal reaction and career deviance: a critical analysis. Sociological Quarterly 12 214–218

Morrell M 2002 Stigma and epilepsy. Epilepsy & Behaviour 3:21–35

Parker R, Aggleton P 2003 HIV and AIDS-related stigma and discrimination: a conceptual framework and implications for action. Social Science & Medicine 57:13–24

Parsons T 1951 The social system. Routledge & Kegan Paul, London

Rhodes T, Singer M, Bourgois P et al 2005 The social structural production of HIV risk among injecting drug users. Social Science & Medicine 61:1026–1044

Scambler G 1989 Epilepsy. Tavistock, London

Scambler G 1990 Social factors and quality of life and quality of care in epilepsy. In: Chadwick D (ed) Quality of life and quality of care in epilepsy. Royal Society of Medicine, London

Scambler G 2004 Re-framing stigma: felt and enacted stigma and challenges to the sociology of chronic and disabling conditions. Social Theory and Health 2:29–46

Scambler G 2006 Sociology, social structure and health-related stigma. Psychology, Health & Medicine 11:288–295

Scambler G, Hopkins A 1986 Being epileptic: coming to terms with stigma. Sociology, Health and Illness 8:26–43

Scheff T 1966 Being mentally ill. Aldine, Chicago

Schneider J, Conrad P 1983 Having epilepsy: the experience and control of illness. Temple University Press, Philadelphia

Scott R 1969 The making of blind men. Russell Sage Foundation, New York

Sontag S 1977 Illness as metaphor. Allen Lane, New York

Thomas C 2007 Sociologies of disability and illness. Palgrave, London

Organization of health services

Origins and development of the National Health Service

Nicholas Mays

The organization and financing of health care varies widely in different countries. Each healthcare system is the product of the social, economic, demographic and technological context, and the political philosophy of the country. All exhibit their own balance of advantages and limitations when judged on criteria such as equity, efficiency, accessibility, acceptability and relevance to needs (see Chapter 19). The history of health care in the UK in the last 150 years mirrors the trend in all advanced western countries towards greater government involvement in health care in response to calls for better access to and coordination of services (Thane 1982). However, the National Health Service (NHS) that emerged from the interplay and conflict between the medical profession, government, experts, public opinion, employees and insurers was unique to the UK, providing services that are predominantly free at the point of use, accessible to all and paid for out of general government taxation. It is perhaps the best-known example of a 'health service' solution to the financing and allocation of health care in which the vast majority of health care is publicly financed and most of it provided through a publicly managed system.

The purpose of this chapter is to place recent changes in the NHS in a historical context by briefly surveying the evolution of health care in the UK since the 19th century and the development of the NHS since its inception in 1948, including the internal market initiated in 1991, before describing and analysing the Labour government's programme of change, which began in 1997.

HEALTH CARE IN THE UK BEFORE THE NATIONAL HEALTH SERVICE

Health care provision in the UK before the NHS comprised a number of disparate elements: general practitioner (GP) services, the voluntary hospitals, municipal hospitals, and local authority public health measures and related services.

General practitioners

In the 19th century, hospitals were used primarily by the poor. They remained dangerous places until the very end of the century when developments in anaesthesia and antiseptic surgery improved the success rate of treatments. For those who could afford it, fee-for-service consultation with a qualified practitioner, either in the surgery or at home, was the main means of obtaining medical care. A variety of insurance schemes, organized by Friendly Societies (non-profit-making, mutual-benefit organizations) and trade unions gradually enabled other groups, mainly skilled workers, to use GPs.

By the end of the 19th century, only about half the working class was covered by these schemes of contributory insurance. In 1911, Britain introduced a National Health Insurance (NHI) scheme, covering manual workers between 16 and 65 years of age whose earnings were below the threshold for payment of income tax. It provided funds for sickness, accident and disability benefits in cash, and access to GP services free of charge. Hospital and specialist care were not included.

NHI improved GP remuneration because it provided additional public funds to subsidize the treatment of many more, poorer patients while still allowing doctors to work for other insurers as fee-for-service private practitioners. By 1939, approximately 40% of the working population had some coverage for GP services through the NHI scheme and about two-thirds of GPs were involved in NHI work (Carpenter 1984). However, the economic recession of the 1930s had caused high levels of unemployment, which had, in turn, led the scheme into financial difficulties.

▮ Hospital services

Hospital care was available from two separate sources: the voluntary hospitals and the municipal or local authority hospitals.

The voluntary hospitals

There were 1100 voluntary hospitals with 90 000 beds in Britain before the Second World War. These were charitable foundations and treated 36% of all hospital patients in 1938 (Abel-Smith 1964). Their consultants offered their services at the hospital without payment so that the hospital could provide free care to patients who could not afford private treatment. In return, they were relatively free to choose to treat the complex and 'interesting' cases. Consultants' incomes were derived from private practice undertaken outside the hospital.

After the First World War, inflation reduced the real value of the income from donations to the voluntary hospitals. Medical science was becoming increasingly complex and expensive. As a result, the voluntary hospitals found themselves with mounting financial problems. They responded by trading on their reputations to raise money from the public – as well as by means testing and charging the growing numbers of more affluent patients who were now using their services as the effectiveness of hospital care increased. Hospitals set up their own contributory prepayment schemes for those who had some money but could not afford to pay directly out-of-pocket when they used services. To raise income, voluntary hospitals also undertook work on contract to local authorities, some of which were extending their provision of hospital care in the 1930s. By 1937, at least one-third of the voluntary hospitals were virtually bankrupt (Political and Economic Planning 1937). The government had given them some money in the 1920s to reduce their deficits but had refused to take on responsibility for their finances.

Despite the prepayment schemes, many middle-class people found that hospital care between the two World Wars was very expensive because the charges they paid also had to subsidise the care of lower-income patients who still generally received free services. However, poor patients brought no income to the voluntary hospitals and so there was an increasing incentive for the hospitals to neglect them, passing responsibility for their care to the municipal hospitals. Both poor and better off people became dissatisfied with this state of affairs.

Municipal (local authority) hospitals

The 19th-century system known as the Poor Law provided public assistance, including long-term hospital care, to the very poorest people and the unemployed. In 1929 the Poor Law hospitals were taken over by the health departments of the elected local government headed by the Medical Officer of Health (MOH). They continued to provide mainly chronic, means-tested care for those unable to obtain treatment in the voluntary hospitals or by private means. By 1939 there were 400 000 beds in public hospitals run by the local authorities: 200 000 in 'asylums' serving the mentally ill and mentally handicapped, and 200 000 in a range of tuberculosis sanatoria and isolation hospitals for infectious diseases.

There were big differences in approach by different local authorities to the public hospital system in their areas, with some simply perpetuating Poor Law standards, particularly outside London. Indeed, the economic depression of the 1930s meant that many lacked the money to invest in hospitals. Although the voluntary and municipal hospitals were, in a loose sense, complementary, there was little liaison or coordination between them.

223

▓ Public health and community health services

The earliest and most significant action to protect the population's health in the 19th century was the public health legislation enacted between 1848 and 1875. This had led to major improvements in water supplies and sewerage, and, ultimately, the control of infectious diseases, which made a far greater impact on the general standard of health than anything in the field of curative medicine up to that time (see Chapter 1). By the end of the 19th century, each local authority was required by law to have a MOH, responsible for environmental health, control of infectious diseases, certification of causes of death and a range of preventive services. By the 1930s, the MOH headed a health department in every local authority, with responsibility for services that were not available under NHI, such as maternity services, child health and welfare (health visiting in modern terminology), the school medical service and services for the support of elderly people in their own homes (e.g. district nursing).

▓ Overview of health care in the UK before the Second World War

Despite a reasonably effective pattern of public health and preventive health services, a series of reports between the two World Wars, both official and unofficial, identified major deficiencies in the other health services:

● financial barriers to the use of health services remained because NHI was not available to more than half the population and it did not cover the dependants of the insured worker;

● NHI did not include hospital care;

● specialists, GPs and hospital beds were unevenly distributed across the country;

● there were wide variations in standards in all services;

● there were mounting financial problems, especially in the voluntary hospitals, and shortages of equipment and skilled staff; and

● the local authority services, the voluntary hospitals and the GP services were uncoordinated.

ESTABLISHING A NATIONAL HEALTH SERVICE

By the late 1930s there was growing support for the idea that everybody should have access to good quality health care, but how this should be accomplished was a matter of hot dispute. Decisions would have to be made about, for example, whether services should be funded from general taxation or local taxes or by extending contributory NHI; whether hospitals should be administered by *ad hoc* bodies or by elected local government; whether doctors should become salaried employees of the state or remain independent contractors; and whether services should be free at the point of use or whether there should be charges and tests of the ability to pay (Webster 1988).

The experience of the Second World War showed how the state could intervene positively in many areas of national life; it also generated demands for a better post-war society. As a result, a national, universally available healthcare system administered by the State rather than the insurance industry was a central plank in Beveridge's famous blueprint for a post-war 'welfare state' (Beveridge Report 1942). Box 14.1 sets out the government's ambitious aims for a comprehensive health service (Ministry of Health 1944).

BOX 14.1 Aims of a comprehensive health service with free treatment paid for from taxes

'To ensure that everybody in the country – irrespective of means, age, sex and occupation – shall have equal opportunity to benefit from the best and most up-to-date medical and allied services available. To provide, therefore, for all who want it, a comprehensive service covering every branch of medical and allied activity.'

'To divorce the case of health from questions of personal means or other factors irrelevant to it; to provide the service free of charge (apart from certain possible charges in respect of appliances) and to encourage a new attitude to health – the easier obtaining of advice early, the promotion of good health rather than only the treatment of bad.'

From Ministry of Health (1944 p. 47).

Yet the NHS could not be established without the cooperation of the medical profession. Between 1942 and 1948 there was continuous negotiation between the government and key interest groups, particularly the representatives of the medical profession, about almost every aspect of the finance, organization and control of a new unified service (Eckstein 1958). The GPs resisted a salaried service to preserve professional autonomy. The hospital specialists refused the proposal for local authority control. Both groups were hostile to anything that hinted at the two 19th century systems of lay control – the Friendly Societies and the Poor Law. The system that finally emerged, established by the National Health Service Act, 1946, was the product of skilful compromises by Aneurin Bevan, the Labour Minister of Health after 1945. Although it was never formally agreed to by the British Medical Association (BMA), it reflected professional concerns to a considerable degree in that:

- GPs remained independent contractors but most were made better off by the NHS;
- hospital consultants were paid for the hospital work they had previously done for nothing;
- consultants were allowed to work part-time in the NHS on good salaries and keep their private practices;
- beds for private patients ('pay beds') were permitted in NHS hospitals;
- a system of distinction (merit) awards controlled by the profession was established for hospital consultants but not GPs;
- doctors were to play a major role in deciding policy at all levels; and
- hospitals were not to be controlled by elected local authorities, but 'nationalized' under the control of local appointed bodies.

From the outset, therefore, despite its apparent radicalism, the NHS represented a compromise between the principles of traditional medical authority and rational public administration (Klein 2006). In terms of overall control, finance and access, however, the system had changed markedly. The NHS was open to the whole population solely on the basis of healthcare need, free at the point of use and funded almost entirely from the general tax revenues of central government. The goal was to secure equality of access throughout the country to a comprehensive range of modern services accessible by referral from a GP except in emergencies.

THE NHS, 1948–74

The NHS, which began in 1948, nationalized the existing pattern of services and therefore inherited many of the strengths and weaknesses of the previous arrangements. The historical divisions between general practice, local authority health services, local authority hospitals and teaching hospitals remained, and no significant steps were taken to tackle inequalities in the geographical distribution of hospital beds, staff and equipment. Thus the new NHS fell far short of the ideal of full integration (see Fig. 14.1 for the

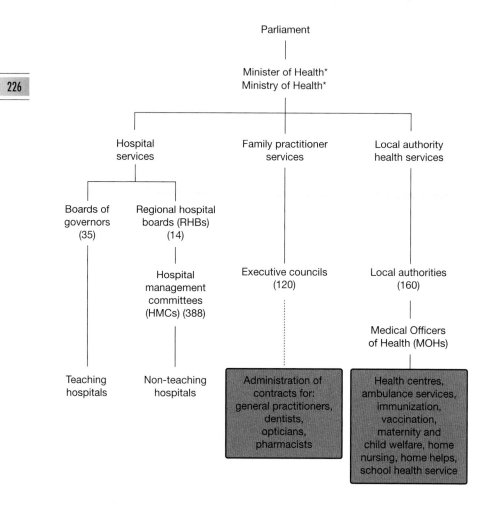

*Secretary of State for Social Services and Department of Health and Social Security (DHSS), respectively, from 1968

—— Direct managerial authority

······ Administrative responsibility

Fig. 14.1 The structure of the NHS in England and Wales, 1948–74.

structure of the NHS in England). Similar but separate structures were created in Wales, Scotland and Northern Ireland.

The NHS was immediately very popular with the public and rapidly proved financially attractive to the vast majority of medical practitioners. However, two main sources of discontent marked the first 25 years: (1) the level of expenditure; and (2) the organization of the service.

The original expenditure estimates were relatively modest and assumed that spending would stabilize rapidly, although Aneurin Bevan was in no doubt that the NHS would be expensive because of previous under funding and a backlog of untreated ill health. The planners had reckoned without the popularity of the NHS, rising public expectations, inflation and post-war developments in technology and drugs; all of which drove up the cost of the service. To limit public spending, charges were introduced in 1951 for spectacles, dentures and, eventually, prescriptions, and have remained ever since.

The demand for health care continued to rise in the 1960s, fed by professional and public aspirations and supported by economic growth. The period 1960–74 was marked by a steady expansion in spending in real terms and in the volume of services provided through the NHS. Spending rose from 3.8% to 5.7% of gross national product. By the second half of the 1970s, economic growth had slowed, and with it the growth in NHS resources. The service was having to face up to the dilemmas imposed by the requirement, which faces all health systems, to reconcile seemingly infinite demand for care with inevitably finite resources (see Chapter 19). One possible solution was to get more from the existing level of resources through a more efficient organization. The prevailing view was that the lack of linkage between the different arms of the NHS (see Fig. 14.1) was preventing continuity of care and the most effective use of resources.

REFORM BY REORGANIZATION, 1974

The NHS was reorganized in 1974. This produced a new, more integrated structure of 14 Regional Health Authorities (RHAs) whose main function was to allocate finance, plan major capital projects and monitor 90 Area Health Authorities (AHAs), which were responsible for both the hospitals and the community health services formerly managed by the local authorities (Fig. 14.2). The GPs remained independent contractors outside the control of the new authorities. A similar reorganization took place in Wales, Scotland and Northern Ireland.

At RHA and AHA levels, a multidisciplinary team comprising an administrator, an accountant, a senior nurse, a public health physician (now employed by the health authority), a consultant and a GP managed the system. This style of management was devised deliberately to incorporate the main professional groups in the decision-making process, and decisions could be taken only when there was a consensus in favour within the team ('consensus management').

The reorganization was designed to facilitate the implementation of an ambitious cyclical process of short- and long-term rational planning and priority setting by region, area and district, which began in 1976. This was accompanied by the introduction of the Resource Allocation Working Party (RAWP) formula to redistribute finance fairly between different parts of the country on the basis of the size and relative needs of the population.

The 1974 reorganization went some way to unifying the NHS and to improving the opportunities for coordination with local authority social services. It failed, however, to reconcile effectively the role of central government in setting policy, overseeing expenditure and monitoring performance, with the requirement for local, delegated authority

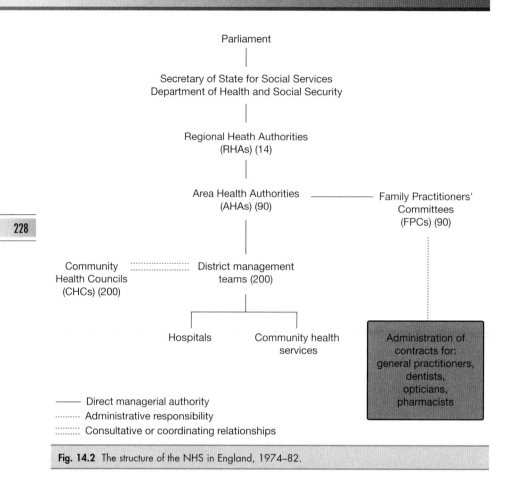

Fig. 14.2 The structure of the NHS in England, 1974–82.

and freedom to implement policy in the light of specific circumstances. The new structure was criticized for having too many tiers of administration, an overelaborate planning system, and too many consultative committees of doctors, nurses and other health workers. Consensus management was said to lead to slow and ineffective decision-making. The effects of redistribution of finance in line with the RAWP formula were particularly painful because redistribution was applied to a now near-static NHS budget.

MANAGERIAL REFORM, 1982–7

From 1979 to 1983 the Conservative government under Margaret Thatcher had encouraged those at the local level in the NHS to take decisions in the light of local circumstances. However, this posed the problem of how to ensure that local managers were using resources efficiently and in line with central policy. There was also a pressing need from the government's perspective to find ways of preventing health authorities overspending their budgets.

Whereas previous enquiries had concentrated on the structure of the NHS, a small team of private-sector managers, led by Roy Griffiths of Sainsburys, was asked in 1983 to undertake an inquiry into its management practices. Griffiths found a lack of individual responsibility and accountability for the attainment of objectives among the senior officers in the consensus teams. He concluded that the NHS needed a stronger, clearer management system (Department of Health and Social Security (DHSS) 1983). At every level in the NHS, the consensus teams were replaced by a single general manager with the power to take executive decisions over the resources under his or her control.

By establishing a hierarchy of general managers on fixed-term contracts and paid according to their performance, the Griffiths reforms enabled central government to exercise greater control over activity at all levels and increased the powers of managers. Managers began gradually to introduce more controls over the way traditionally autonomous clinicians used the resources available to them. For example, clinicians became increasingly accountable for delivering an agreed workload efficiently within a set budget through systems of 'resource management' (Packwood et al 1991).

Overall, far greater emphasis was placed on considerations of efficiency and 'value for money' than ever before. The traditional, professional viewpoint that medical services could and should not be susceptible to measurement, external evaluation and control was increasingly challenged (see Chapter 18 for more on this). For example, to ensure that resources had been spent effectively and in line with objectives, a system of quantitative performance indicators (PIs) was developed to measure and compare the activity and costs of each district and unit. The government established a limited list of drugs of proven effectiveness that GPs were allowed to prescribe on the NHS; instituted competitive tendering for support services (e.g. catering, cleaning, portering and security) involving the private sector; implemented new cost–benefit methods for assessing new building schemes; and brought in strict cash limits linked to compulsory 'cost improvement programmes' to generate savings for new services.

THE NHS REVIEW, 1988

Despite the emphasis on greater efficiency in the later 1980s, the NHS still faced the familiar problem of reconciling increasing demand for its services, generated by rising expectations and the availability of new treatments, with the available funds. Total spending was higher than ever in real terms, and more patients were being treated, but, by the autumn of 1987, the NHS, and especially its acute hospitals, had entered one of its periodic financial and waiting list crises. In January 1988, the Prime Minister, Margaret Thatcher, announced a wide-ranging, confidential review of the NHS by a Cabinet committee.

The review team was forcibly reminded in the course of its work of the advantages of the existing arrangements, particularly the ability to control the level of expenditure (the lack of such control was a problem in most western countries) and the cost-effectiveness of the GP system, which allowed many health problems to be dealt with inexpensively without recourse to hospital care. These led to a comparatively low level of overall health spending by international standards (6.5% of the gross domestic product for most of the 1980s). Nevertheless, the whole population was given equitable access to a comprehensive range of high-quality services, regardless of the ability to pay, and with low administrative costs. Although this situation was the envy of many countries: 'the very success of the government in controlling expenditure ... had turned the NHS into a source of political aggravation. Ministers were being constantly (and successfully) pilloried by the medical profession and the political opposition for their failure to fund the NHS adequately' (Klein 1995, p 803).

The most influential economic critique was that the NHS was badly flawed because there were no incentives for healthcare providers to become more efficient (Enthoven 1985).

229

It was argued that the near-monopoly position of the NHS in the healthcare market had allowed a paternalistic, professionally dominated and inflexible system to develop with limited patient choice, and managers and clinicians who were insensitive to consumer views (Butler & Pirie 1988). At the same time, studies that demonstrated big variations in patterns of clinical activity (e.g. referral rates to hospital (Andersen & Mooney 1990)) were said to prove that resources were not being used as well as they could be (see Chapter 18). In response, US economist, Alain Enthoven (1985) had proposed the creation of an 'internal market' that would introduce explicit incentives to efficiency into the seemingly monolithic NHS. The basic idea was that it was desirable to separate the role of health authorities as purchasers of health care from their role as providers (see Box 14.2 for the key features of such an arrangement within a publicly financed service).

'WORKING FOR PATIENTS' (1989) AND THE NATIONAL HEALTH SERVICE AND COMMUNITY CARE ACT (1990)

Although the NHS White Paper of 1989 'Working for patients' (Secretaries of State 1989) was the result of a review by a radical Conservative administration in response to a perceived funding crisis, it was notable that the main changes concerned the means of delivery of health care and not general tax financing or the level of funding (Klein 2006).

Despite concerted opposition from the BMA and other NHS trade unions, the main elements in the White Paper became law in the NHS and Community Care Act, 1990, and were implemented rapidly. There were four main areas of change covering: the internal or quasi-market; professional accountability; the management hierarchy; and the development of general practice.

The internal market was introduced in the NHS from April 1991, based on the separation of the roles of purchaser and provider along the lines suggested by Enthoven (1985). The aim was to bring to the NHS the benefits of competition between suppliers, together with business management, without jeopardizing its basic principles. The purchaser-provider relationships are set out schematically in Fig. 14.3 (with the purchasers shown at the top of the Figure and the range of providers of services to the NHS at the bottom). District Health Authorities (DHAs), or Districts, became the main purchasers, financed according to the needs of their populations by a variant of the former RAWP formula, and were free to buy hospital and community health services from any provider, whether in the public, private or voluntary sector (though the vast majority of NHS

BOX 14.2 Key features of an 'internal' or quasi-market in public services

- Between the extremes of a fully private, free market and a bureaucratic 'command and control' economy (fully planned hierarchy)
- Some separation of the demand (purchasing) and supply (providing) functions within a service which is still largely publicly financed
- Creation of a network of buyers and sellers linked by more or less binding contracts or service agreements specifying the nature of the service to be provided, to whom, the volume and the timescale
- Purchasers tend not to be individuals (e.g. patients) but agencies acting on behalf of groups (e.g. health authorities) – hence the term 'quasi-market'
- Usually some competition between providers or at least the potential for competition if a provider does not perform well
- Variants were developed in 1980s in UK in state education, public housing, community care and the NHS

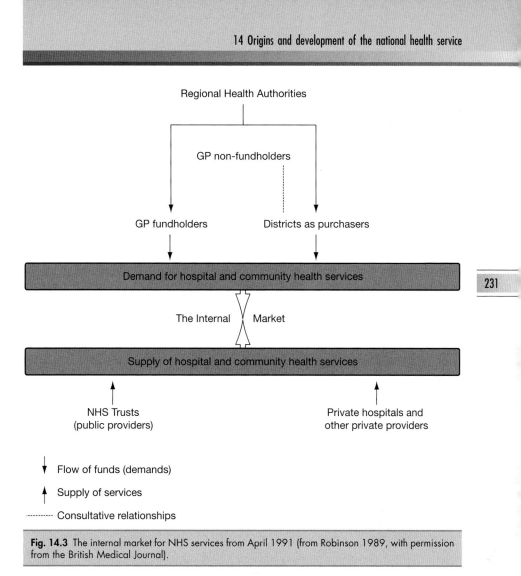

Regional Health Authorities

GP non-fundholders

GP fundholders   Districts as purchasers

Demand for hospital and community health services

The Internal   Market

Supply of hospital and community health services

NHS Trusts   Private hospitals and
(public providers)   other private providers

↓ Flow of funds (demands)

↑ Supply of services

------- Consultative relationships

Fig. 14.3 The internal market for NHS services from April 1991 (from Robinson 1989, with permission from the British Medical Journal).

services continued to be provided by the public sector). Major NHS acute hospitals and other NHS providers (e.g. of mental health services) became 'Trusts' free from DHA control. Providers such as hospitals were funded on their ability to win contracts to undertake an agreed amount of work for a DHA at a locally negotiated price. The theoretical incentive for providers, therefore, was to minimize costs and maximize quality in order to stay in business.

At the same time, larger GP practices were encouraged to become 'GP fundholders' and to take control of their own budgets for the non-emergency hospital outpatient, diagnostic and pharmaceutical care of the patients on their lists. They were expected to act as informed agents on behalf of their patients and to place contracts, for example for elective surgery, with those providers offering a good standard of service at a reasonable price in line with patients' wishes. It was also believed that fundholders would be more likely to challenge providers to produce better services than staff in health authorities.

Medical audit (the systematic analysis of the quality of clinical care) was made compulsory in hospitals and general practice. Hospital consultants were to have job descriptions that explicitly set out their clinical time commitments in the NHS. General managers were to be involved in the appointment of new consultants and in the allocation of merit awards.

The Griffiths management reforms were extended, with further change towards a private sector corporate model. Health authorities lost their remaining local authority and professional representatives, were slimmed down to 10 members, and became managerial bodies akin to the boards of directors of private companies. Senior managers became members of the new health authorities in their own right. A Chief Executive was appointed to run the NHS in England, including family practitioner services. Figure 14.4 gives the structure of the Service a few years later (this is a more conventional organizational chart of the internal market relationships shown in Figure 14.3). Chief Executives were also appointed to run the NHS in Wales, Scotland and Northern Ireland through separate management structures.

General practice reforms included a new NHS general practitioner contract to: encourage more preventive activities such as screening by GPs; promote a degree of competition between practices for patients; and improve the cost-effectiveness of services delivered in primary care. GPs were required to provide more information about the services they offered and were allowed to advertise their services, and it was made easier for patients to change GP. A higher proportion of GP remuneration was to come from capitation (from 46% to 60% on average) to encourage them to keep their patients healthy. Other elements of GP pay were linked to the attainment of activity targets set by the government (e.g. achieving specified rates of take-up for child immunization and vaccination and cervical cytology). All GPs were given an official indication of the amount they should be spending on drugs to exert downward pressure on their expenditure. High-prescribing GPs were given advice on how to reduce costs without denying patients the drugs they needed. Family Practitioner Committees (FPCs), which had administered family practitioners' contracts, were renamed Family Health Services Authorities (FHSAs) and given greater powers to audit and monitor the work and spending of family practitioners. FHSAs were merged with the Health Authorities in April 1996 (see Fig. 14.4 for the structure of the NHS after April 1996).

THE IMPACT OF THE NHS INTERNAL MARKET, 1991–7

Despite the government's radical intentions, the NHS internal market did not produce the degree of measurable change predicted by proponents and feared by opponents (Mays et al 2000). The principal explanation lies in the way the internal market was implemented: the incentives were too weak and the constraints too strong (Le Grand et al 1998, p 130). Central government strictly controlled competition between providers in case the potential efficiency gains from, for example, restructuring hospitals, threatened other goals such as equality of access to services, or caused politically embarrassing closures. As long as the NHS remained publicly financed and the Secretary of State for Health was accountable to Parliament for events within it, it proved impossible to allow competition to take its course. In fact, with the exception of GP fundholders, who were given more freedom to make significant shifts in the pattern of services they purchased, the NHS was driven at least as much by central directives (e.g. on reducing waiting times) as by the forces of the internal market.

In terms of efficiency, the internal market had complex effects. There was some evidence that the costs of providing hospital services fell faster than in the previous decade (Mulligan 1998) and that productivity (the ratio of outputs to inputs) rose (Soderlund et al 1997), but management and administrative costs increased as both purchasers'

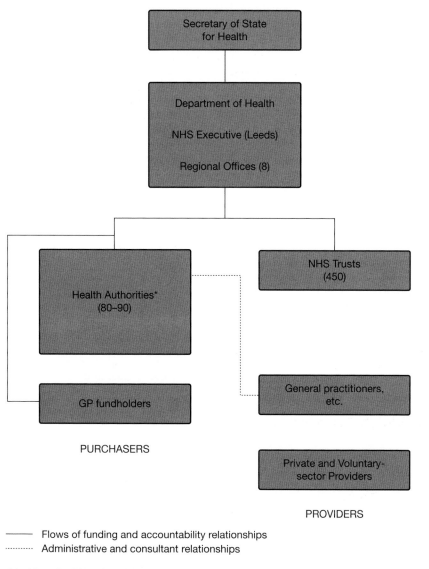

Fig. 14.4 Structure of the NHS in England in April 1996.

and providers' roles entailed activities that had not previously existed (e.g. negotiating contracts for services).

In terms of equity, there was little sign of the discrimination against chronically ill or high-cost patients that had been feared by critics of the internal market. However, there is little doubt (though little good research) that a 'two-tier' system (the preferential treatment of fundholding GPs' patients over patients whose services were purchased by the health authority) did operate in many places. Indeed, it was implicit in the policy that fundholding practices would be able to obtain advantages for their patients through controlling their own budgets for elective treatments. GP fundholders used their budgets to provide more accessible services for their patients within their own premises and negotiated shorter hospital waiting times on average than health authorities (Dusheiko et al 2004). However, waits for inpatient treatment (especially long waits over 18 months) fell for all NHS patients during the 1990s.

There was little evidence on the quality of care and no obvious signs of harm to standards of patient care in general, but studies found an increase in deaths of patients admitted with heart attacks associated with the internal market (Propper et al 2004). Public dissatisfaction with the NHS is another proxy measure of quality. Dissatisfaction with the NHS rose before the introduction of the internal market, fell during the early 1990s as more money was put into the system and resumed its previous upwards trend in the later 1990s.

On choice and responsiveness to the demands of individual patients – another of the goals of the internal market – the system was designed to empower the purchasers (e.g. fundholding GPs) to act as agents for patients rather than patients themselves as in a more conventional market. Methods of expressing patient 'voice' were little altered by the 1991 system and remained relatively weak.

Whatever else the internal market might have failed to achieve, it did change fundamentally the operating culture of the NHS and the balance of power both between managers and healthcare professionals, and between hospital providers and GPs. Providers had to be far more aware than in the past of the quality and cost of what they provided. Purchasers, after a slow start, came to question traditional ways of providing services and encouraged providers to think of new forms of service more relevant to the needs of patients (e.g. development in specialist 'outreach' services in the community, early discharge schemes, shared and intermediate forms of care between hospital and general practice, use of skilled nurse practitioners rather than medical staff and so on). Managers in NHS trusts gained greater influence over the pattern of clinical work than before 1991, although this shift in power should not be exaggerated: managers remained dependent on clinicians to make the contractual system work, and specialists retained substantial cultural and social authority and autonomy (Griffiths & Hughes 2000). GP fundholding, however, significantly increased the ability of GPs with budgets for hospital care to influence the way in which hospital specialists provided care to their patients. It also increased the degree of communication between primary and secondary care (Glennerster et al 1994). The experience of fundholding profoundly increased the role of primary care professionals in the system.

The internal market also exposed long-standing issues of priority-setting (Klein 2006). For example, the purchaser–provider separation and the requirement to contract for specific groups of services drew increasing attention to the fact that purchasers had finite budgets and an ever-lengthening list of demands for services. At the same time, cost-conscious NHS trusts and health authority purchasers came to ask harder questions about where the responsibilities of the NHS for continuing care should end and those of the local authority social services should begin (see Chapter 16).

'NEW LABOUR', NEW NHS?

Eighteen years of Conservative government were brought to an end with the Labour Party's victory in the 1997 General Election. The self-styled 'New Labour' government, determined to find a novel 'third way' between market ideology and old-style socialism, was critical of many of the changes to the NHS made by its Conservative predecessors under the broad banner of the internal market. In particular, the Labour government argued that the emphasis on markets and incentives to shape the behaviour of providers had undermined the public service ethos of the NHS and had led to an excessive focus on performance measured in terms of the numbers of services delivered rather than the quality or outcomes of care (see Chapter 18 on measuring outcomes). The government resolved to sweep away the internal market and replace it with a system based on 'partnership' and 'collaboration' (Klein 1998a, Secretary of State for Health 1997). The government was also developing proposals for devolution from the national Parliament at Westminster to Assemblies in Wales and Northern Ireland and a Parliament in Scotland. From 1999, these bodies took responsibility for the NHS in their respective territories although continuing to receive funds from Westminster. The developments in the NHS in England are described in detail in the rest of this chapter.

First, and perhaps surprisingly, the purchaser–provider separation was maintained, although longer-term contracts between purchasers and providers (for 3 years or more) were introduced to help tackle the alleged short-termism of the internal market.

235

Second, fundholding by individual GP practices was abolished, but replaced by a collective form of fundholding for all GPs. All the GPs in an area became members of the local Primary Care Trust (PCT), which holds the budget for most of the health services used by the patients on their lists and undertakes most of the healthcare commissioning (the new term for purchasing, involving developing new types of services as well as buying what is already available). This shift of resources to budgets controlled by primary care professionals continued the process begun under GP fundholding of increasing the influence of GPs on the direction of the NHS. For the first time, PCTs are responsible for the funding of both general medical services (i.e. general practice), and the commissioning of hospital and community health services. The integration of budgets was intended to improve the coordination of services in and out of hospitals, and to improve the overall use of resources (e.g. by encouraging extensions of the scope of primary healthcare services and the development of alternatives to costly hospital care).

The retention of the purchaser–provider separation and primary care-based purchasing suggests that, despite rhetoric to the contrary, the government was prepared to learn from the experience of the internal market (Le Grand 1999). The changes were designed to build on the positive aspects of purchaser–provider separation and fundholding, and to deal with the negative.

The third main set of early Labour changes was designed to ensure greater consistency in the availability and quality of services across the NHS. A number of widely publicized cases of unacceptably poor quality clinical care, most notably at Bristol Royal Infirmary (Report of the Public Inquiry into Children's Heart Surgery at the Bristol Royal Infirmary 1984–1995 2001), had demonstrated the need to bolster the systems of professional self-regulation and clinical audit, and to establish accepted external standards against which to measure clinical care:

● The National Institute for Clinical Excellence (NICE) was set up in March 1999 to synthesize the best available evidence on the effectiveness and cost-effectiveness of treatments, drugs and technologies, particularly new ones, and to produce official guidance on whether they should be funded as part of the NHS. In 2005, its remit was extended to include interventions to improve public health and it was renamed the National Institute for Health and Clinical Excellence.

● In a related initiative, expert groups were commissioned by the Department of Health to develop evidence-based National Service Frameworks (NSFs) for the main diseases and fields of care to identify 'best practice' and optimum service design for use by local purchasers and providers.

● A new and independent inspectorate, the Commission for Health Improvement (CHI), began work in April 2000 to: monitor the quality of services in each NHS Trust; scrutinize local efforts to assure and improve quality; publish the reports of its investigations; and intervene in 'failing' NHS providers if the Secretary of State should decide that serious or persistent problems need to be resolved. The inspectorate also assessed the performance of NHS Trusts against the government's targets for improvement. CHI, now called the Healthcare Commission, investigates, in particular, to see how well NHS Trusts, including PCTs, have implemented the concept of 'clinical governance', which is the shorthand for each NHS organization's responsibility for assuring the quality of its services. Although subject to a number of differing interpretations, 'clinical governance' is probably best defined as 'a system through which NHS organizations are accountable for continuously improving the quality of their services and safeguarding high standards of care by creating an environment in which excellence in clinical care can flourish' (Scally & Donaldson 1998) (see Box 14.3). As an example, the chairperson and chief executive of each NHS trust are statutorily responsible not only for the financial state of the organization, but also its ability to provide high quality care.

● A National Performance Framework was developed to broaden the basis of quality assessment from activity levels and crude measures of productivity to include indicators of the quality and effectiveness of the services delivered by NHS providers. Currently, the Healthcare Commission assesses NHS and independent sector healthcare organizations (since these now provide increasing amounts of care to NHS patients) against a set of standards and national targets, with an emphasis on ensuring that progress is being sustained (see Box 14.4). This results in an annual 'health check' of each organization.

These changes to the NHS in England also applied, to varying degrees, to Wales and Northern Ireland, but subsequently, policies in Scotland, and to a lesser extent in Wales, have increasingly diverged from policy in England.

BOX 14.3   Clinical Governance

What is it?
● The responsibility of all NHS organizations that deliver health services to ensure that their clinical services are of good quality
● Duty of doctors and other clinicians to ensure that their colleagues are enabled to practise well

Elements at provider level
● A focus on evidence-based practice
● Facilities for continuing professional development
● Clinical audit of care against explicit standards and monitoring of patient outcomes
● The use of quality assurance techniques
● Risk management
● Formal, regular appraisal and re-accreditation of clinicians
● Identification and remedy of poor clinical performance

Elements at national level in England
● National Institute for Health and Clinical Excellence (NICE)
● Commission for Health Improvement (CHI) – now the Healthcare Commission
● National Service Frameworks
● Adverse events monitoring and reporting system
● Modernization Agency - now part of the NHS Institute for Innovation and Improvement
● National Clinical Assessment Authority (NCAA) - now part of the National Patient Safety Agency

MAKING THE NHS MORE ACCESSIBLE AND USER-FRIENDLY

One of the Labour government's most frequently articulated desires for the NHS in its first term (1997 to 2001) was to 'modernize' the service. This comprised efforts to make the NHS more responsive to the needs of its users, often regarded as the main weakness of public services delivered by powerful professional groups where competition is limited. The argument runs that with private service industries like banks, supermarkets and travel agencies now accessible on-line, at call-centres or through extended opening hours 24 hours a day, seven days a week throughout the year, the NHS should become more user-friendly in the same way. The main response was in the field of primary or first contact health care with the establishment of NHS Direct (a national, nurse-led telephone help-line) and the emergence of NHS Walk-in Centres designed to supplement the services provided by ordinary NHS general practices by providing quick, initial treatment to patients who cannot visit their family doctor conveniently (e.g. because of work commitments).

237

The management of waiting lists was also influenced by rising public expectations and by models from other service industries. For example, targets were set and achieved to increase the proportion of patients given a booked date for admission to hospital for elective surgery rather than being called for treatment at the convenience of the hospital. As a result, the surgical waiting list shifted from an uncertain queuing system towards a more predictable system of reservations. Similarly, the target wait for patients urgently referred for suspected breast cancer was reduced to 2 weeks from GP referral to specialist assessment.

THE NHS PLAN, 2000

Despite the focus on improving service quality and accessibility, the NHS continued to attract adverse publicity in the later 1990s. Further clinical scandals involving unacceptably low standards of care in individual units were uncovered. Research was reported that appeared to show that patient survival rates after common cancers were lower in the NHS than in other European countries. This was attributed to both the organization of services and the level of resources in the NHS. It was popularly argued, not for the first time in its history, that the NHS was in 'crisis' due to long-term underinvestment in staffing and infrastructure.

The government, and particularly the Prime Minister, Tony Blair, concluded in 2000 that something must be done to reverse the 'crisis' and to rebuild public confidence in the NHS. In a bold initial move, the Prime Minister promised to bring the level of funding of the NHS as a percentage of national income to the average level enjoyed elsewhere in Europe so as to remedy what he interpreted to be the 'underfunding' of the NHS over many years. At the time, the UK's combined public and private spending on health care was approximately 7% of its gross domestic product, whereas the average for the European Union was 8%. The government committed itself to 7.5% per year growth in real terms (i.e. after allowing for inflation) in NHS spending over the period 2000–8. This was more than twice the previous long-term rate of increase.

With such an unprecedentedly large increase in NHS spending in view, it was important to plan how to use the new resources. The 'NHS plan' for England (Secretary of State for Health 2000) offered a significant increase in resources in exchange for a tougher regime of modernizing targets, rewards and sanctions, backed up by regulation and inspection, to improve the performance of the NHS over a 10-year period. At the core of the Plan were more staff and more hospital beds, and a range of performance targets

---

BOX 14.4 Examples of standards and targets used in the Healthcare Commission's annual 'health check' of health care organizations (Healthcare Commission 2006)

Standards and targets	Examples
Core and developmental standards	
● Patient safety	Organizations have systems to ensure that the risk of health care-acquired infections is reduced, with particular emphasis on high standards of hygiene, achieving reductions in MRSA (core standard)
● Clinical and cost effectiveness	Organizations conform to National Institute for Health and Clinical Excellence (NICE) technology appraisals and take into account nationally agreed guidance when planning and delivering treatment and care (core standard)
● Governance	Organizations apply principles of sound clinical and corporate governance (see box 14.3 on clinical governance) (core standard)
● Patient focus	Patients receive information when they need and want it on treatment and other services, and are encouraged to express their preferences and supported to make choices and shared decisions about their own health care (developmental standard)
● Accessible and responsive care	Organizations enable all members of the population to access services equally, and offer choice in access and treatment equitably (core standard)
● Care environment and amenities	Health care is provided in well-designed environments that are appropriate for the effective and safe delivery of treatment, including the effective control of health care associated infections (developmental standard)
● Public health	Organizations promote, protect and demonstrably improve the health of the community and narrow health inequalities by cooperating with one another and with local authorities and other organizations (core standard)
National targets (from 2006/07)	
● Priority 1: improve the health of the population	Reduce mortality rates from heart disease and stroke by at least 40% in people under 75, with a 40% reduction in the inequalities gap between the fifth of areas with the worst health and the rest of the population, by 2010 Tackle the underlying determinants of ill health and health inequalities (see Chapter 8) by halting the year-on-year rise in obesity among children under 11 by 2010 (joint target with Department for Education and Skills, and the Department of Culture, Media and Sport)
● Priority 2: supporting people with long-term conditions	Improve outcomes for people with long-term conditions by offering a personalized care plan for vulnerable people most at risk, and to reduce emergency bed days by 5% by 2008 through improved care outside hospital
● Priority 3: access to services	Ensure that by 2008 no one waits more than 18 weeks from GP referral to hospital treatment
● Priority 4: patient/user experience	Halve the MRSA bacteraemia infection rate by 2008

---

relating particularly to outpatient and elective surgery waiting times and focusing effort on priority areas such as cancer and heart disease (Box 14.4 gives examples of some of the current targets being pursued by the Service). The first annual report on the implementation of the Plan provided some evidence that progress was being made (e.g. there had been a 25% increase in critical care beds, 10 000 more nurses and the number of people waiting for more than 15 months for inpatient treatment had fallen by more than a third (NHS Modernisation Board 2002)). Better performers against the performance targets were given higher 'star' ratings in a system akin to restaurant and hotel 'stars' and were rewarded with greater autonomy (e.g. over their use of resources) and allocated part of a discretionary performance-related fund.

Consistent with the government's wider commitment to 'what works' rather than to old Left hostility to the private sector, the NHS Plan included a 'Concordat' with the private sector that more strongly encouraged NHS purchasers to use spare private capacity for their patients if this enabled them to meet the government's performance targets (e.g. to reduce waiting times for elective surgery) more quickly or cost-effectively than relying on NHS hospitals. The Plan included positive support for public–private partnerships (PPPs) in the NHS; for example, in the case of major hospital building projects. Critics were concerned that such moves were part of a gradual dismantling of the NHS or that they risked leaving the NHS with all the most difficult and costly cases.

239

Although recognizing the role of the private sector when this could support the achievement of NHS goals, the Plan also made it clear that the government would reduce the influence of the private sector in contrary circumstances. For example, the Plan proposed stronger inducements for hospital specialists to work full-time in the NHS and tighter restrictions on the degree to which specialists could work simultaneously in the public and private sectors in order to minimize any perverse incentives for consultants to favour their private practices over their NHS commitments.

The final strand in the Plan reflected the continuation of the government's desire to strengthen both professional self-regulation and external clinical accountability for national standards of care, particularly in medicine, by introducing new systems to ensure the clinical competence of doctors and other health workers throughout their careers (see Chapter 15 for a discussion of the health professions). The Plan included proposals for the periodic revalidation of doctors' qualifications, and changes to the powers and functioning of the General Medical Council, which deals with the registration (entry into the profession and right to practise) and disciplining of doctors. It also introduced a system for the reporting and monitoring of adverse events and 'near-misses' in clinical practice run by the National Patient Safety Authority (NPSA) (see Box 14.3). This aims to prevent clinical errors in future by identifying current errors comprehensively, learning about what causes them and developing methods of working to avoid them occurring again. Inspired by the safety culture of the aeronautical industry, the focus is on redesigning systems rather than blaming individual practitioners when things go wrong. A National Clinical Assessment Authority (NCAA) (now part of the NPSA) was established to help NHS employers assess the small number of 'poorly performing' doctors and make recommendations about whether and under what circumstances they can continue to practise in the NHS.

Whereas the medical profession is subject to increasing external scrutiny, in return, politicians in Britain are increasingly supportive of the idea that clinicians should become more directly involved in the design of services at all levels and the Department of Health less so (Milburn 2001). In a number of high-profile clinical areas, such as cancer services, mental health and emergency care, senior clinicians (the so-called clinical 'tsars') have been appointed with nationwide authority to implement changes to entire systems of service delivery in the hope that this will secure more rapid progress than change led by civil servants and managers.

The final strand in the government's efforts to improve performance in this period was the negotiation of a new NHS national GP contract that included a radical 'pay for performance' element. Practices are rewarded for delivering care exhibiting particular features

> **BOX 14.5** The four main elements in the 2003 NHS GP contract quality and outcome framework (QOF)
>
> 1. Clinical standards for the care of people with ten conditions:
>   - coronary heart disease,
>   - stroke or transient ischaemic attacks,
>   - hypertension, diabetes,
>   - chronic obstructive pulmonary disease,
>   - epilepsy, cancer,
>   - mental health problems,
>   - hypothyroidism
>   - asthma.
> 2. Organizational quality standards (in five areas)
> 3. Experience of patients (consultation length and results of patient surveys)
> 4. Provision of additional services (in four areas – cervical screening, child health surveillance, maternity services and contraceptive services).
>
> There are 146 indicators, including structure, process and outcome indicators, to measure practice performance in relation to the four elements of quality.
>
> A points system (maximum score 1050) links achievement of quality standards to payments. The maximum number of points achievable for each indicator is related to the workload associated with it.
>
> The clinical indicators account for 52% of the total number of points achievable by a practice. Most points are available for ischaemic heart disease (n = 121), hypertension (n = 105) and diabetes (n = 99).

deemed to be associated with clinical and organizational quality (Roland 2004). The contract addresses quality in two ways. First, it states a set of quality-related requirements which have to be fulfilled by providers in order to be contracted to the NHS (e.g. having an information leaflet for patients, a system to handle patient complaints, safety policies and a system to enable quality assurance). Second, a system of financial incentives for clinical and organizational quality has been designed. Traditionally, NHS funding of GPs was largely (though there were exceptions such as target-driven payments for cervical cancer screening and child immunisations) on the basis of the number of patients registered with a practice. Now, quality rewards make a substantial part of the funding (25% typically) in addition to capitation and infrastructure payments (e.g. to support information systems in practices). Performance is measured using an outcomes and quality framework especially developed for this purpose (known as the 'QOF') (see Box 14.5).

THE REINTRODUCTION OF MARKET COMPETITION

The NHS plan had encouraged NHS commissioners of services (PCTs) to make greater use of private sector providers in order to speed up their ability to meet NHS targets. In 2002, the government published *Delivering the NHS Plan* (Secretary of State for Health, 2002) which went much further in encouraging a more diverse range of providers of services to NHS patients and a greater emphasis on patient choice of provider. At the same time, government Ministers and the Department of Health began to decentralize responsibility for service improvement to the local level and to downplay the significance of national targets and upward accountability to the centre.

In what can now be seen in retrospect as part of a gradual process leading towards the revival of a more market-like NHS, so called Foundation Trusts were created in 2003. These are high-performing NHS Trusts that have successfully applied to become free-standing, non-profit making, 'public benefit corporations'. Foundation Trusts remain part of the NHS but have greater financial and managerial freedoms (e.g. they can borrow from the private sector up to limits set by the regulator and develop joint ventures with the private sector). Unlike ordinary NHS Trusts, Foundation Trusts cannot be directed by the Secretary of State for Health. Instead, their behaviour is regulated by an independent economic regulator known as Monitor established in 2004. Foundation Trusts are, however, subject to quality inspections by the Healthcare Commission. The intention is that all NHS Trusts should eventually achieve Foundation status. By the end of 2006/07, there were 62 Foundation Trusts.

If Foundation Trusts were controversial among Labour's supporters and its MPs, the decision that followed to procure additional elective surgical treatment capacity from the private sector was even more radical. The government was determined that the additional funds flowing into the NHS should increase capacity, particularly for services such as waiting list surgery and routine diagnostics where waiting had been a problem. From 1999, it had gradually developed NHS 'treatment centres' in response. These are standalone centres on NHS hospital sites specializing in high volumes of low risk, straightforward operations that do not require a hospital admission. By the end of 2005, there were 32 NHS treatment centres. However, acquiring additional services from new independent sector treatment centres (ISTCs) as well as existing private hospitals became government policy in 2004/05. Bids were invited from private providers to set up ISTCs to provide extra surgery to NHS patients. Around 10% of NHS procedures were carried out in the independent sector in 2008.

As the range of providers of services to the NHS became more diverse (the 'supply side' of the emerging market), the government acted to alter the way in which services were commissioned (the 'demand side' of the emerging market). PCTs remained responsible for commissioning NHS services from a budget allocated in relation to the relative needs of their populations (though their numbers were reduced from 300 to about 100). However, they were required to further devolve their budgets and decisions to general practices (called practice-based commissioning), thereby allowing GPs once again to shape the pattern of local services as under the former GP fundholding scheme (see above). PCTs negotiate contracts on behalf of practices in line with their wishes to avoid the increase in transaction costs observed under the Conservatives' quasi-market of the 1990s. More specialized services are commissioned by PCTs or even groups of PCTs. Some PCTs also have responsibility for social care, previously the responsibility of local authorities, and are known as Care Trusts (see Fig. 14.6).

The final, crucial element in the changes affecting the relationships between commissioners, patient and providers was the introduction of a new provider payment mechanism known as 'Payment by Results' (PbR) designed to improve the efficiency and quality of services (Fig. 14.5 shows how the four main reform mechanisms are supposed to come together). In fact, PbR is a system of paying for each service or treatment delivered according to a national set of prices based on the NHS average and is not payment for patient outcomes ('payment for activity' would be a more accurate title). The aim is that providers of all types (public and private) compete on level terms to attract patients on the basis of the accessibility and quality of their services since there is no price competition (unlike the 1990s internal market). However, there is pressure on providers with costs above the national tariff to become more efficient (though equally they may stop providing certain services rather than work to improve their efficiency).

A key part of the new financial framework for the NHS, is the right of individual patients rather than PCTs or even practice-based commissioners to choose where they go for their treatment. The aim is that patients' choices will drive the PbR system in large part. Thus from January 2006, where care can be planned, NHS patients have to be offered at the point of referral a choice of five providers of which at least one must be from

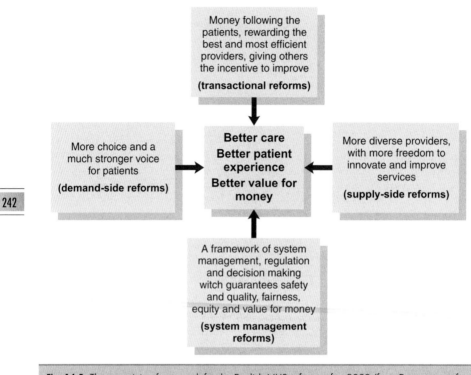

Fig. 14.5 The organizing framework for the English NHS reforms after 2002 (from Department of Health 2005, page 9).

the independent sector. It is argued that the offer of hospital choice is feasible given that most people in England already have an extensive potential choice of hospital (Damiani et al 2005). The absence of similar policies of choice and competition in the other parts of the UK can be attributed, in part, to their greater rural populations who have limited choice of hospitals, though there are also political and ideological differences between the Westminster government and the devolved governments outside England. English policy makers were perhaps also influenced by a rather different pilot project in London in which patients who had already waited several months after referral were offered treatment at another hospital with a guaranteed shorter wait. Not surprisingly, two-thirds of those offered this choice, took it (Dawson, Gravelle, Jacobs, Martin and Smith, 2007). It remains to be seen whether choice of provider at the point of referral is as popular with patients in future, particularly if NHS elective waiting times remain short.

Figure 14.5 depicts the NHS market that has gradually developed since 2002. Taken together the changes represent the most radical alteration of the NHS since its inception in 1948, despite the fact that the underlying principle of care free at the point of use available to all on the basis of need remains firmly in place. Figure 14.6 depicts the organization of the English NHS market system.

Why did the Labour government reinvent a more fluid, competitive version of the quasi-market introduced by the Conservatives in the 1990s and mostly abolished by New Labour after 1997? There are a number of reasons. Ministers and their advisers concluded that 'command and control' in the shape of target setting and enforcement from

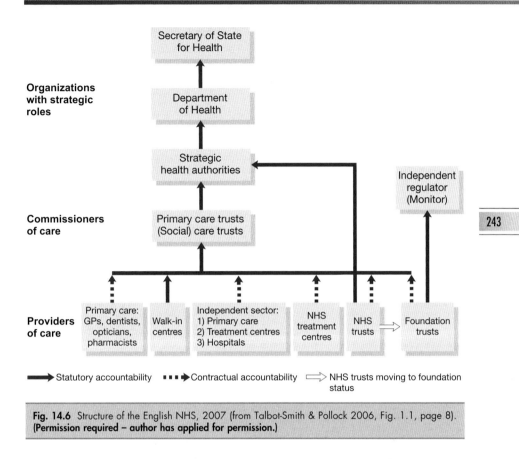

Organizations with strategic roles

Secretary of State for Health

Department of Health

Strategic health authorities

Independent regulator (Monitor)

Commissioners of care

Primary care trusts (Social) care trusts

Providers of care

Primary care: GPs, dentists, opticians, pharmacists

Walk-in centres

Independent sector: 1) Primary care 2) Treatment centres 3) Hospitals

NHS treatment centres

NHS trusts

Foundation trusts

➡ Statutory accountability ∎∎∎➤Contractual accountability ⇨ NHS trusts moving to foundation status

Fig. 14.6 Structure of the English NHS, 2007 (from Talbot-Smith & Pollock 2006, Fig. 1.1, page 8). **(Permission required – author has applied for permission.)**

the centre could only produce improvements in services for a time before inducing demoralization and resistance. Also there were still poorly performing parts of the NHS despite average improvements. More ambitious performance targets, such as the current goal that no patient should wait more than 18 weeks from GP referral to treatment (see Box 14.4), were increasingly seen as requiring a 'self-improving' NHS rather than one that had to be constantly chivvied by politicians, civil servants and managers. Furthermore, by the mid-2000s, the very large investment in new staff and infrastructure was largely in place. What was needed were the incentives throughout the system to make best use of the new resources for the benefit of patients; hence the attraction of a system in which a wider range of providers competed to provide NHS-funded services to PCTs, practice-based commissioners and individual patients, and were, in turn, rewarded for the work they undertook.

TOWARDS A BALANCE SHEET OF NHS REFORMS SINCE 1997

While the 1980s and 1990s were seen at the time as a period of major change in the NHS, the period since the election of the first Blair government in 1997 has seen, if anything, even more rapid and more extensive change driven by a series of activist, reforming Labour governments. The political importance for a government of being seen by the media and thus by the public as presiding over an improving NHS has increased in recent years. So how should the period since 1997 be judged?

Achievements

There has undoubtedly been very significant improvement in the NHS. The Service is probably closer to meeting its original highly ambitious goals of a universal, comprehensive service free at the point of use (Box 14.1) than it ever has been (Oliver 2005). Spending increased between 1997 and 2007 by 6.6% per year (7.8% since 2000/01 when Labour began the process of reaching the European Union average). This compares with the 3.4% average in the period, 1949–2000 (Thorlby & Maybin 2007). By the end of 2007/08, NHS spending had trebled in nominal terms since 1997/98 to over £90 billion. Total health spending in the UK is at or near to the EU average (and likely to remain so, even though the annual rate of spending increase was planned to be nearer the long-term average from 2008), so low spending is no longer an excuse for poor performance. Between 1997 and 2006, there was a 26% increase in whole-time equivalent NHS nurses, a 56% increase in consultants (specialists) and 20% increase in GPs. Pay also increased markedly, especially for GPs and consultants.

Access to services improved, particularly in terms of reduced waiting times in accident and emergency departments and GP surgeries, and for elective operations. The NHS Plan targets were achieved by the end of 2005. The maximum wait for an outpatient appointment was reduced from more than 6 months in 2000 to 3 months and for inpatient treatment from 17 months in 2000 to 6 months. These improvements appeared sustainable in that by the end of April 2007, the median waiting tme for a first outpatient appointment was 3.3 weeks and for inpatient treatment was 6.4 weeks (Department of Health 2007a). Figure 14.7 shows the reduction over time in the maximum waiting times.

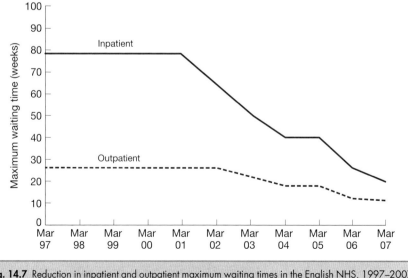

Fig. 14.7 Reduction in inpatient and outpatient maximum waiting times in the English NHS, 1997–2007 (from Department of Health 2007b, Fig. 3.1, page 41).

In 2004, the government set the most ambitious target yet – to reduce to 18 weeks the maximum wait from GP appointment to treatment, including the previously unacknowledged waits for diagnostic tests and decisions to treat in outpatients. At the end of 2006, only 35% of inpatients were treated within the 18-week target. A very significant part of the extra resources put into the NHS has been used to try to achieve the 18-week target (e.g. spending more on diagnostic tests and re-organising diagnostics).

The clinical quality of care improved, particularly in the fields where National Service Frameworks (NSFs) were established (mental health, coronary heart disease, cancer, etc.). Both the independent reviews of the heart disease and cancer NSFs reported substantial progress towards better outcomes as a result of shorter waits, more staff, improved prevention and wider implementation of clinical 'best practice'. For example, the percentage of heart attack victims given thrombolysis within 30 minutes of arrival at hospital had increased from 38% in 2000 to 83% in 2005/06 (Department of Health Coronary Heart Disease Policy Team 2007) and cancer survival rates have been increasing. In addition, NICE has been recognized world-wide as one of the leading attempts to encourage a public health system to devote its resources to the most cost-effective new treatments. The Healthcare Commission is now established as a quality inspectorate capable of assessing and reporting on the quality of NHS services as well as intervening where system failures are suspected.

Since 1998, there has been a large scale patient survey programme in England covering experiences of primary and hospital care, as well as specific patient groups (those with stroke, heart disease, mental health problems and cancer). Overall, the surveys have shown that the quality of NHS care is improving from the perspective of users, particularly in areas that have been the subject of concerted action (e.g. waiting times, cancer care, coronary heart disease and cancer) (Coulter 2005). In the 2006 survey of hospital inpatients, more than nine out of ten rated their care as 'excellent', 'very good' or 'good' (Healthcare Commission 2007). On the other hand, patients still reported wanting more information about their medicines, more involvement in decisions that affected them and better support for self-care. Transitions between different providers of care were also not always well coordinated. By contrast, the general public's perceptions of the NHS tend to be unrelated to either patients' experiences or trends in 'objective' measures of performance, instead reflecting the wider political fortunes of the government and media coverage of the NHS.

Weaknesses

Perhaps the greatest weakness in the English NHS in the period was that the substantial increase in resources, staff, wages and treatment capacity did not appear to increase productivity, as conventionally measured, at least in the short term. Between 2000 and 2005, the ratio of inputs to outputs declined, though the downward trend was less marked and could even be seen to be rising if the increasing quality of services (e.g. better outcomes) was taken into account (Office for National Statistics 2006). However, it is the accepted view of measurement experts that there is currently no definitive way of measuring NHS productivity (Martin et al 2006).

Large variations in the use of resources remained; for instance, in the efficiency of use of operating theatres. The new contracts for hospital specialists and general practitioners raised their incomes greatly, but the gains for patients and in terms of productivity were less obvious, particularly since the generosity of the contracts led to some doctors working fewer hours for the NHS. The government was increasingly under pressure from the media to show that the extra resources were being well used.

The increase in capacity and of new, more accessible services, accompanied by greater competition between providers and a more transparent way of paying for services (PbR) revealed endemic financial weaknesses in certain providers as well as showing that there was excess provision of hospital services in some parts of the country. Attempts to respond by 'reconfiguring' hospital services led to public and staff campaigns of resistance. Implementation of change was further slowed by the inflexibility inherent in many of the public–private partnerships that have been used to build new hospitals under the Private Finance Initiative (PFI).

Another weakness related to the tensions, some would say contradictions, between different strands of Labour's NHS policy, all of which remained in play; in particular, between the need for commissioners and providers of service to compete in certain circumstances (e.g. provision of routine elective surgery), while collaborating in others (e.g. reconfiguration of highly specialized services), and between individual patient choice and the decisions of PCTs and practice-based commissioners of services (Paton 2007). Added to this, the 'top-down' targets which drove the system in the late 1990s and early 2000s were still in place much later, albeit fewer in number, yet in a system which was supposed to be locally 'self-improving'. Another potential tension was between efforts to improve access to a wider range of less centrally managed services while still keeping the Service within its budget. This tension will become more acute in future since after 2008 the NHS is likely to return to its long-run rate of increase of spending – roughly half the rate of increase seen in the previous seven years.

FUTURE CHALLENGES FOR THE NHS

Like all health systems in high income countries, the NHS faces the major challenge of helping people maintain and improve their own health against unhealthy lifestyle trends in the opposite direction such as excessive food and alcohol consumption. As elsewhere, the Service will have to adapt to the fact that an increasing proportion of the population is likely to live for longer with a number of inter-related long-term conditions that are best managed largely outside hospital by coordinated, multi-disciplinary teams working with patients over years. The days of predominantly acute illness requiring episodic care are in the past. Ironically, the market-style NHS reinvented by New Labour since the mid-2000s is arguably better suited to the responsive provision of episodic care such as elective surgery than to the management of long-term conditions.

As well as facing epidemiological challenges, the government faces a challenge of its own making in reconciling the potential dynamics of the English NHS market with its remaining political accountability for the NHS as an equitable, universal service. For example, if, as a result of PbR and individual patient choice, some NHS hospitals 'fail' or get into severe financial difficulties in the new market, how easy will it be politically for ministers to argue that this is not their responsibility and that as long as services are available from other providers, all is well? If one way out of financial difficulties is for NHS trusts to merge and/or be 'reconfigured' (i.e. radically change the pattern of services they provide), will this be permitted to occur piecemeal, or will regional planning have to be reintroduced to encourage coordinated reconfiguration?

Markets in health care are different from conventional markets (Edwards 2005). The English NHS market operates with largely fixed prices and a range of social objectives including ensuring equitable access to services. In the early years (2001/02–2004/05), it appears that the incentives of PbR on provider Trusts to increase activity and compete on quality had relatively little measurable effect (Farrar et al 2006), though it is too soon to know what pattern of benefits and costs the fully-fledged market will eventually generate.

Experience elsewhere suggests that there are likely to be complex trade-offs; for example, between increased costs of regulation and improvements in the responsiveness of services to users (see Table 14.1 for a summary of the possible costs and benefits of market-like health systems). Much of the evidence about the effects of markets in health care is contested and it relates only to hospital services. One reading of the international evidence suggests that competition between providers of health care where prices are fixed centrally can improve quality (Gaynor 2006), but only with appropriate market regulation (e.g. to prevent differential treatment of patients depending on the severity of their conditions, or to encourage competition to prevent local monopolies developing) (Propper et al 2006). The government faces a significant challenge in determining where and how more market-like policies are likely to be beneficial and where other approaches should be retained.

CONCLUSION: HOW HAS THE NHS CHANGED AND HAS IT A FUTURE?

There are three basic ways of organizing public services – through hierarchies, markets and peer networks (see Box 14.6 for definitions of these terms). There is evidence that all three organizational forms have coexisted, to differing degrees, throughout the life of the NHS. For example, Exworthy et al (1999) argue that although the NHS appeared to be a hierarchy up to the 1980s, the centre had very limited control over the periphery where services were delivered and policy was largely made through professional networks. Later, one of the paradoxes of the 1990s quasi-market period was that hierarchy became more prominent as the government regulated the extent of competition it had created to prevent political embarrassment (see discussion of the impact of the internal market, above) and professional networks adapted to the new world of purchaser–provider contracts rather than being eroded. Similarly, the NHS after 1997 used strong elements of hierarchical control (e.g. the greater emphasis given to a national framework

TABLE 14.1	Costs and benefits of markets in health care
Costs	**Benefits**
Likely increased costs of marketing, transactions and patient search	Increased user choice
Increased regulatory costs since incentives to 'gaming' the system are stronger	Increased responsiveness of providers to needs and wants of users
Need for spare capacity so that choice and competition can occur	Likely to increase the rate of innovation
Risk of 'cream skimming' (i.e. avoiding costly patients) or skimping unless payment system and regulation are highly sophisticated	Generates comparative information on performance
May reduce professional motivation	Can improve quality and efficiency under certain conditions and with appropriate regulation – poor quality providers may leave the market
Can lead to fragmentation of care	Greater flexibility (e.g. of use of staff and buildings)
Can encourage supplier-induced demand for services	
Requires good information about quality of different providers	
Difficulties in altering highly specialized services requiring critical mass (e.g. trauma)	

> **BOX 14.6**   Hierarchies, markets and networks as different forms of coordination
>
> - Hierarchy: tends to be associated with bureaucracies, typified by a high degree of centralization of policy making and resource allocation; often described as 'command and control'; coordination is by administrative instruction
> - Market: form of coordination derived from the exchange between buyers and sellers of a good or service in which quantity and quality determine price, which determines the pattern of consumption. Associated with the notion of the 'invisible hand', which brings supply and demand into balance through rational factors responding to market signals; coordination is by price and quality competition
> - Network: form of coordination based on linkages between individuals, often informal and based on a common outlook on life that involves relationships based on trust and reciprocity. Associated with professional groups; coordination is through trust and cooperation

of performance measurement and targets) even as the potential for competition was being widened (e.g. the opportunity for private hospitals to bid against NHS hospitals to undertake elective surgery). After 2002, the emphasis shifted towards markets and competition more obviously, but despite this, hierarchical performance targets remained in place.

So much for the past of the NHS, but what of its future? At the beginning of this chapter it was noted that the NHS still represents the purest example, worldwide, of a health system in which central government pays for health services for the entire population from general tax revenue, still owns most of the facilities and employs most of the staff who deliver care, despite an increasing role in provision for the private sector (see Chapter 19). Although it is unlikely that the NHS would be set up in the same way as in the 1940s were it to be invented from scratch today, two leading American commentators have argued strongly that, despite its problems, the fundamental principles of the NHS – universal coverage, general tax financing and the ability to plan nationally – remain correct (Leatherman & Berwick 2000).

By contrast, Rudolf Klein, a long-time observer of the NHS, is more pessimistic about the ability of such a system to meet the aspirations of an increasingly diverse, demanding society and to manage the inevitable conflict between what health professionals believe they should do for their patients and the resources available from taxes to pay for this. Klein (1998b) argues that the NHS continues to be attractive to governments because it enables the costs of health care to be controlled on behalf of tax payers in ways that other countries struggle to achieve (see Chapter 19), but that the increased frequency of restructuring and cycles of attempted devolution followed by return to centralization are indicative of the difficulty of managing central financing and accountability against a background of rising expectations (e.g. for choice) and burgeoning technologies. As long as the NHS remains very largely financed from general taxes, it is unlikely that any Secretary of State for Health will ever succeed in becoming distanced from what happens in all parts of the NHS. This is despite repeated calls for the NHS to be run at arm's length from government (Edwards 2007, King's Fund 2002). As a result, Klein's hunch is that future governments will continue recent trends towards a system that is more pluralistic and diverse in the distribution of responsibility for the delivery of health care (e.g. making more use of independent suppliers of health services and less of publicly owned providers), but also begin to experiment with sources of finance other than taxation. Such a system might be more in tune with a society that has less faith in central planning and professional paternalism than was the case in 1946, but it would still need to ensure a reasonably fair pattern of access to services across the population, because the public continues to value fairness in health services. Combining greater pluralism, choice and flexibility with a high degree of fairness in financing and access will not be an easy task.

References

Abel-Smith B 1964 The hospitals 1800–1948. Heinemann, London

Andersen TF, Mooney G (eds) 1990 The challenge of medical practice variations. Macmillan, London

Beveridge Report 1942 Interdepartmental Committee on Social Insurance and Allied Services. Cmnd 6404. HMSO, London

Butler E, Pirie M 1988 Health management units. Adam Smith Institute, London

Carpenter G 1984 National health insurance: a case study in the use of private non-profit making organizations in the provision of welfare benefits. Public Administration 62:71–89

Coulter A 2005 Trends in patients' experience of the NHS. Picker Institute, Oxford

Damiani M, Propper C, Dixon J 2005 Mapping choice in the NHS: cross-sectional study of routinely collected data. British Medical Journal 330:284- doi:10.1136/bmj.330 7486.284

Dawson D, Gravelle H, Jacobs R et al 2007 The effects of expanding patient choice of provider on waiting times: evidence from a policy experiment. Health Economics 16:113–128 doi:10.1002/hec

Department of Health 2005 Health reform in England: update and next steps. Department of Health, London
http://www.dh.gov.uk/en/Publicationsandstatistics/Publications/PublicationsPolicyAndGuidance/DH_4124723 Accessed 22 June 2006

Department of Health 2007a Statistical press notice: NHS inpatient and outpatient waiting times figures, April 2007. News Release 2007/0142. Department of Health, London
http://www.gnn.gov.uk/environment/fullDetail.asp?ReleaseID=288665&NewsAreaID=2&NavigatedFromDepartment=False Accessed 22 June 2007

Department of Health 2007b Departmental report 2007. Cm 7093. The Stationery Office, London
http://www.dh.gov.uk/en/Publicationsandstatistics/Publications/AnnualReports/DH_074767 Accessed 22 June 2007

Department of Health Coronary Heart Disease Policy Team 2007 Shaping the future progress report 2006: the coronary heart disease national service framework. Department of Health, London
http://www.dh.gov.uk/en/Publicationsandstatistics/Publications/PublicationsPolicyAndGuidance/DH_063168 Accessed 22 June 2007

Department of Health and Social Security (DHSS) 1983 NHS management inquiry. The Griffiths Report. DHSS, London

Dusheiko M, Gravelle H, Jacobs R 2004 The effect of practice budgets on patient waiting times: allowing for selection bias. Health Economics 13:941–958

Eckstein H 1958 The English health service. Harvard University Press, Cambridge, MA

Edwards B 2007 An independent NHS: a review of the options. Nuffield Trust, London
http://www.nuffieldtrust.org.uk/publications/detail.asp?id=0&PRid=275 Accessed 22 June 2007

Edwards N 2005 Using markets to reform health care. British Medical Journal 331:1464–1466

Enthoven AC 1985 Reflections on the management of the National Health Service. Nuffield Provincial Hospitals Trust, London

Exworthy M, Powell M, Mohan J 1999 The NHS: quasi-market, quasi-hierarchy and quasi-network? Public Money and Management Oct–Dec:15–22

Farrar S, Yi D, Scott A et al 2006 National evaluation of payment by results: interim report – quantitative and qualitative analysis. Health Economics Research Unit, University of Aberdeen, Aberdeen
http://www.abdn.ac.uk/heru/documents/PbR%20interim%20report%20feb%2007.pdf Accessed 22 June 2007

Gaynor M 2006 What do we know about competition and quality in health care markets? Working Paper 12301. National Bureau of Economic Research, Cambridge MA
http://www.nber.org/papers/w12301 Accessed 10 August 2006

Glennerster H, Matsaganis M, Owens P, with Hancock S 1994 Implementing GP fundholding. Open University Press, Buckingham

Griffiths L, Hughes D 2000 Talking contracts and taking care: managers and professionals in the British NHS internal market. Social Science and Medicine 51:209–222

Healthcare Commission 2006 The annual health check in 2006/2007: assessing and rating the NHS. Healthcare Commission, London http://www.healthcarecommission.org.uk/_db/_documents/The_annual_health_check_in_2006_2007_assessing_and_rating_the_NHS_200609225143.pdf Accessed 22 June 2007

Healthcare Commission 2007 The views of hospital inpatients in England: key findings from the 2006 survey. Healthcare Commission, London http://www.healthcarecommission.org.uk/_db/_documents/Inpatient_survey_briefing_note.pdf Accessed 22 June 2007

King's Fund 2002 The future of the NHS: a framework for debate. Discussion paper. The King's Fund, London

Klein R 1995 Review of Ray Robinson and Julian Le Grand (eds) Evaluating the NHS reforms. Journal of Health Politics Policy and Law 20:802–807

Klein R 1998a Why Britain is reorganizing its National Health Service – yet again. Health Affairs 17:111–125

Klein R 1998b Economic and political costs of the NHS: a changing balance sheet? In: Macpherson G (ed) Our NHS: a celebration of 50 years. BMJ Books, London, p 106–111

Klein R 2006 The new politics of the National Health Service: from creation to reinvention, 5th (revised) edn. Radcliffe, Oxford

Leatherman S, Berwick D 2000 The NHS through American eyes. British Medical Journal 321:1545–1546

Le Grand J 1999 Competition, cooperation, or control? Tales from the British National Health Service. Health Affairs 18:27–39

Le Grand J, Mays N, Dixon J 1998 The reforms: success or failure or neither? In: Le Grand J, Mays N, Mulligan J-A (eds) Learning from the NHS internal market. King's Fund Publishing, London, p 117–143

Martin S, Smith PC, Leatherman S 2006 Value for money in the English NHS: summary of the evidence. The Health Foundation, London. http://www.health.org.uk/qquip/ Accessed 22 June 2007

Mays N, Mulligan J-A, Goodwin N 2000 The British quasi-market in health care: a balance sheet of the evidence. Journal of Health Services Research and Policy 5:49–58

Milburn A 2001 Shifting the balance of power in the NHS. Speech delivered on 25 April 2001. Online. Available: http://tap.ccta.gov.uk/doh/intpress.nsf/page/2001-0200

Ministry of Health 1944 A National Health Service. Cmnd 6502. HMSO, London

Mulligan J-A. 1998 Health authority purchasing. In: Le Grand J, Mays N, Mulligan J-A (eds) Learning from the NHS internal market: a review of the evidence. King's Fund, London, p 20–42

NHS Modernisation Board 2002 The NHS Plan: a progress report. Department of Health, London

Office for National Statistics 2006 Public service productivity: health. Economic Trends 628, March: 26–57 http://www.statistics.gov.uk/articles/economic_trends/ET628_Productivity_Heath.pdf Accessed 22 June 2007

Oliver A. 2005 The English National Health Service: 1979–2005. Health Economics 14:S75–S99

Packwood T, Keen J, Buxton M 1991 Hospitals in transition: the resource management experiment. Open University Press, Milton Keynes

Paton C 2007 New Labour's state of health: political economy, public policy and the NHS. Ashgate, Aldershot

Political and Economic Planning 1937 Report on the British Health Services. PEP, London

Propper C, Burgess S, Green K 2004 Does competition between hospitals improve the quality of care? Hospital death rates and the NHS internal market. Journal of Health Economics 21:227–252

Propper C, Wilson D, Burgess S 2006 Extending choice in English health care: the implications of the economic evidence. Journal of Social Policy 4:537–557 doi:10.1017/S0047279406000079

250

Roland M 2004 Linking physicians' pay to the quality of care – a major experiment in the United Kingdom. New England Journal of Medicine 351:1448–1454

Report of the Public Inquiry into Children's Heart Surgery at the Bristol Royal Infirmary (1984–1995) 2001 Learning from Bristol. Cmnd 5207. HMSO, London

Robinson R 1989 New health care market. British Medical Journal 298:437–439

Scally G, Donaldson LJ 1998 Clinical governance and the drive for quality improvement in the new NHS in England. British Medical Journal 317:61–65

Secretaries of State for Health, Wales, Northern Ireland and Scotland 1989 Working for patients. Cmnd 555. HMSO, London

Secretary of State for Health 1997 The New NHS: modern – dependable. Cmnd 3807. HMSO, London

Secretary of State for Health 2000 NHS plan: a plan for investment – a plan for reform. Cmnd 4818. The Stationery Office, London

Secretary of State for Health 2002 Delivering the NHS plan. Cmnd 5503. The Stationery Office, London

Soderlund N, Csaba I, Gray A et al 1997 Impact of the NHS reforms on English hospital productivity: an analysis of the first three years. British Medical Journal 315:1126–1129

Talbot-Smith A, Pollock AM 2006 The new NHS: a guide to its funding, organization and accountability. Routledge, London

Thane P 1982 The foundations of the welfare state. Longman, London

Thorlby R, Maybin J 2007 Health and ten years of Labour government: achievements and challenges. King's Fund, London

http://www.kingsfund.org.uk/publications/briefings/health_and_ten_1.html Accessed 22 June 2007

Webster C 1988 The health services since the war. Volume 1: problems of health care, the National Health Service before 1957. HMSO, London

The health professions

Iain Crinson

INTRODUCTION

The post-war popular demand for the development of a national health service providing health care provision for all, free at the point of use, created the basis for the establishment of the NHS in 1948 in Britain. Despite these democratic foundations, an unaccountable self-regulated professional group was able to assume, with the support of the state, a position of dominance within this new publicly-financed health service. Doctors were given the power and authority to determine individual and community health need, to allocate healthcare resources, and to control the day-to-day activities of other health professions. The medical profession was able to consolidate this position of dominance for the next half century. This position was maintained through extensive organizational and structural change within the NHS, the raising of public expectations and demands, and the development of new technological innovations in the diagnosis and treatment of disease (see Chapter 14).

One of the defining features of the process of 'modernization' that has occurred within the NHS over the past decade has been the development of new structures of clinical regulation and performance management, overseen by empowered local health service managers, which has made significant inroads into the autonomy of the medical profession. Davies has asserted that these developments represent the most fundamental challenge to the working practices of the health professions that has occurred in the 60-year history of the NHS:

'For many people working inside the NHS, the 1980s and early 1990s felt like a period of total revolution in health care. New vocabularies of business management pervaded thinking. Markets and managerialism came to the fore, and competition and contracting were the order of the day. Yet, despite the new words and employment relations, the division of labour in delivering patient care remained much the same....(however) the real revolution came later, after 1997, when New Labour began not just to reshape once again the overall organizational arrangements of healthcare, but to redesign the workforce. Assumptions about the professional autonomy of doctors, about the hierarchies and divisions of labour between and among other health professions that had survived successive health service reorganizations of earlier decades began to be cast aside. The workforce of the future seemed set to look remarkably different from the workforce of the present.' (Davies 2003, page 1)

Alongside the impact of these organizational changes, the ruling bodies of the medical profession, and in particular the General Medical Council (GMC), have experienced a sustained criticism for failing to protect the public. This follows the recent history of high-profile cases of malpractice and negligence, in which the apparent inability of the GMC to enforce a robust regulation of the practice of its registered members is generally recognized as having led to a decline in public trust. This ultimately prompted the direct intervention of government, which in 2007 published its White Paper on reforming the regulatory structure of the health professions (Cm 7013 2007).

This chapter will examine the historical and social processes that led to the medical profession assuming a position of dominance within the healthcare system. It will also examine why nursing has historically failed in its attempt to gain a comparative professional status. It will then move on to consider the challenges to this authority and autonomy now faced by the medical profession, and will conclude with an examination of the impact of the on-going processes of modernization on the future structure of the healthcare workforce.

WHAT CONSTITUTES A PROFESSION?

Before embarking on an analysis of the processes of change affecting the health professions in modern healthcare systems, it is useful to be clear about what distinguishes professional work from the work of other occupations. Friedson (2001) has set-out an 'ideal-type' of professionalism which forms a useful starting point. Although ideal-types are by definition static constructs, they have an important analytical function as heuristic tools and are routinely utilized within the social sciences as the basis for the assessment of real world processes of variation and change.

Friedson (2001) constructs his comprehensive ideal-type model of professionalism on the premiss that the historically-recognized professions are occupations, and like all occupations cannot exist without gaining an income which is dependent upon their position as workers within the marketplace. On this basis, he argues that the ideal-typical professional occupation is associated with the possession of specialized skills rooted in a knowledge base founded upon abstract concepts and formal learning. However crucially, these *skills and knowledge* must also be linked to the right to discretion, wherein an occupation is sufficiently trusted by the public at large and the state to be given control over the use of these skills and knowledge (2001, page 34). This 'discretionary specialization' operates within a structure of social relationships best described as a *division of labour*.

Friedson (2001) goes on to contrast the institutions associated with the ideal-typical profession with those structured by the operation of the free market, and those that characterize bureaucratic organizations. The division of labour as it operates within the free market serves to socially organize or regulate the type and task content of the specializations required by the economy. In Adam Smith's classic economic model, as described in the *Wealth of Nations*, this is very much a fluid process which is dependent upon the demands of consumers as well as the availability of these specialized skills in a 'free market'. For Karl Marx, on the other hand, the historical form taken by the division of labour within the market reflects the development of capitalist commodity production, and its ever increasing need for greater specialization in the tasks required of workers. The development of the modern institutions of the nation state and of large multi-national corporations in the 20th century can be seen to reflect the emergent process described by Max Weber as 'rational-legal authority'. These new social and economic structures added a further level of complexity to the social division of labour, requiring as they did the development of large bureaucracies to organize their activities. The division of labour within these bureaucratic organizations is composed of jobs or positions which reflect a hierarchical division of tasks defined by written rules (job descriptions). These first two forms of the division of labour are contrasted with the 'occupational division of labour of professionalism', where specializations become 'stabilized as distinct occupations' whose members have the exclusive right to perform the tasks connected with them. Functionally related occupations, as for example the health-care professions, negotiate with each other to 'determine the relationship of the specialization of each to the other'. The occupations themselves determine what qualifications are required to perform particular tasks as well as the criteria for legally licensing members to practise, enforced through the state (Friedson 2001, page 56).

Divisions of labour are sustained and organized through *labour markets*, which bring together the occupations with the consumers of their relative knowledge and skills. Entry to jobs or positions within the bureaucratic labour market is determined by specified impersonal criteria of competence which specify prior training and status. Applied to positions in the lowest level of the bureaucracy this can amount to little more than basic secondary education, but for those positions with a more defined career path, higher education and other forms of cultural capital are a key requirement. By contrast, entry to the occupationally controlled labour market of professionalism is determined by the organized occupational groups themselves, who have the exclusive right to determine the qualifications and the nature of the tasks to be performed by individuals. Professional labour markets are therefore structured by a process which sociologists describe as 'social closure' (which is expanded upon below). Recruits to the profession are selected on the basis of what is believed to be their capacity to learn how to perform these tasks. The nature of the *training* is specified by the profession itself which oversees its delivery within institutions which are usually attached to universities. Upon completion of training a credential is awarded by the institution which serves as the only entry point to the labour market for the professional occupation. These institutions also serve to legitimize the practical work activities of the profession, they are also the primary source of the status of its members, as well their personal and public identities; 'It also contributes to the development of commitment to the occupation as a life career and to a shared identity, a feeling of community or solidarity among those who have passed through it' (Friedson 2001, page 84).

THE HISTORICAL RELATIONSHIP BETWEEN THE MEDICAL PROFESSION AND THE STATE

In order to utilize Friedson's (2001) ideal-typical model as the basis for the analysis of variation and change in the role of professionals, the model needs to be situated within a social-historical context. While sociological assessments of the role of the medical profession universally recognize that doctors enjoy a position of pre-eminence within the health-care system, the question for analysis is what were the social and historical processes that contributed to this outcome?

Johnson's (1982) historical account of the development of the professions in the 19th century emphasized the importance of the 'trade-off' between the state and newly developing occupational groups such as doctors. In return for the profession applying its socially valued body of knowledge and expertise to the practice of medicine ('the medical model'), the state extended the profession's influence, so increasing its membership. In Britain, the Medical Act of 1858 established the device of registration for those completing an approved training qualification and conferred the title of 'doctor'. The General Medical Council (GMC) was established by the Act and was given the role of approving the registration of doctors and upholding ethical standards. This legislation was 'both instrumentally and symbolically the sign that state power now stood behind those who controlled the Council' (Moran 2004, page 29). In effect, the British state had created a monopolistic labour market structure within the emerging system of health care in the late 19th century which served to secure the institutional arrangements for the long-term dominance of the profession. Over the course of the next 90 years up until the founding of the NHS in 1948, the medical profession gradually developed its role as 'a publicly mandated and state-backed monopolistic supplier of a valued service' (Elston 1991, page 58).

The establishment of the NHS was initially opposed by the doctors' representative body, the British Medical Association (BMA), fearing that it would extend greater state regulation over the activities of general practitioners and consultants; however, this turned out to be a misplaced fear. The newly created universal health care system depended upon the clinical knowledge and skills of doctors to deliver services; this enabled the BMA to negotiate favourable terms for their participation in the new service with Aneurin Bevan, the Minister of Health in the post-war Labour government. This bargain gave doctors effective control over the everyday allocation of resources, while the role of the state was confined to deciding the level of overall state funding allocated to the NHS. Doctors, who already enjoyed a high degree of (clinical) autonomy in the pre-NHS health-care structures, were now able to extend this authority in their new role as 'gatekeepers' within the new state healthcare system. Thus, '(t)he medical profession gained money, status and the power to protect its privileges, (while) the state gained a healthcare system to protect and regulate its populace' (Salter 1998, page 98).

However, this medical dominance with the NHS ultimately led to a situation whereby the clinical needs of individual patients became prioritized over the long-term health of the population. The power given to the medical profession meant they were able to shape the new system to reflect their own professional concerns, but this resulted in the creation of a national *medical* service rather than a national *health* service.

This state–professional regulatory bargain first came under threat during the changing economic circumstances of the mid-1970s, when as a result of a crisis of profitability in the UK economy and subsequent rising unemployment, state resources began to be squeezed in all directions. By the 1980s, the rising cost of the health service had led the Department of Health to seriously assess how to best manage the performance of

255

the system and so maximize the use of limited state health resources. This process led to a detailed examination of the work of doctors and proposals to improve their 'efficiency and effectiveness'. This inevitably led on to attempts to dismantle the system of self-regulation and limit the discretionary power of the profession.

ANALYSING THE DOMINANCE AND AUTONOMY OF THE MEDICAL PROFESSION

The sociology of the professions has for a long period been dominated by those working within a Weberian tradition built around the assumption that society is made up of individuals pursuing their own interests and that this results in the formation of more or less collectively conscious groups. In furthering their common interests these collective groups then engage in 'social closure' strategies which are designed to prevent others from their group from usurping their privileges. Professions are seen as the archetypal example of groups which use these strategies to develop and maintain occupational boundaries.

Closely tied to the concept of social closure is the notion of the 'professional project'. Larson (1977) uses this term to focus attention on the need for occupations to work at bringing their professional status into being, and then maintain and enhance that status within a division of labour (this process is discussed in relation to the history of nursing below). In developing the notion of the 'project', Larson (1977) draws on Friedson's earlier influential work, *The Profession of Medicine* (1970), which had focused attention on the nature of professional power. Friedson argued that the power of medicine in modern societies did not derive from a social consensus around a professional gatekeeping role serving to legitimate sickness, but rather rested on two essentially self-serving pillars. The first was its 'autonomy', or the ability of the profession to control its own work activities. The second related to the control the profession exercised over the work activities of other healthcare occupations within the division of labour of healthcare systems, namely its 'dominance'. Friedson argued that while the professional training of doctors emphasized abstract ethical principles concerning the various traits required of the 'good doctor', in the real world of practice the profession was engaged in maintaining and developing its power and autonomy. This 'power approach' was to become the orthodoxy in sociological analyses of the professions for the next decade and more.

The model of professional dominance became subject to increasing criticism in the 1980s, as sociologists attempted to describe and explain the apparent decline in the autonomy of the professions as a whole. Two alternative perspectives achieved some prominence. The first was the 'proletarianization' thesis associated with the work of McKinlay and Arches (1985). This identified two key changes as being responsible for the medical profession's perceived loss of dominance within the healthcare system. First, the then recent development of 'managerialism' within healthcare systems which was seen to have reduced doctors' control over clinical decision-making. The second was the process of deskilling in the face of increased specialization and technological developments within the medical field. Together, these processes were seen as having 'technicized' the role of doctors, in that they were recognized as increasingly becoming just another group of employees (albeit one with a high degree of expertise) within the health-care system.

The second model of professional decline termed 'deprofessionalization' was associated with the work of Haug and Lavin (1983). In this model it was argued that the knowledge gap between doctors and patients has narrowed, and that consequently there has been a shift in power towards the healthcare consumer. Haug and Lavin argued that this general trend was leading to a diminishing of the cultural authority and health knowledge-monopoly of medicine. However, more than two decades on, the trajectory of decline in the autonomy and dominance of doctors identified by these two models would appear to have been somewhat overblown.

More recent work is hesitant in drawing general conclusions about any long-term loss of power and authority experienced by the medical profession. Elston (1991) develops Friedson's (1970) rather limited notion of professional autonomy and identifies three distinct dimensions: 'economic autonomy' as the ability to determine remuneration, 'political autonomy' as the ability to influence policy choices, and 'clinical autonomy' as the profession's right to set its own standards and to control clinical performance. Elston argued that a decline in one of the forms of medical autonomy does not necessarily effect change in other areas of autonomy and status. On this basis she maintains that while the 1990 internal market reforms within the NHS challenged the post-war political consensus over the fundamental way in which the NHS should be structured, and therefore represented a decline in the political autonomy of medicine, it did not significantly impact on clinical autonomy, as the profession continued to retain clinical control over health resources. (see Chapter 14).

Friedson (1994) also shifted his position over the years on the relative power of the medical profession. He has argued that professional dominance is best understood by an assessment of the actual work of doctors within the context of the healthcare division of labour; what might be termed the micro-level of power. Friedson identifies what he terms a 'zone of discretion' specific to medical work, and at this level the professional monopoly over certain skills ensures that even rank-and-file doctors are able to maintain considerable discretion in their daily work vis-à-vis other health workers. These discretionary powers, Friedson argues, usually enable doctors to prevent encroachment upon their clinical autonomy, whether that comes from managerialist attempts to monitor their performance or from the nursing or midwifery professions in taking on aspects of work doctors regard as being within their prerogative.

THE PROFESSIONAL PROJECT OF NURSING

Health and social care occupations such as nursing, physiotherapy, radiography, and medical social work have all attempted to emulate the medical profession's route to professional authority; 'however, lacking the doctor's distinctive combination of a highly-regarded body of expertise and skills with a high degree of cohesion and a tradition of forceful political organization, they were unable to achieve the same status' (Langan 1998, page 10).

The long-standing pursuit of professional status is arguably the defining feature of the history of modern nursing;

> Nursing has pursued its professional project for over a century, striving to achieve some autonomy and jurisdiction of its own. Its professional milieu is one which the powerful forces of medicine and the hospitals constantly seek to control, or to change the metaphor, they represent the upper and nether millstones between which nursing has always been ground (Macdonald 1995, page 143).

Sociologists recognize the existence of a distinct knowledge base as the epistemological basis for the establishment of any profession. In the context of nursing's striving for professional status this is especially pertinent given the frequent criticism of nursing knowledge as being 'indeterminate' because it is 'practice-based'. The origins of this issue have been attributed to the 'Nightingale movement' of the 1870s which emphasized the female 'virtues' of nursing practice over the development of a more esoteric knowledge base in order to ensure women's control over nursing as an occupation. This approach is a particular example of Weber's concept of social closure: men were to be excluded from the occupation by making the indeterminate aspects of nursing impossible for men to acquire. This was the opposite case to that of the medical profession at the time, which excluded women by making it virtually impossible for them to acquire the technical and scientific knowledge necessary to enter the profession. Florence Nightingale's position was opposed by the other strand of late 19th century nursing led by Mrs Bedford-Fenwick. The objective of the latter group was statutory registration of nursing, the aim being the establishment of an occupational professionalism for nursing with its own knowledge base.

Developing this application of the concept of social closure, Witz (1992) has argued that combining the two strategies of exclusion and usurpation, amounted to a 'dual closure' approach. Creating the new occupational field of nursing required that areas of healthcare practice hitherto controlled by medicine as the dominant exclusionary profession be usurped, together with the gendered exclusionary strategy which prevented men from becoming nurses. This strategy appeared to achieve success with the passing of the 1919 Nurses' Registration Act which established the General Nursing Council (GNC); this, however, subsequently came to be seen as a Pyrrhic victory. The GNC was not a self-regulatory body nor did it contain a majority of nursing members. The original aim of having only the one-portal entry system to nursing was not achieved, and many entry points to the occupation remained (represented by the branches of nursing, general, paediatric, mental health). Over the next 70 years, nursing's strategy for achieving professional status achieved very little progress largely because of the continuing dominance and control of the medical profession over the work of nurses, and the 'inaccessibility' of hospital organizational decision-making structures for nurses. This was also the case even after the formation of the NHS which reinforced the conception (originally championed by Florence Nightingale) that the organization of the hospital rather than professional concerns should constitute the locus of nurses' knowledge (Macdonald 1995).

Witz (1992, 1994) has persuasively argued that this dual closure approach has historical continuities with contemporary nursing's 'professional project'. Nursing, having traditionally sought to achieve occupational authority through its efforts to institutionalize a distinctive knowledge base hailed the major reform of nurse education in the late 1980s (termed *Project 2000*) as a successful outcome of its usurpationary strategy. The integration of the training of nurses into the system of higher education met the occupation's aim of uncoupling the historical ties between training and the organizational demands of the healthcare system at the organizational level, while also enabling the development of a distinct knowledge base that would 'epistemologically demarcate nursing from medicine' (Allen 2001, page 10). The new academic nursing departments now acted as advocates for a new 'holistic approach' to care delivery. This would require the individual nurse to move away from a primary concern with the biological functions of their patient towards a more direct engagement, seeing patients as subjective beings, as individuals with their own subjective experience of illness and care. The nurse–patient relationship was to be reformulated on a more equal basis, with nurses encouraged to promote healing rather than treating patients instrumentally. However, in the decade and more following the introduction of *Project 2000* there has been widespread and consistent criticism, particularly at the local level of hospital and primary care NHS Trusts, concerning the ability of newly-qualified nurses to fit in with the needs of service. Increasingly, the university-based system of training was seen by the government as reflecting an overly theoretical education programme which lacked relevance and practical experience for student nurses. Dingwall & Allen (2001) have concluded that this organizational devaluing of holistic care has resulted in 'professional demoralisation', because nurses in practice are not actively engaged in the work they are trained to value.

In summary, the attempt to construct a 'new nursing' framework of theory and practice as the basis for the 'professionalizing' of nursing has in many ways been undermined by the reality of practice, where the care provided by nurses has to be coordinated with the needs of a complex organization (Allen 2001). While historically the 'bundle of tasks' which comprise nursing work has always been fluid, the role that nursing plays as an adjunct to the medical profession in the healthcare division of labour has remained largely unchanged (Porter 1996).

CHALLENGES TO THE CONTINUED AUTHORITY AND AUTONOMY OF THE MEDICAL PROFESSION WITHIN THE NHS

▊ Governance in the modernized NHS

The notion of 'governance' is increasingly deployed to conceptualize the changing relationship of authority that exists between the key 'actors' within the healthcare system: the state, the health professions, and the service users themselves. Governance draws attention to: '(t)he arrangements by which authority and function are allocated, and rights and obligations established and regulated and through which policies and practices are effected' (Gray 2004, page 6). Within the health service, these organizational 'arrangements' have been subject to considerable change over the past decade, particularly following the New Labour government's programme of 'modernization' set out in *The NHS Plan* (Department of Health 2000a).

The role of the state in these changing forms of healthcare governance is in theory to resolve the tensions that exist between the clinical decision-making autonomy exercised by medical professionals, and the demands for a greater role in the management of their care and treatment by service users. However, the state is not a neutral player in this process. In nearly all developed countries, healthcare systems now face profound challenges in meeting the new demands which arise from demographic and technological changes. At the same time, the attempt is being made to restructure the delivery of medical services so as to achieve greater effectiveness and efficiency in the use of health resources (see Chapter 19). In this evolving context, the British state has a direct interest in effecting a change in the relations of governance that exist between service providers, health professionals and service users. As Moran has argued: 'changes in the government of the medical profession reflect the outcome of the struggles about these issues. The government of doctors, in other words, is a function of the government of medicine' (Moran 2004, page 27).

New challenges to the traditional relationship of governance within the NHS which privilege the clinical autonomy of the medical profession arise from a series of interconnected developments that have occurred over the last decade. These include the introduction of new regulatory structures and mechanisms designed to raise the performance of local healthcare provider organizations and the working practices of health professionals in line with the principles of greater efficiency in use of resources; the promotion of 'patient-centred care' reflecting the desire for greater service user involvement; and the emergence of 'evidence-based medicine' (EBM) reflecting the goal of more effective and safer medical interventions. In the following sections, these developments will be examined in the context of changing professional practice and relationships.

▊ Regulation, trust and patient safety

Public trust in the medical profession has been severely diminished following the outcome of the public inquiries into the Shipman murders (Shipman 2004) and children's heart surgery at Bristol Royal Infirmary (Kennedy 2001), and has led the government to the point of finally ending self-regulation. The Kennedy Inquiry (2001) pointed to the ways in which the dominance of senior doctors within an institution can lead to a 'club culture' and an imbalance of power between medical and other members of staff. This was recognized as contributing to a lack of team-working and the failure to work together in the best interests of the patient.

In 2007, the government published a White Paper which set out its programme of reform to the system for the regulation of health professionals, with its primary concern being to ensure patient safety and quality of care (Cm 7013 2007). Many of the proposals will require primary legislation, including the restructuring of the GMC, and new licensing arrangements for doctors.

The promotion of an 'evidence-based practice' was the central pillar of the clinical governance framework introduced as a key element of the modernization programme for the NHS in 1998 (see Chapter 14). At a theoretical level, the medical profession has generally embraced the criticisms of routine-based interventions as leading to unsafe and ineffective practice; however, integrating evidence into practice is another matter. There are important barriers to doctors delivering evidence-based care, not least of which are the demands associated with keeping abreast of an ever-widening literature.

Managing the performance of health professionals

Across all levels of healthcare activity, the NHS was largely free of any form of external regulatory intrusion until the late 1980s, the organization being directly accountable through a traditional bureaucratic hierarchy to central government. Although the Audit Commission and National Audit Office were created in the 1980s, their regulatory objective was essentially to ensure public money was spent as Parliament intended, and to improve financial control within public service organizations.

The Conservative government reforms of the NHS (Department of Health 1989) resulted in an organizational restructuring which gave a greater role to the new professional managers in healthcare resource decision-making, but as previously discussed, this essentially left the medical profession's control over its own standards and activities of work unchallenged. Although a new process of clinical audit was introduced, the profession was allowed to manage this process internally. The New Labour government did not set out initially to overtly regulate the work of doctors on coming into power in 1997, but it did introduce the 'clinical governance framework', a new professional accountability and quality assurance structure. This framework was introduced in part to get doctors to think in wider strategic terms about the efficient use of healthcare resources, the prevailing view of government being that the medical profession had historically only been able to conceive of clinical need at the level of the individual patient. However, the development of this framework, together with the capacity of the Department of Health to monitor local clinical outcomes, both in relation to the new national performance standards and to further the commissioning process for local service purchasers, has enabled local and national managers to achieve a much greater measure of scrutiny over the day-to-day work of doctors (Crinson 2004).

There is an increasing use of regulatory instruments to control the performance of the healthcare professions within the health service. The National Institute for Clinical Excellence (NICE) was created in 1999 and charged by the Department of Health with appraising a particular drug or 'medical technology' where its use may have a 'significant impact on

NHS resources', or where 'there is confusion or uncertainty over its value' (NICE 2002). This development has significantly diminished the ability of doctors to prescribe medicines they judge to be the most clinically effective, on grounds of cost. The introduction of a set of National Service Frameworks (NSF) for different medical conditions has also played an important role in regulating clinical work through the setting of incentivized (through the new GP Contract) clinical guidelines.

The challenge of patient-centred care

The term 'patient-centred care' is not a precise one, but indicates an approach to the organizing of healthcare services that centres on addressing the expressed needs of patients and directly involving them and their families in the treatment decision-making process. This approach is often contrasted with the 'disease-centred' approach which is seen to privilege the health professional's own agenda (see Chapter 4). This move away from a paternalistic model of clinical decision-making can be seen as reflecting the shift in the relationship of healthcare governance described above. Encouraged by the evidence that higher degrees of patient-centredness are related to higher patient satisfaction rates, these principles are now a core element in the curriculum taught to medical students.

However, studies of doctor-patient communication in practice do vary in the extent to which they recognize patient-centredness as being the norm rather than the exception in medical practice. Stevenson et al (1999) looked specifically at the extent to which doctors in primary care welcomed patient participation in treatment decisions. It was found that GPs' perceptions of both their own role and of the behaviour of their patients reduced the likelihood of shared decision-making being initiated by clinicians themselves. The explanation offered by GPs who participated in the study as to why they had not engaged in shared decision-making included lack of time and other organizational pressures in general practice. It was also suggested that patients expect their problems to be solved, and that the solution should include a treatment prescription; that is, a belief that patients lack the will or ability to participate in treatment decision-making. The study concluded there was no basis on which to build a consensus about the preferred treatment and reach an agreement on which treatment to implement. More recent research concurs with these findings. A study by Rogers et al (2005) of patients self-managing their chronic condition and their relative satisfaction with the support received from their doctor suggested that a number of factors served to inhibit effective patient-centred consultations. These included the failure of doctors to fully incorporate the expressed need relevant to people's self-management activities, and an interpretation of patient self-management as compliance with medical instructions.

One of the important contributions of these sociological papers is the finding that professional culture still plays an important role in perpetuating certain core beliefs, for example the idea that the doctor knows what is in the best interests of the patient, which act to hinder the development of a truly patient-centred healthcare service. Such values can be still found to underpin the professional cultures of not just doctors but all the health professional groups (National Primary Care Research and Development Centre 1997). The recognition that a cultural shift is required was highlighted in a recent commentary in the *British Medical Journal*. Donald Irvine, the former president of the General Medical Council, argued that unless there was a 'wholehearted commitment' by doctors as a collective group to a 'patient-centred culture of medical professionalism' then the profession would not be able to 'regain the public trust and respect' that it was argued it had lost following the medical scandals described above (Irvine 2006).

WHAT IS THE FUTURE FOR THE HEALTHCARE PROFESSIONS?

The 'modernization' programme for the NHS was predicated on the assumption that the goal of greater resource efficiency and wider choice for patients could not be achieved with the existing health workforce structure and traditional forms of professional practice. Derek Wanless's report on the future of the health service produced in 2001 and commissioned by the Treasury stated that: 'the number and mix of staff in the health service is a major determinant of the volume and quality of care...a health service without the right number of people, with the right skills, in the right locations will not deliver a high quality, comprehensive service to patients over the next two decades' (Wanless 2001).

The *Agenda for Change* policy (Department of Health 2004) was introduced in order to develop a new pay and incentive system that would give the NHS employers this 'flexibility' to design jobs around the needs of patients rather than around grading definitions, and to define the core skills and knowledge they wanted staff to develop in each job. Alongside this development, the Department of Health has sought to engage in a critical reappraisal of the types of roles and expertise needed for the healthcare workforce of the future. This concern has found expression in the 'Care Group Workforce Teams' (CGWT) that have been set up by the Department of Health in order to identify national staffing issues affecting particular services and form plans on how they should be addressed. Recommendations have now been produced on the skills and competencies that will be required to deliver on all the National Service Frameworks (NSF), in the areas of cancer, maternity and gynaecology services, coronary heart disease, long-term conditions including diabetes, mental health, and services for older people (Department of Health 2002). Associated with the work of CGWTs is the organization known as *Skills for Health* (SfH). This body was first established in 2002 and was licensed by DfES as the UK Sector Skills Council (SSC) for health in May 2004; it is part of the NHS, hosted by a Trust but with its own Board and management. Its function is to 'develop solutions that deliver a skilled and flexible UK workforce in order to improve health and healthcare'. This has involved developing frameworks termed 'National Occupational Standards' (NOS) and 'National Workforce Competences' (NWC). These are statements of competence describing good practice and are written precisely so as to measure performance outcomes.

Complementary to this process, the Department of Health (2000b) has for some time been encouraging the development of shared learning in the education and training of new health and social care professionals (including medical students). Recent shifts in health service workforce planning have sought to focus on integrated inter-professional or inter-agency working rather than on traditional profession-centred planning. Following the recommendation of Wanless's Final Report (2002), nurses are now increasingly being encouraged by the Department of Health to take on aspects of doctors' work, especially within primary care ('enhanced roles'). All these developments clearly represent a significant challenge to the traditional clinical autonomy of the medical profession within healthcare teams, and the hegemony of the profession in overall healthcare planning.

CONCLUSION

This chapter has sought to focus attention on the ways in which the traditional autonomy and dominance of the medical profession has been challenged by a range of recent developments. However, it has also been argued that the primary driver is the necessity for the state to ensure greater control over the efficient use of health resources in the face of rising demands for health care and raised public expectations about the quality of medical interventions. These developments are leading to a reconfiguration of the NHS workforce that will undoubtedly have a fundamental impact on the role of the health professional in the future.

References

Allen D 2001 The changing shape of nursing practice. Routledge, London

Cm 7013 2007 Trust, assurance and safety – the regulation of health professionals in the 21st century (white paper) The Stationery Office, London

Crinson I 2004 The politics of regulation within the 'modernised' NHS: the case of beta interferon and the 'cost-effective' treatment of multiple sclerosis. Critical Social Policy 24(1):30–49

Davies C 2003 Introduction: a new workforce in the making? In: Davies C (ed) The future health workforce. Palgrave, Basingstoke, p 13

Department of Health 1989 Working for patients. HMSO, London

Department of Health 2000a The NHS Plan. HMSO, London

Department of Health 2000b A health service of all the talents: developing the NHS workforce: a framework for lifelong learning for the NHS. Department of Health, London

Department of Health 2002 Getting the right skills to deliver the CHD NSF – a guide for meeting workforce needs. Department of Health, London

Department of Health 2004 Agenda for change - final agreement. Department of Health., London

Dingwall R, Allen D 2001 The implications of healthcare reforms for the profession of nursing. Nursing Inquiry 8(2):64–74

Elston MA 1991 The politics of professional power: medicine in a changing health service. In: Gabe J, Calnan M, Bury M (eds) The Sociology of the Health Service. Routledge, London, p 58–88

Friedson E 1970 The profession of medicine: a study in the sociology of applied knowledge. University of Chicago Press, Chicago

Friedson E 1994 Professionalism reborn. Polity Press, Cambridge

Friedson E 2001 Professionalism: the third logic. Polity, Cambridge

Gray A 2004 Governing medicine: an introduction. In: Gray A, Harrison S (eds) Governing medicine: theory and practice. Open University Press, Maidenhead, p 5–20

Haug M, Lavin B 1983 Consumerism in medicine: challenging physician authority. Sage, Beverley Hills

Irvine D 2006 Success relies on winning hearts and minds. British Medical Journal 333:965–966

Johnson T 1982 The state and the professions: peculiarities of the British. In: Giddens A, MacKenzie G (eds) Social class and the division of labour. Cambridge University Press, Cambridge

Kennedy I 2001 The Report of the Bristol Royal Infirmary Inquiry London. The Stationery Office, London

Langan M 1998 Rationing health care. In: Langan M (ed) Welfare: needs, rights and risks. Routledge, London, p 35–80

Larson MS 1977 The rise of professionalism: a sociological analysis. University of California Press, Berkeley

Macdonald K 1995 The Sociology of the professions. Sage, London

McKinlay J, Arches J 1985 Towards the proletarianization of physicians. International Journal of Health Services 18:191–205

Moran M 2004 Governing doctors in the British regulatory state In: Gray A, Harrison S (eds) Governing medicine: theory and practice. Open University Press, Maidenhead, p 27–36

National Primary Care Research and Development Centre 1997 Cultural differences between medicine and nursing: implications for primary care Manchester. NPCRDC, University of Manchester

NICE 2002 About NICE – background. www.nice.org.uk/article.asp

Porter S 1996 Breaking the boundaries between nursing and sociology: a critical realist ethnography of the theory-practice gap. Journal of Advanced Nursing 24:413–420

263

Rogers A Kennedy A, Nelson E, Robinson A 2005 Uncovering the limits of patient-centredness: implementing a self-management trial for chronic illness. Qualitative Health Research 15(2): 224–239

Salter B 1998 The politics of change in the health service. Macmillan, Basingstoke

Shipman Inquiry 2004 Safeguarding patients: lessons from the past, proposals for the future (chair Dame Janet Smith). Stationery Office, London

Stevenson F, Barry C, Britten N et al 1999 Doctor–patient communication about drugs: is shared decision-making possible? Social Science and Medicine 50:829

Wanless D 2001 Securing our future health: taking a long-term view. Interim Report. The Stationery Office, London

Wanless D 2002 Securing our future health: taking a long-term view. Final Report. The Stationery Office, London

Witz A 1992 Professions and patriarchy. Routledge, London

Witz A 1994 The challenge of nursing. In: Gabe J, Kelleher D, Williams G (eds) Challenging medicine. Routledge, London, ch 2, p 23–45

CHAPTER

16 Community care and informal caring

Fiona Stevenson

WHAT IS COMMUNITY CARE?

Community care has been a goal of government policy in the United States, Britain and the rest of Europe since the late 1950s. The overarching aim of a policy of community care is to shift the emphasis of care for dependent groups such as the elderly, chronically ill, people with learning difficulties and those with disabilities, wherever possible, from institutional care to community or home based settings.

The term community care is used both in a prescriptive sense to relate to how people should meet the health and social needs of dependent people and also as a description of the set of services that are currently provided.

THE POLITICS OF COMMUNITY CARE

Cowen (1999) suggested that in Britain there was a contrast in the 'spirit of the age' in the period between 1948 and 1978, which he described as the classic welfare state, and the period between 1979 and 1997, which was the period of the new right (or neoliberal) Conservatism. Thus after the election of the Conservative government in 1979 there was a move from the idea of formal care *in* the community to an emphasis of care *by* the community; that is care by family, relatives, neighbours and friends (informal care) and by voluntary organizations. This emphasis has continued to the present day.

On the surface the ideology of community care appears good and humane; however, when examined at a deeper level the meanings and objectives of community care are associated with confusion and ambiguity. In particular, there is a tension between acting in the interests of vulnerable people in society and the view that successive governments have of community care, in particular care by the community with a heavy reliance on the use of informal care, as a way of controlling the financial cost of caring for those who are less able to care for themselves. This leads to debates around the interface between informal and formal services.

THE EFFECTS OF COMMUNITY CARE POLICIES

The vast majority of dependent people have always lived outside of institutions, cared for informally at home, usually by family, relatives or friends. In 1986 the Audit Commission investigated the extent to which there had been a change in the balance of care in the previous 15 years, notably the replacement of institutional care by community care. The report concluded that progress had been limited. It suggested that the policies had proved poor value for money in terms of those still in institutions, while people in the community may not be getting the support they need (Audit Commission 1986).

Obstacles to the implementation of community care centre on a lack of resources and managerial difficulties. There is also the problem of the coordination between social and health services. The introduction of Primary Care Groups and Trusts in April 1999 combining GP and community health services gives GPs and social services new avenues of cooperation to support carers (Simon 2001). Lewis (1999), however, argued that the continued dominance of general practice in primary care policy may continue to be an obstacle to the integration of community care and primary care. As an initial measure, GPs, members of primary care teams and social services staff were required to have systems in place for identifying carers by April 2000 (Department of Health 1999). Yet, Simon & Kendrick (2001) found that there was a wide variation in the recording of carer status in the notes of carers. They also identified a gap between the expected role envisaged by government and carers' organizations and the actual roles of GPs and district nurses in the support of carers. Simon (2001) provided a list of measures that GPs could take to improve the quality of life of informal carers, such as listening to them, asking their opinions and providing them with information. In essence, treating them as a part of the care team.

LEGISLATION

A summary of the key aspects of both legislation and policy documents in relation to carers is presented in Box 16.1.

The NHS and Community Care Act 1990 requires local authority social services and the NHS to work together to prepare, publish and monitor packages of care in concert with other agencies and users. The historical division between health (NHS) and social care (local authorities) has been marked since the inception of the NHS. Collaboration between health authorities and social services departments is traditionally low as they not only have different organizational structures, but are also based on different ideologies, resulting in conflicting perspectives (Cowen 1999). The NHS and Community Care Act also requires local authorities to involve and consult with users, carers and local organizations. Cowen (1999), however, suggested that there has been little advance in real citizenship rights or in the reconfiguring of traditional power relationships in which managers maintain control.

BOX 16.1   Key aspects of legislation and policy documents in relation to carers

NHS and Community Care Act 1990
- Implemented in full in April 1993
- Requires local authority social services and the NHS to work together to prepare, publish and monitor packages of care
- Local authorities also have to involve and consult with users, carers and local organizations
- The active role of the voluntary sector is encouraged
- Local authorities have to take the needs of carers into account when undertaking assessments

The Carers (Recognition and Services) Act 1995
- Made the requirement to take the needs of carers into account when undertaking assessments a legal right
- Defines a carer as someone who provided or intends to provide 'a substantial amount of care on a regular basis'
- What is meant by 'substantial' and 'regular' is not defined
- There is no right to services
- Assessments have to be done at the same time as an assessment of the cared-for person

Carers and Disabled Children's Act 2000
- Carers have a right to a separate assessment
- There is a requirement for local authorities to provide services to carers to meet their assessed needs

The Report of the Royal Commission on Long Term Care (March 1998)
- Primarily concerned with financing long-term care for elderly people
- Suggested that services to people with a carer should be 'carer blind'
- Recommended the Government should consider a national carer support package
- Contained a note of dissent arguing that more emphasis needs to be placed on help for informal carers, in particular the provision of respite care

Caring about Carers: A National Strategy for Carers (1999)
- Carers should receive information, support and care
- A central aspect of the care provision was for short breaks from caring. A special grant of £140 million over 3 years was announced
- Identified the need for flexible working practices from employers
- Identified the need for special help for young carers

Activity within the voluntary sector, for example the National Association for Mental Health (MIND) and the National Schizophrenic Fellowship (NSF), has been encouraged as a result of the Act and the amount of services they deliver has directly increased. However, Cowen (1999) argued there is a conflict of interests, raising doubts as to the appropriateness of training and the extent to which voluntary agencies should substitute themselves for professional health services.

There has been growing concern expressed for the well-being of carers. The NHS and Community Care Act 1990 requires local authorities to take the needs of carers into account when undertaking assessments. The Carers (Recognition and Services) Act 1995 (Carers Act) made that requirement a legal right. Yet the definition given in the Act of a carer as someone who provided or intended to provide 'a substantial amount of care on a regular basis' is ambiguous. In practice it is left to the discretion of local authorities to determine what constitutes 'regular' and 'substantial' care.

There were a number of problems with the Carers Act. Under the terms of the Act assessments of carers had to be done at the same time as the assessment for the cared-for person; if the cared-for person refused an assessment then the carer could not be assessed. Crucially no extra funding was provided to enable assessments and even once assessed there was no right to services. The Carers and Disabled Children's Act 2000 has since addressed the right to a separate assessment. This Act also contains a requirement for local authorities to provide direct services to carers to meet their assessed needs. However, as the Department of Health has indicated that any additional costs are expected to be contained within local authorities' existing allocation (Arksey 2002), it is unlikely that much change will be evident. Indeed Seddon & Robinson (2001) argued that separate carer assessments are not an established feature of care management practice and care managers lack an explicit framework to direct the assessment of carers' needs. Moreover, Arksey (2002) showed how carers are filtered out of the assessment process in line with the imperative to remain within budget.

POLICY DOCUMENTS

In 1999 the government published Caring about Carers: A National Strategy for Carers, containing a package of measures to support carers consisting of three elements: information, support and care. A central aspect of the 'care' provision was for short breaks from caring and a special grant of £140 million over 3 years was announced. The following statement from the document Caring about Carers provides an understanding of the approach. 'Helping carers is one of the best ways of helping people to help themselves' (Department of Health 1999, page 6).

The Royal Commission on Long Term Care, which was established by the government in 1997, published its report in March 1999. The primary concern of the Royal Commission was financing long-term care for elderly people. It suggested that services to people with a carer should be improved and the provision of services should be 'carer blind', thus the existence of a carer should not affect the services provided. It also recommended that the Government consider a national carer support package.

The Royal Commission report also contained a note of dissent by two members of the committee. The note of dissent argued that more emphasis needed to be placed on help for informal carers than was given in the Royal Commission's report, in particular on the provision of respite care. They recommended a budget of £300 million a year to support carers.

The National Service Framework for Older People (2001) also considered the centrality of the role of carers for older people, and outlined the importance of involving carers in decision-making at all levels in shaping services as well as individual care packages.

The change in terminology from the report published in 1989 entitled Caring for People and the publication of Caring about Carers in 1999 demonstrates a shift in government thinking with an increased focus on carers (Pickard 2001). This shift is further illustrated by the inclusion for the first time of the following question in the 2001 census: 'Do you look after, or give any help or support to family members, friends, neighbours or others because of long-term physical or mental ill-health or disability, or problems related to old age? Do not count anything you do as part of your paid employment'.

THE IMPLICATIONS OF POLICY DOCUMENTS

Pickard (2001) argued that Caring about Carers and the note of dissent, on the one hand, show concern with the interests of carers per se, yet there is also an instrumental concern arising from an interest to ensure that caring continues. The Royal Commission, in contrast, focused on the cared-for. Support for the carer is on the grounds of fairness and to relieve carers of the 'burden' of caring by providing support to the person they care for. Thus it is possible following this model that informal caring can be at least partially substituted by formal caring. This is a new departure for social policy in the UK and contrasts with the Government White Paper 'Growing Older' in 1981 which stated that it was the role of public authorities to sustain and where necessary develop but never to displace informal care.

Pickard (2001) pointed out that exclusive focus on the interests of carers might have major drawbacks if pursued at the expense of the person being cared for. For example, a common suggestion for the support of carers is the introduction or increase in the availability of respite care. This, however, might prove traumatic for the cared-for person, and therefore also the carer, particularly with regard to mentally alert older people who are cared for by their spouse. Thus carers may be badly served by overarching policies which fail to take account of individual needs and preferences.

The Royal Commission focused on the interests of the cared-for person on the understanding that such support has advantages for the carer. Aside from concerns about the financial costs of such a policy, it also fails to account for the fact that the cared-for person may want to be cared for by family and family (McGarry & Arthur 2001), raising the issue of the proper boundary between family and state (Pickard 2001).

These two examples, that respite care does not suit everyone and preferences for informal care, demonstrate the necessity of considering the effects of proposed schemes on all parties concerned and of recognizing that carers and cared-for people are individuals and their needs and wants are likely to vary.

THE RELATIONSHIP BETWEEN THE FORMAL AND INFORMAL SECTORS

Pickard and Glendinning (2002) argued that care in the community has been constructed on the basis of professional support for lay carers, who are expected to take on the main responsibility for caregiving. Services are predominately structured around the cared-for person rather than the carer and there is confusion over the way the relationship between social care agencies and informal carers should be perceived (Twigg 1989). Twigg (1989) argued that carers occupy an ambiguous position within the social care system. Carers are on the margins of the social care system, therefore concern with carer welfare has something of an instrumental quality to it. Twigg (1989) condensed the relationship between social care agencies and carers into three ideal types: carers as resources, carers as co-workers and carers as co-clients (Box 16.2).

BOX 16.2	Three models of carers

1. Carers as resources

Represents the 'given', or the taken for granted reality against which formal services are structured.
The informal sector exists prior to and quite separate from formal services.
Social care agencies, like social services, thus operate, with regard to carers, an essentially
   residualist model in which the agency responds to the deficiencies of the informal care network.
The availability of carers remains beyond the influence of agencies.
Agencies cannot control or influence carers' decisions about whether or not to take up caregiving.
The model places its central focus on the dependant. Although agencies may be concerned to
   understand caregiving they are not concerned with the subjective interests of carers.

2. Carers as co-workers

Agencies work in parallel with the informal sector, aiming at a cooperative and enabling role.
There are difficulties due to the different normative bases that underpin the formal and informal
   sectors.
The model encompasses the carer's interest and the carer's morale within its concerns, but based
   on what is essentially an instrumental motive.

3. Carers as co-clients

The general criteria whereby carers do or do not become defined as clients are complex. In
   practice, the usage tends to be focused on the 'heavy end' of caregiving and on the most
   heavily stressed individuals.
Carers' status as clients is never a fully equal one and they remain at best secondary clients rather
   than fully co-clients.
The aim is the relief of carer strain.

Adapted from Twigg (1989).

Carers can be perceived as resources when social care agencies operate a model in which the agency responds to the deficiencies of the informal care network. Thus the informal sector is perceived as the backdrop to formal provision. In this model of care agencies are not concerned with the welfare of carers given that they have little control over their supply or activities (Twigg 1989).

In the carer as co-worker model agencies work in parallel with the informal sector, aiming at a cooperative and enabling role. The formal and informal sectors are interdependent (Qureshi and Walker 1986) and complementary (Bulmer 1987). There are, however, crucial differences between the two systems, meaning they do not mesh easily or happily together (Twigg 1989, Bulmer 1987). The co-worker model encompasses the carer's interest and the carer's morale within its concerns, but based on what is essentially an instrumental motive, as maintaining high carer morale and involvement represents an intermediate outcome on the way to the final outcome of increased welfare for the dependent person.

In the carer as co-client model the general criteria whereby carers do or do not become defined as clients are complex. In practice, this model tends to be focused on the 'heavy end' of caregiving and on the most heavily stressed individuals. Even here, however, carer status as client is never a fully equal one, and carers remain at best secondary clients rather than fully co-clients. The aim is the relief of carer strain.

The interface between formal and informal care is complex (Pickard & Glendinning 2002). Interaction between the formal and the informal sectors varies according to which model is adopted. In the carer as resources model agencies have no obligation towards the informal sector. In the carer as co-worker model agencies relate more actively to the informal sector but in an essentially instrumental way. In the model of carers as co-clients carers become fully integrated into the concerns of the agency (Twigg 1989). In terms of how legislation operates, financial constraints mean it is mainly in terms of carers as resources. Policy introduced in the 1990s, such as Caring about Carers and the note of dissent to the report of the Royal Commission on Long Term Care, presents a move towards carer as co-worker, while the Royal Commission report itself advocates a model of carer as co-client. However, although there has been an increased focus on carers, change has not been seen in the mainstream services that all the evidence suggests support carers best (Parker 2002).

THE PROVISION OF CARE

▓ Who cares?

Around 6 million people (11% of the population aged 5 or over) provide informal care (HMSO 2006) (Fig. 16.1).

Informal caring rests on personal ties, those of kinship, friendship and neighbourliness (Bulmer 1987). Caring may be a source of satisfaction and add a positive and valued dimension to carers' lives (Arber & Ginn 1992). However, there are also potential problems. Care by families can be problematic due to the generally unequal gender division of caring responsibilities and the past history of the relationship (Qureshi & Walker 1986). Caring can be problematic in friendship because the notion of equivalence tends to be built into the relationship, with a parity of contribution that may be difficult to maintain in a caring relationship (Bulmer 1987). The support offered by neighbours is likely to be general support and social contact rather than more involved care.

Finally, some people have no personal ties and therefore no access to informal care (Bulmer 1987), forcing reliance on formal care. The amount of formal care provided by local authorities has increased markedly in recent years (HMSO 2006).

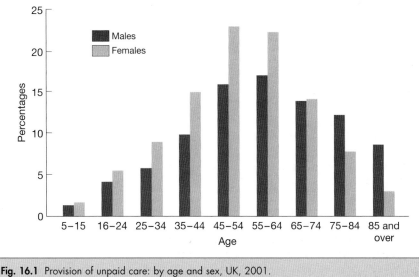

Fig. 16.1 Provision of unpaid care: by age and sex, UK, 2001.
Reproduced with permission from National Statistics Website (http://www.statistics.gov.uk)

Why people care

People may become carers by force of circumstance, a sense of family obligation or as a return for past care and support (Rhodes & Shaw 1999). McGarry & Arthur (2001) reported that some carers saw the support of family members as part of their duty and an expected obligation. Moreover, practical help from the family was preferred to help from formal services that was perceived as help from 'strangers'.

Proctor et al (2001) conducted a study to provide an in-depth understanding of the process of hospital discharge. They suggested that where the experience of illness is new both the patient and family members may not have understood the implications of the illness for the carer role. In established illness family members or the patient may not acknowledge, or be in a position to comply with, the obligations commonly associated with the role of informal carer. Only 11 out of 30 patients in their study at risk of an unsuccessful discharge were willing or able to name an informal carer. Thus carers became defined by the social context of the situation, rather than through personal choice. Having been defined as a carer by either the patient or professionals, it was then morally difficult for individuals to challenge the obligations associated with the role. When the carer did not conform to professional expectations, they sensed that professionals questioned their moral integrity, thus creating a highly coercive environment within which care was given and received.

Finch & Mason (1997) explored people's perceptions of caregiving and reported that most people thought help should be offered to the older generation, yet there is less agreement about what people should actually do. The views expressed as to the type of help that should be offered did not always follow gender stereotypes but there were some normative judgements, for example that sons should provide money and that daughters should care for elderly women (Finch & Mason 1997). Although a poor relationship was not perceived to be a reason for not offering help, the needs of the younger generation were generally seen to take precedence over those of the older generation.

Finally, it is worth noting a possible consequence of shifting care into the community demonstrated in Hubert's (1997) work examining the lives of carers of young adults with challenging behaviour. She discussed how by keeping these young adults in the community, families as a whole, but mothers in particular, may become cut off from the community, leading to social isolation. Thus care in the community may lead to isolation from the community.

Defining a carer

Arksey (2002) pointed to the reluctance of people to identify themselves as carers, instead seeing themselves as spouses, sons or daughters whose care work reflects marriage vows, family obligations and duty. Rose & Bruce (1995) argued that the term 'care' is rescued from the language of work and reclaimed by spouse carers as 'natural'. Thus, particularly among elderly people caring for spouses, the longevity and quality of the relationship prior to the onset of caring means that the boundaries are blurred between caring as part of a close relationship and caring as a more formal role (McGarry & Arthur 2001).

Arber & Gilbert (1989) described the change in the relationship between couples that were over 65 as moving from reciprocity to dependency. The trend is similar in adult children living with their parents. The transition, they argued, is perceived to be natural. They contrasted the situation with that in which an elderly person moves in with married relations where there is not the same drift into care.

Morris & Thomas (2001) suggested that 'carerhood' is a process rather than a fixed state, and one in which competing needs vie for recognition. Caring cannot necessarily be broken down into a series of identifiable tasks (Martin et al 1995) and is not organized along dichotomous lines; for example, the carer and the cared-for, or women care and men don't (Orme 2001). Thus in Thomas et al's (2002) study of the care given by informal carers to people with cancer, 35% of the carers surveyed had a long-standing illness or disability of their own. The study demonstrated the ways in which reciprocity and co-dependency between people with cancer and carers changed in the context of illness. There was greater reciprocity at earlier critical moments in the cancer journey, but greater dependency during periods when patients were undergoing active treatments or were at the palliative care only phase.

Alongside the type of illness or disability for which care is required it is also necessary to consider the wider context in which care occurs. Rose & Bruce (1995) focused on caring within a marital relationship and provided examples in which the cared-for person performed tasks, such as peeling potatoes or repotting plants, that meant more work for the carer in terms of setting the task up and clearing away afterwards, but was important in maintaining at least a show of reciprocity in the relationship. Thus caring and the tasks associated with it should be viewed within the context of the relationship within which they occur. Interestingly, Rose & Bruce (1995) also provided examples to demonstrate how even when the cared-for person is very dependent they may still exert their influence.

Finally, it is important to recognize that caring can consist of emotional but not physical support. Thus Thomas et al (2002) divided care into care work and emotion work. Their data suggested that the management of emotions is a crucial aspect of what informal carers do in relation to cancer. They discussed how carers, particularly in spousal relationships, managed the patient's emotions through taking on the illness mantle and symbolically sharing the illness.

■ The needs of carers

Carers are individual people and their responses to caring situations and their needs will vary; thus, for example, in conditions that affect cognitive function, spouse carers may be mourning the loss of their partner as they have known them as well as coping with physically caring for them and may need psychological support (Addington-Hall et al 1998). Addington-Hall et al's (1998) study concerned the quality of care received in the last years of life by stroke patients, including informal care. They concluded that there was a need for improved support for informal carers, especially for spouses and for those caring for people who are depressed or anxious. Although they pointed out that the data on which the study were based were collected before the implementation of the National Health and Community Care Act (1990), a more recently published study also reported the significant unmet needs of carers. The focus here was a wide range of cancer patients. Needs clustered around aspects of managing daily life, emotions and social identity. Over one in four carers (28%) had three or more significant unmet needs (Soothill et al 2001). Carers with significant unmet needs were more likely to be those where the relationship to the patient was not that of partner or spouse, where the carer had other caring responsibilities, and where the carer did not have friends or relations to call upon for help. They were also likely to be in poor health themselves and caring for a patient who was in the palliative only stage (Soothill et al 2001). Thus those who are already socially disadvantaged are less likely to have all their important needs met. These studies suggest carers still have unmet needs despite legislation and government policy focusing on carers.

Carers put the needs and interests of those they care for above their own and therefore are only likely to take up support services if they feel this will not divert resources and attention away from those for whom they care (McGarry & Arthur 2001, Morris &

273

Thomas 2001, Thomas et al 2002), so even if services are offered to carers it may be necessary to provide reassurance before they will accept.

Caring in the future

Rhodes & Shaw (1999) underlined the importance of stable communities, strong social networks, and local kinship networks, including both immediate and extended kin, for the provision of informal care. Underlying this was the importance of a stable employment base, both in terms of individuals' ability to care and in sustaining the community networks and resources on which they can draw. They discussed the implications of the move away from a stable industrial base towards a more flexible and uncertain employment market associated with an increasingly mobile society, all of which raise worrying questions about patterns of informal caring in the future (Qureshi & Walker 1986). Much of the concern about future informal care has centred on the ageing population; however, the vast majority of elderly people care for themselves without help or only minimal support. It is only those in late old age who begin to decline in terms of self care (Qureshi & Walker 1986). Concern has also been voiced about the adverse effect on informal caring of married women's increasing involvement in the labour market; this has, however, been countered by Hirst (2001), who suggested that having a job often increases mobility and other resources and therefore might enable informal care to be carried out 'at a distance'.

The implications of caring on work outside the home

Figure 16.2 presents the percentage of people aged 16 to 74 who identified themselves as carers in April 2001, organized according to their economic activity status. Of the 13 % of

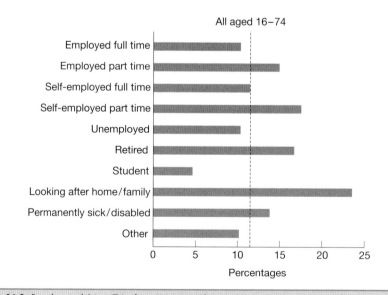

Fig. 16.2 People aged 16 to 74 who were carers: by economic activity status, April 2001, England and Wales.
Reproduced with permission from National Statistics Website (http://www.statistics.gov.uk)

people aged 16 to 74 who provided unpaid care for other people, 12 % of people in work provided care, compared with 15 % who were not in work. Part-time workers were more likely to provide care than full-time workers. Self-employed people were slightly more likely to provide care than people who were employees. Of people not in paid work, those who looked after the home and/or family were the most likely to provide care. Retired people were more likely than average to be carers and there was a substantial provision of care among people who were themselves permanently sick or disabled (HMSO 2004).

The mothers of severely disabled young people are half as likely as their counterparts in the general population to be in paid work. Yet mothers with responsibility for a less than severely disabled young person are just as likely to be working as mothers in the general population. Moreover, when mothers do go out to paid work the severity of their son or daughter's condition makes no difference to the kind of job they do and the number of hours they work (Hirst 1992).

Caring can be unpredictable, which makes it hard to manage, particularly for those with other responsibilities such as childcare and employment. Paid employment can have important social and psychological benefits (Glendinning 1992). However, caregiving may have an effect on paid employment. This needs to be taken into account in assessing the overall 'costs' of community care policies (Glendinning 1992).

There may be economic consequences of constraints on carers' employment at a time when resources are likely to be required for costs such as additional heating. Moreover, caring is likely to have an adverse effect on actual and future employment opportunities and pension provision. These constraints can be substantial and far reaching, although they vary according to factors such as the carer's age, gender, marital status, occupation and amount of time spent caring. The potential long-term effects of a period of restricted labour market participation or withdrawal because of care commitments are of concern as these are likely to occur at a later stage in the life-cycle when there may be greater loss of seniority and less time to 'catch up' before retirement (Glendinning 1992). Glendinning (1992) argued that there is a need for opportunities to work part time or share a job without loss of responsibility, seniority or rate of pay. There is also a need for flexibility. The need for flexibility in the workplace and offering unpaid leave for family emergencies has been taken up in Caring about Carers (Department of Health 1999).

Both men and women experience workplace and personal costs associated with involvement in the caring role, but gender differences are apparent. Martin et al (1995) found that when employment and the provision of personal care were combined both men and women were significantly more likely to experience job effects, career costs and personal costs than their peers without informal caring responsibilities or those only providing instrumental care. Yet women providing personal care experienced more effects than men.

Informal caring varies according to gender, social class, ethnicity and age, all of which affect the likelihood both of caring and receiving support from the formal sector.

The specific implications of gender for caring

Women dominate both formal care work (Peace 1986), including that as paid volunteers (Cowen 1999), and informal service provision (see Fig. 16.1). Under the age of 65 a larger proportion of women than men are carers (HMSO 2006).

Cowen (1999) argued that community care policies are formulated on the basis that women's caring will automatically support formal caring. Care has traditionally been viewed as coming from the nuclear family, although this has been challenged both by feminists in terms of an assumption of the 'natural' caring role of women and by those who present the reality of who does the caring.

Many of the stresses and strains and economic costs associated with caring remain unaccounted for. Relatives act as the main carers in a largely unpaid capacity with women frequently carrying out care in highly stressful situations, frequently lacking 'know how' and without adequate financial support (Cowen 1999). Feminist arguments in particular have focused on the effects on women's physical and psychological health but also on their long-term employment prospects and future pensions.

Invalid Care Allowance for carers was introduced in 1974 but married women were excluded from receiving the benefit. Campaigning by feminists altered this ruling and married women have been able to claim Invalid Care Allowance since 1986. Yet the focus on getting this allowance may in fact have secured women's place as tied to caring, further entrenching a traditional caring role for women (Annandale 1998). There is a general consensus among feminists that community care is resourced through women's unpaid labour, and this consensus is reflected both in empirical studies and theoretical papers (Graham 1997). The arguments have not moved on and continue to present women carers and those they care for as homogeneous. There is a failure to consider the differences and divisions among women, thus masking 'race' and class, sexuality and disability and ignoring the perspective of the cared-for (Graham 1997).

Caring by men and women may be perceived differently. Thus what is perceived as admirable in a man may be perceived as the natural duty of a woman (Rose & Bruce 1995). Caring responsibilities may be allocated by default or lack of power or resources, therefore men are more able to resist the caring role (Martin et al 1995). Annandale (1998), however, cautions against focusing just on women's experience and the idea that it is a priori different to the experience of men, suggesting that this may unintentionally reinforce the idea that caring is women's work. Orme (2001) stressed that a focus on the difference between men and women may have negative consequences for both, while Fisher (1997) suggested there should be a focus on the similarities between men and women in terms of caring.

The focus on women has meant that the role of male carers, particularly as spouse carers, has been ignored. Among older people traditional gender roles are likely to diminish in importance, with tasks divided according to ability (McGarry & Arthur 2001, Rose & Bruce 1995). Interestingly, the balance of power within the relationship may, however, remain as before (McGarry & Arthur 2001).

An analysis of Canadian statistics of informal caring found little gender difference in the amount of informal caring between men and women, but that women provided more personal care, while men provided more instrumental care. Thus the conceptualization of caregiving directly influences the estimate of gender differences in the provision of informal care. The broader the definition the more likely men are to be included in estimates of informal caregiving (Martin et al 1995).

Arber & Gilbert (1989) investigated gender difference in the amount of support carers received. They found that if the level of disability is controlled for then the major source of variation in the amount of support received from formal services was by type of household. People who lived alone received the most from the formal services, followed by people living with a spouse or other elderly person. Those living with a younger married couple received the least support, although they may need support due to pressures such as young children and employment. Male carers in most households received more help than women, but the difference was very small for elderly married couples.

It has been argued that there is an assumption that women will undertake a caring role as part of informal care. However, although more women than men are informal carers and women are more involved in personal care, many factors, such as marital status, the nature of their sibling network and social class, intersect with gender to determine the likelihood of taking on the role of carer (Martin et al 1995).

■ The specific implications of social class for caring

The percentage of people aged 16 to 64 providing unpaid care does not vary greatly by social group, although there is clear variation across the social groups in the number of hours of care provided. Over a fifth of carers in routine occupations, and nearly two-fifths of carers who have never worked or are long-term unemployed, provide 50 hours or more of care per week. This compares with less than one in ten of carers in the higher managerial and professional groups (HMSO 2006) (Fig. 16.3).

Class inequality in informal care reflects the socially structured nature of ill health in British society, since the greatest ill health and disability is suffered by those on the lowest rungs of the class structure. Such families face the greatest burden, providing the greatest number of hours, while at the same time possessing fewer material, financial and cultural resources to ease their caring burden (Arber & Ginn 1992). In addition, the need for informal care is not fixed but conditioned by factors that are intimately bound up with class (Arber & Ginn 1992). The possession of material, financial and cultural resources reduces a physically impaired person's need to rely on informal carers (Arber & Ginn 1992).

The poorer health status of the working class leads to working-class women being disproportionately disadvantaged by the burdens of informal care provision compared to middle-class women (Arber & Ginn 1992). A higher proportion of lower working-class than middle-class mothers have to contend with caring for a chronically sick or disabled child. In adulthood the poorer health of semi-skilled and unskilled men requires

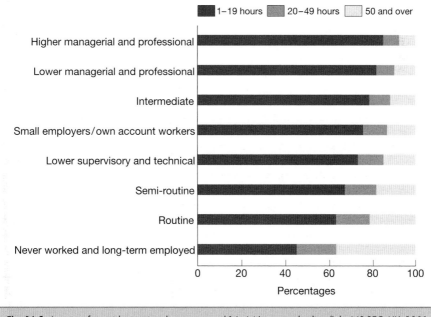

Fig. 16.3 Amount of unpaid care given by carers aged 16–64 (age standardized): by NS-SEC, UK, 2001. *Reproduced with permission from National Statistics Website (http://www.statistics.gov.uk)*

correspondingly greater care, generally provided by their wives (see Arber & Ginn 1992). The difference in timing of the need for this care, with middle-class women more likely to be caring in their 60s and working-class women caring in their 40s, can have profound implications for the development or re-establishment of women's careers (Arber & Ginn 1992).

If co-resident and extra-resident care are examined separately then significant and opposing class differences emerge. Working-class families are more likely than middle-class families to provide care to an impaired or elderly person in the same household. Co-resident care is more time intensive than extra-resident care and is more likely to constrain the life of a care-giver (Arber & Ginn 1992). Working-class people, however, have fewer financial and material resources such as car ownership and this increases their likelihood of being a co-resident carer. Moreover, fewer resources also means less space and less opportunity to manage caring in a way that suits both the carer and the cared-for person (Arber & Ginn 1992).

Arber & Ginn (1992) argued that as the market becomes a more important mechanism in the provision of residential and social care, class may become a key determinant in access to formal private care services, with correspondingly greater burdens of informal care falling on the lower social classes.

Finally, class and gender interact, with a stronger class gradient in caring for men than for women. Higher middle-class men are the least likely to be co-resident carers, while semi-skilled and unskilled men are as likely as women in these classes to be co-resident carers (Arber & Ginn 1992).

■ The specific implications of ethnicity for caring

Figure 16.4 presents the percentage of people caring by ethnic group and time spent caring per week.

In summary, people from White British and White Irish backgrounds, together with Indian people, are most likely to provide informal care to relatives, friends or neighbours. In the census in April 2001 10% each of these groups in Great Britain reported providing informal care. Those least likely to be providing informal care were people from Mixed backgrounds (5.1%), Black Africans (5.6%) and the Chinese (5.8%) (HMSO 2004).

This pattern to some extent reflects the different age structures of the different ethnic groups, as informal care is most likely to be provided by people aged 50 to 60. The White groups have older age structures and are therefore more likely to both provide and need care.

The amount of time that people spend caring differs by ethnic group. Groups most likely to provide very substantial amounts of care (50 hours per week or more) tend to be the same groups who provide care in the first place. The White Irish (2.5%), Bangladeshi (2.4%), Pakistani (2.4%) and White British (2.2%) groups were most likely to report spending 50 hours a week or more caring. Indian, Pakistani, Bangladeshi and Other Asian groups were more likely to report spending 20 to 49 hours a week caring (1.5% or slightly more for each group).

Gunaratnam (1997) suggested that the literature about caring is ethnocentric with little about how ethnicity can shape a caring relationship. Shaky assumptions are adopted about extended family networks supporting elderly and disabled people (Cowen 1999, Gunaratnam 1997). There is variation between the experiences of different ethnic groups as well as within groups. Experiences are affected by class, migration history, gender and the disability of the person needing care (Gunaratnam 1997). Thus there is a need to explore the nature and meaning of care within individual black and ethnic minority communities.

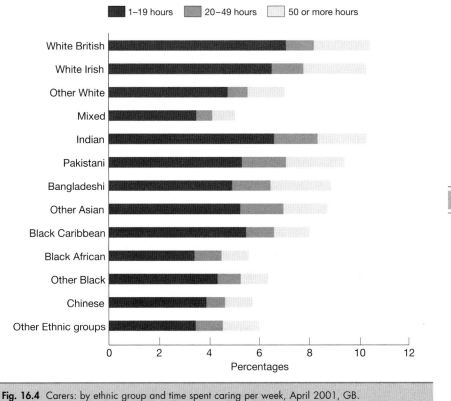

Fig. 16.4 Carers: by ethnic group and time spent caring per week, April 2001, GB.
Reproduced with permission from National Statistics Website (http://www.statistics.gov.uk)

Black and Asian carers figure among the least supported. Diminishing overall family size in Asian communities exacerbates the situation (Cowen 1999). Family care is still strong in British Jewish communities, while occupational and social mobility means the Chinese extended family is diminishing (Cowen 1999). The absence of family networks has shaped the domestic lives and health experiences of many black women in Britain (Graham 1997). Family networks govern access to care within the community, yet such resources are not universally available. Poor employment prospects and tightening immigration controls leave many black elders without access to kin (Graham 1997). Although there are voluntary organizations aimed at specific minority communities, not only does family care vary but so does the capacity of such organizations to support family care (Cowen 1999).

Minority ethnic groups experience exclusion from quality public services and community care, regardless of the introduction of anti-racist legislation and the promulgation of anti-racist charters. This may be because of a fear of uncovering demand in an already stretched service (Gunaratnam 1997). Take up of formal services is low due to a lack of knowledge about services, affected by the inability of some elders to speak English and compounded by illiteracy in their own language (Gunaratnam 1997). There are also insensitivities that alienate minority ethnic elders, for example a lack of dietary awareness, a lack of interpreters and under-representation of minority staff within formal services. Crucially there may be a lack of familiarity among ethnic minority communities with both the word and concept 'carer' (Gunaratnam 1997). Therefore the figures in Fig. 16.4 which rely on self-identification of caring status may require caution in interpretation.

Low social class and poverty are associated with restricted access to informal sources of help (Graham 1997). The wider social and economic position of minority communities in terms of class, gender, poverty and racism within employment can interact with ethnic identity to shape the needs of minority carers (Gunaratnam 1997).

▓ The specific implications of age for caring

Figure 16.3 presents data on carer status organized according to age.

The idea that elderly people are a care burden not only fails to take account of the fact that most elderly people do not require care, it also denies the amount of support that older generations provide for younger, for example in terms of childcare. Thus there is reciprocity in patterns of intergenerational caring (Martin et al 1995). Given this reciprocity, it is important not to ignore the experiences of those who receive care, as denial of reciprocity in the caring relationship can make caring oppressive (Orme 2001).

Thirteen per cent of people over the age of 65 provide some form of informal care (Rowlands 1998). Increasing longevity and demographic changes, combined with the continued emphasis on community care, mean greater numbers of older people both giving and receiving care in the future (McGarry & Arthur 2001). Far from being a burden on service resources, older people provide a substantial amount of informal care, often alone and with very little formal support (McGarry & Arthur 2001). Of older people in Britain who had help with domestic tasks, 80% relied exclusively on informal help, 10% on both informal and formal sources and 10% on exclusively formal services (Pickard 2001). Hirst's (2001) secondary analysis of the British Household Panel Survey confirmed that spouse care increased more than any other caring relationship during the 1990s, more so for men than for women. As male life expectancy increases, men are now more likely to survive to an age where their spouse or partner needs informal care. By the end of the 1990s as many men as women were spouse carers.

Many older people meet the demands of being a carer alongside managing their own health difficulties. McGarry & Arthur (2001) in their study of the experiences of informal carers who were aged 75 and over found that both carers and care recipients were aware of the precarious nature of the relationship. A change in circumstances for either the carer or the care recipient could force the intricate nature of the relationship to collapse.

At the other end of the age continuum, the contributions of children to caregiving have been relatively under-researched (Fox 1998). Fox (1998) reported that children are involved in a range of care activities and often there is a strong emotional component to this caregiving. In April 2001, 109 000 children under the age of 16 in Great Britain were providing some informal care. Indian, Bangladeshi and Pakistani children were the most likely to be carers, around 1.5% of each group. Black African children were least likely to provide care, at 0.7%. Among White British children, 0.9% were providing some unpaid care (HMSO 2004). Many of these young people receive no support at all from statutory or voluntary services. Fox (1998) suggested that there is a need to acknowledge the practical contribution to informal care that young people are making within the private spaces of family life. The policy document Caring about Carers (Department of Health 1999) contained a chapter on young carers and proposed measures to ensure that these carers receive both recognition and support.

CONCLUSIONS

This chapter has focused on informal care; however, as has been demonstrated, neither care nor informal care are necessarily clear cut and easy to define. There is a blurring of the notion of carer as people may 'drift into care', particularly spousal care. The dominance of women in both formal and informal care may also serve to blur the distinction between the two, particularly as formal carers may develop a more personalized relationship with individual clients (Qureshi & Walker 1986). Moreover, the increase in medical technologies which can be administered at home means private space is violated as the home becomes more like the hospital (Kirk & Glendinning 1998, Rhodes & Shaw 1999), further blurring the distinction between formal and informal care.

There is a rhetoric about carers that has yet to be fulfilled. Legislation has provided carers with the right to an independent assessment of their needs; however, the legislation has not been accompanied by additional resources and it is unlikely that assessments for carers will receive priority within a system which is already financially stretched. Resources have been made available for respite care, on the basis that this was effective for carers of people with Alzheimer's and related disorders. Yet caring situations are individual and this may not be the most appropriate way of supporting all carers, particularly people caring for their spouse. It can be argued that the recent policy initiatives are instrumental as they support carers to ensure that they continue to care, thus reducing the burden on formal services. Therefore, although the ideology behind policy initiatives appears good and humane, they can also be seen as a way of controlling the financial costs of caring at the expense of informal carers.

References

Addington-Hall J, Lay M, Altmann D, McCarthy M 1998 Community care for stroke patients in the last year of life: results of a national retrospective survey of surviving family, friends and officials. Health and Social Care in the Community 6:112–119

Annandale E 1998 The sociology of health and medicine. Polity Press, Cambridge

Arber S, Gilbert N 1989 Men: the forgotten carers. Sociology 23:111–118

Arber S, Ginn J 1992 Research note. Class and caring: a forgotten dimension. Sociology 26:619–634

Arksey H 2002 Rationed care: Assessing the service needs of informal carers in English social services authorities. Journal of Social Policy 31:81–101

Audit Commission 1986 Making a reality of community care. HMSO, London

Bulmer M 1987 The social basis of community care. Allen and Unwin, London

Cowen H 1999 Community care, ideology and social policy. Prentice Hall Europe, London

Department of Health 1999 Caring about carers: a national strategy for carers. Department of Health, London

Finch J, Mason J 1997 Filial obligations and kin support for elderly people. In: Bornat J et al (eds) Community care: a reader, 2nd edn. Open University, Basingstoke

Fisher M 1997 Older male carers and community care. In: Bornat J et al (eds) Community care: a reader, 2nd edn. Open University, Basingstoke

Fox NJ 1998 The contribution of children to informal care: a Delphi study. Health and Social Care in the Community 6:204–208

Glendinning C 1992 Employment and 'community care': policies for the 1990s. Work Employment and Society 6:103–111

Graham H 1997 Feminist perspective on caring. In: Bornat J et al (eds) Community care: a reader, 2nd edn. Open University, Basingstoke

Gunaratnam Y 1997 Breaking the silence: black and ethnic minority carers and service provision. In: Bornat J et al (eds) Community care: a reader, 2nd edn. Open University, Basingstoke

Hirst M 1992 Employment patterns of mothers with a disabled young person. Work Employment and Society 6:87–101

Hirst M 2001 Trends in informal care in Great Britain during the 1990s. Health and Social Care in the Community 9:348–357

HMSO 2004 National Statistics (http://www.statistics.gov.uk)

HMSO 2006 National Statistics (http://www.statistics.gov.uk)

Hubert J 1997 At home and alone: families and young adults with challenging behaviour. In: Bornat J et al (eds) Community care: a reader, 2nd edn. Open University, Basingstoke

Kirk S, Glendinning C 1998 Trends in community care and patient participation: implications for the roles of informal carers and community nurses in the United Kingdom. Journal of Advanced Nursing 28:370–381

Lewis J 1999 The concepts of community care and primary care in the UK: the 1960s to the 1990s. Health and Social Care in the Community 7:333–341

McGarry J, Arthur A 2001 Informal caring in late life: a qualitative study of the experiences of older carers. Journal of Advanced Nursing 33:182–189

Martin Matthews A, Campbell L 1995 Gender roles, employment and informal care. In: Arber S, Ginn J (eds) Connecting gender and ageing. Open University Press, Buckingham

Morris SM, Thomas C 2001 The carer's place in the cancer situation: where does the carer stand in the medical setting? European Journal of Cancer Care 10:87–95

Orme J 2001 Gender and community care. Palgrave, Basingstoke

Parker G 2002 Guest editorial: 10 years of the 'new' community care: good in parts? Health and Social Care in the Community 10:1–5

Peace S 1986 The forgotten female: social policy and older women. In: Phillipson C, Walker A (eds) Ageing and social policy. Gower, Aldershot

Pickard L 2001 Carer break or carer-blind? Policies for informal carers in the UK. Social Policy and Administration 35:441–458

Pickard S, Glendinning C 2002 Comparing and contrasting the role of family carers and nurses in the domestic health care of frail older people. Social Care in the Community 10:144–150

Proctor S, Wilcockson J, Pearson P, Allgar V 2001 Going home from hospital: the carer/patient dyad. Journal of Advanced Nursing 35:206–217

Qureshi H, Walker A 1986 Caring for elderly people: the family and the state. In: Phillipson C, Walker A (eds) Ageing and social policy. Gower, Aldershot

Rhodes P, Shaw S 1999 Informal care and terminal illness. Health and Social Care in the Community 7:39–50

Rose H, Bruce E 1995 Mutual care but differential esteem: caring between older couples. In: Arber S, Ginn J (eds) Connecting gender and ageing. Open University Press, Buckingham

Rowlands O 1998 Informal carers. Results of an independent study carried out on behalf of the Department of Health as part of the 1995 General Household Survey. ONS, London

Royal Commission on Long Term Care 1999 With respect to old age: long term care – rights and responsibilities. HMSO, London

Seddon D, Robinson CA 2001 Carers of older people with dementia: assessment and the Carers Act. Health and Social Care in the Community 9:151–158

Simon C 2001 Informal carers and the primary care team. British Journal of General Practice 51:920–923

Simon C, Kendrick T 2001 Informal carers – the role of general practitioners and district nurses. British Journal of General Practice 51:655–657

Soothill K, Morris SM, Harman JC et al 2001 Informal carers of cancer patients: what are their unmet psychological needs? Health and Social Care in the Community 9:464–475

Thomas C, Morris SM, Harman JC 2002 Companions through cancer: the care given by informal carers in cancer contexts. Social Science and Medicine 54:529–544

Twigg J 1989 Models of carers: how do social care agencies conceptualise their relationship with informal carers? Journal of Social Policy 18:53–66

CHAPTER

17 Public health and health promotion

Judith Green

PUBLIC HEALTH

▪ What is public health?

Chapter 2 discussed the growing recognition of the social causes of disease and health. Individual behaviours, economic conditions and the material environments in which we live have a powerful impact on the overall health of populations and the inequalities in health within and between them. Public health is the speciality concerned with these broader determinants of health, and with the health of populations, rather than with individuals as patients. In 1988, Acheson defined public health as:

'The science and art of preventing disease, prolonging life and promoting health through the organised efforts of society' (Acheson 1988)

As this definition suggests, the interests of public health have many overlaps with those of medical sociology, given the importance of understanding social conditions both to understand how diseases are distributed through society, and how to effect change in order to improve health. Indeed, many departments of Public Health in the UK still use the title 'Social Medicine'. One of the main 'sciences' that contributes to public health is epidemiology, which is the study of the distribution and causes of diseases in populations. However, modern public health departments also include a range of other disciplines, including sociologists, economists and statisticians as well as those trained in medicine. In the UK, the Faculty of Public Health (http://www.fphm.org.uk/) describes public health as a multi-disciplinary exercise, which addresses three overlapping domains (see Box 17.1): health protection; health improvement; and health and social care quality.

This is a large and disparate range of activities, and two challenges are immediately obvious. One is that few activities in these domains lie solely within the remit of the health sector: any effective action requires work from a range of other agencies and professionals outside the healthcare arena. For emergency planning, for instance, the responses of the health services are only one element of a coordinated effort needed in the event of a terrorist attack or natural disaster. To address the health effects of poor housing, public health specialists can do little other than research and monitor effects:

they are reliant on social housing providers, local government officials, and the social benefits and taxation systems to address damp conditions, overcrowding or homelessness. Modern public health is, then, of necessity a collaborative discipline. To address effectively the major determinants of health in the 21st century requires partnerships with local government, the education sector, the police, and other statutory, non-governmental and even private agencies, as well as healthcare providers and purchasers.

The second, related, issue is that there is some ambiguity about what the role of medicine in general, and public health professionals in particular, is in addressing many of the broader determinants of health. Injuries, which are a major cause of mortality and morbidity, are one example. Medicine clearly has a role in the treatment of injury and the rehabilitation of those injured, but the role of medicine in public health activity, such as prevention, is less obvious (Green 1999). If the determinants of health lie largely within the remit of professionals such as traffic engineers, whose decisions affect the speed and volume of traffic and thus the likelihood of pedestrian injury, or health and safety inspectors, who can reduce workplace hazards, what is the role of the public health specialist? Should they be advocates for public health, engaged in political activities designed to raise awareness of road traffic injuries, or restrict their role to researching the epidemiology of injury, leaving advocacy to others?

Contemporary public health is marked by these ongoing debates about its proper boundaries and location. Should it be properly part of the healthcare system, as a 'medical' speciality? Or it does it belong more appropriately as part of local government, alongside social housing, education, refuse collection and all the other departments that contribute to the health of a local population? Should public health professionals be primarily 'scientists', focusing on the epidemiology of disease, or is their role more usefully that of the 'activist', generating pressure for healthier public policy?

As the Faculty of Public Health recognizes, a large range of professionals contribute to the three domains of public health. These include healthcare professionals whose

---

BOX 17.1 The domains of public health

- *Health protection*: including the control of infectious disease, radiation, chemicals and poisoning, emergency response, environmental hazards
- *Health improvement*: including reducing inequalities in health, housing, education, lifestyles
- *Health and social care quality*: including clinical effectiveness, clinical governance, service planning and evaluation, efficiency of health services

Source: Faculty of Public Health http://www.fphm.org.uk/.

primary job is related to public health practice, such as community nurses and health promotion advisers, but also those who have a broader role that can underpin health improvement, such as transport planners, housing officers and teachers. Public health consultants, who are the specialists in public health, are usually medically trained doctors, but increasingly are specialists who have trained in other disciplines. These functions are, at the beginning of the 21st century, spread around the healthcare and other systems in the UK. Each Primary Care Trust (PCT) has a Director of Public Health on the Board of the PCT, which is charged with improving the health of the community. The Health Protection Agency is responsible for surveillance and control of communicable diseases, and environmental hazards. The Health Development Agency, founded in 2000, is concerned with the evidence base for public health practice. Its functions were transferred to the National Institute for Health and Clinical Excellence (NICE) in 2005.

These tensions in contemporary public health (the extent of its remit, where it should be located, and who should do it) have historical roots in the ways in which the speciality emerged (see Box 17.2).

The emergence of modern public health

The roots of modern public health lie in the sanitary movement of the 19th century, when the impact of poor environments on the health of, particularly, the urban poor, became a political concern. Armstrong (1993) argues that this represented the point at which disease became seen as residing in places, or specific environments, rather than something that came from 'outside' and needing quarantine to keep out. Environments consisted of soil, water, meteorological conditions and buildings, all of which could put health at risk. A key figure from this period was the campaigning reformer Edwin Chadwick, who was a utilitarian concerned at the large numbers admitted to the workhouses. He published his *Report . . . on an Enquiry into the Sanitary Condition of the Labouring Population of Great Britain* in 1842, and as one of the Directors of the Board of Health between 1848 and 1854, his campaign to improve conditions led to the 1848 Public Health Act. This established a central Board of Health, and allowed Local Boards of Health to take control of local drains and sewage – an important enabler of local government intervention for the public health. The second Public Health Act of 1872 required that local authorities appoint a medical officer who would be responsible for sanitation.

The story of John Snow and the Soho cholera outbreak of 1854 is an iconic one in the story public health tells of its own origins (Vandenbroucke et al 1991). Snow mapped the cases of cholera, noticing that two affected people who lived far from Soho were still drinking water from a pump in Broad Street, in the vicinity of the main outbreak, but that brewery workers who lived nearby were unaffected. It transpired that they did not use water from the local pump, but drank beer instead. Snow not only solved the 'mystery', in identifying that contaminated water was the cause of the epidemic, but also provided an early example of public health advocacy, in his activism in getting the handle of the Broad Street pump removed to stop the epidemic at source. The story of Snow and the pump handle not only illustrates this mixture of 'science' (in early epidemiology) and the 'art' of activism, but more significantly perhaps, marks the moment when medicine saw itself as integral to the business of public health.

The sanitary movement of the 19th century, argues Armstrong (1993), was replaced in the 20th century by a new understanding of public health that focused on hygiene instead of sanitary science. Hygiene was orientated more towards individuals than environments, and this period in public health saw the beginnings of medical surveillance of physical bodies in such settings as the school and the clinic, as it was human bodies and the spaces between them that emerged as the place of risk. To some extent, over the course of the 20th century, the environment was relegated to a background role. Indeed, public health in general became somewhat marginalised in medicine, with increasing focus on curative hospital services, and faith in medical progress as the route to improving health through such technical innovations as antibiotics, organ transplant surgery, and vaccinations.

The 'new' public health and global health

After the mid-20th century, faith in medicine's ability to find cures for all ills began to wane. By the 1970s, there was a resurgence of interest in the social determinants of health, and the idea that medicine alone could not address the necessities for health. The emphasis moved to the idea of building healthy public policy, rather than addressing narrow questions of preventing disease. A key moment in this shift was the publication of the Lalonde report by the Canadian government in 1974 (Lalonde 1974), which is often cited as the beginning of a move towards a more collaborative, less medicalized vision for public health. Lalonde suggested the idea of the *health field*, which included four domains that shaped individual health, as shown in Fig. 17.1.

The World Health Organization enshrined this commitment to inter-sectoral action at its first International Conference on Primary Health Care, in Alma Ata in 1978. The Declaration of Alma Ata (WHO 1978) reaffirmed that health was a fundamental human right, and that inequalities in health were a proper concern. The declaration spurred the slogan *Health for All by the Year 2000*, based on the conference's call to action to ensure that the preconditions of this be met. These included better use of the world's resources, peace and the effective introduction and development of primary care systems worldwide.

In the UK, these movements towards a more integrated vision for public health were heralded by Ashton & Seymour (1988) as the 'New Public Health', which they distinguished from what had gone before in terms of the move away from what they called the 'downstream' causes of ill health, to the more 'upstream' determinants. To some extent this was merely restating the environmental and social causes that had been core

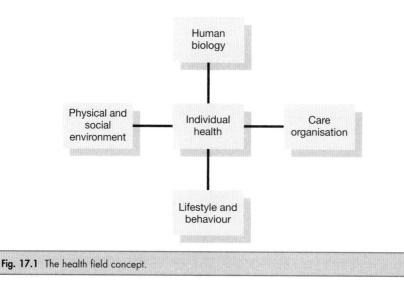

Fig. 17.1 The health field concept.

to 19th century sanitary movements, after a period of the dominance of hospital medicine. However, some commentators, such as Baum (1998), writing on similar shifts in Australia, argued that the 'new' part of the New Public Health was the focus on social justice and healthy public policy, particularly in terms of a global sensibility that addressed international inequalities and the impact of globalization on health.

This is evident in some of the more recent shifts in public health that have begun to link concerns about the health of the planet with concerns about the health of populations (Beaglehole 2003). Some have argued forcefully that the key issues for public health in the 21st century will be those linked to issues of sustainable development in the face of threats such as global warming. Not only is global warming likely to have direct impact on health, through, for instance, causing increasingly extreme weather and changing the distribution of disease-bearing vectors such as mosquitoes, but there are a range of indirect effects that public health practitioners should be concerned about. These issues were first highlighted on the policy agenda by the 1992 Earth Summit in Rio de Janeiro in Brazil, on how to protect the environment. One outcome of this was *Agenda 21*, a commitment to sustainable development at a local level. Local authorities were encouraged to work in partnership with communities to develop plans that reduced environmental pollution and protected natural habitats, but in ways which improved the quality of people's lives. In areas such as transport, waste disposal and energy use, sustainable development was seen as a goal that was to be aligned with public health, in its broadest sense.

Transport is one field in which these global links have been made. Roberts (2004) points to the ways in which transport, industry, global conflict and injuries are related. The cheap international road and air transport needed to sustain a globalized economy, he argues, puts people at further risk of transport injuries, but also from war, made more likely as first world countries struggle to control oil supplies. These kinds of links have led some to claim that health professionals have a duty to advocate for policy change around issues such as global warming. As Stott put it: 'promoting carbon rationing could be your most important contribution to patients' health' (Stott 2006, page 1385). Reducing carbon emissions through reducing air and road transport has a broad impact on public health, in that we reduce air pollution, increase the amount of (healthier) active transport and also rebuild communities that are becoming increasingly isolated by major roads and residents living far from where they work.

▓ Tensions in public health

Public health addresses, then, complex health problems that require coordinated action across different sectors. This inevitably generates some tensions in practice, given that there are a range of political, social and moral values that shape professionals' views of how to do this. Action on smoking provides one illustration. Tobacco smoking has been associated with lung cancer since the 1950s, and there are now over 40 diseases recognized as linked to smoking, including cancer of the bladder and oesophagus, cardiovascular diseases, chronic obstructive pulmonary disease and peptic ulcer disease (US Department of Health and Human Services 2004). There are also inequalities in the harm caused by smoking. Internationally, tobacco companies have extended their markets into low-income countries, where the burden of disease is now growing and it is estimated that by 2030 around 70% of smoking-related deaths will be in low and middle income countries (Gilmore et al 2005). Within the UK, smoking rates are higher for those in routine or semi-routine occupations (35% of men, 32% of women) than they are for those in professional occupations (20% men, 18% of women) (National Centre for Social Research 2004). As Gilmore and colleagues put it, tobacco use raises some urgent issues for public health because:

'there have been ethical debates around the methods that can be appropriately used to control its use...[tobacco control] highlights the key challenges globalization poses for public health, the complex relationship between trade and health, the potential conflicts of interest that tobacco control raises for governments and the difficulties of enacting effective public health policies that are opposed by transnational companies' (Gilmore et al 2005, page 174)

Controlling the effects of involuntary exposure to environmental smoke is one such issue, with many countries and regions now introducing bans on smoking in enclosed public spaces. Such bans generate public debate, with some arguing that they are unjustified state interference with personal choice, and others that such paternalism is justified to protect the public health. Other tobacco control policies include raising taxes on tobacco products, legislating to remove advertising and, particularly in the United States, using litigation against tobacco companies. The latter, argue Gilmore et al (2005) has been effective in forcing the release of tobacco industry documents which have shed light on how the industry has moved into new markets and attempted to control public debate.

These 'upstream' social policies to address a public health issue illustrate the broad coalitions needed for action. This raises a question of whether it is the role of the public health specialist to be overtly partisan in their practice in, for instance, campaigning against tobacco production or for different transport systems, or even aligning themselves with social goals such as poverty eradication. Although such goals may have broad support, some epidemiologists argue that we often have too little knowledge about the causal pathways linking 'upstream' conditions to health outcomes to make firm predictions about what will impact on health (Rothman et al 1998), and that the job of the epidemiologist should not be that of a 'social engineer', however much the eradication of tobacco smoking or poverty is a worthwhile goal. Rothman and colleagues (1998) focus on the role of public health as a science, not a social project, and one in which epidemiologists have a primary obligation not to work for social justice but to study disease processes and improve our understanding of risk factors at the individual level, where we can conduct relatively good studies on effectiveness. In contrast, Beaglehole and colleagues (2004) argue that to be effective public health practice should be as 'upstream' as possible, and directed at poverty itself, and global environmental change, which are the root causes of ill health.

HEALTH PROMOTION

▓ The development of health promotion

Health promotion is an approach that can be seen as part of the emergence of the 'new public health' in the 1980s and 1990s (Macdonald & Bunton 1992). It was distinguished as a new approach through the contrast with what had gone before: health education. Health education was based on a narrow model of informing the public about health risks, and attempting to change behaviour at the individual level. Until the middle of the 20th century, health education largely consisted of mass information campaigns around issues such as avoiding infection (particularly sexually transmitted diseases) and staying healthy. Traditionally, health education was directed at one or more levels of preventative activity (see Table 17.1). These are based on a medical model of disease, in which health effects are conceptualized as a series of risks to be managed (Tones & Green 2004).

This public information function is still an important element of health promotion, but it is now recognized that simply telling people how to lead healthier lives is not

TABLE 17.1	The levels of prevention	
Level of prevention	**Definition**	**Examples**
Primary	Prevention of onset of disease or injury	• Immunization for measles • Traffic calming to prevent serious injuries to pedestrians and cyclists • Campaign to get children eating more fruit and vegetables
Secondary	Early detection and treatment of disease or risk factors for it, in order to prevent morbidity or mortality	• Screening for cervical cancer • Wearing cycling helmets to reduce impact of crashes • Monitoring blood pressure
Tertiary	To minimize disability or morbidity from disease or injury	• Medication to reduce blood pressure • Rehabilitation to improve mobility

particularly effective, as it ignores both the structural causes of ill health and the constraints on individual choice. A simple model of health behaviour based solely on information also ignores the complex role of attitudes and health beliefs on health behaviours. A good example here is information about the risks of smoking. Graham (1987), in a study of why mothers on low incomes smoked, found that all were aware of the health risks of smoking and more education was unlikely to have any impact on behaviour. Smoking was associated with patterns of coping with stress: one 'adult' activity that women could do that provided 'time out' of a busy day.

Health promotion theory has developed more sophisticated approaches for understanding how people change behaviour. An early one was the health belief model (Becker 1974) which suggested that the likelihood of an individual behaving in a certain way (for instance getting immunized or increasing their level of exercise) was a function of their assessment of the likely risks and benefits of that action, their beliefs about the seriousness of the threat to their health of not taking the action, and how far they believe the action will address that threat. Health promotion can thus be directed at any of these elements. An immunization campaign could increase people's awareness of the threat of measles, could inform them about the effectiveness of immunization or could minimize the 'costs' of the action, such as the inconvenience of clinic hours.

In contrast to health education, the health promotion approach is designed to enable people to make healthy choices through empowerment, and also to address the social and environmental causes of unhealthy behaviour. This could include anything from a transport system that makes walking more difficult than driving, to the relative financial cost of healthy food, to the availability of fulfilling employment. As Tones & Green (2004, page 14) put it:

> The scope of health promotion can therefore be summed up in a simple formula:
> health promotion = health education × healthy public policy

To 'promote health', rather than merely prevent disease, contemporary models of health promotion draw on the developments in international health policy discussed above, which take a more holistic view that is in line with the World Health Organization's well known definition of health from its first constitution in 1946:

> A state of complete physical, social and mental wellbeing, and not merely the absence of disease or infirmity

This definition has been a cornerstone of many international and national policies directed at public health and health promotion and the WHO has had a key role in shaping definitions and understandings of health promotion. A 1984 discussion document (WHO 1984) outlined key principles of health promotion as follows:

- Health promotion involves the population as a whole in their everyday life

- Health promotion is directed at the determinants of health

- Health promotion contains diverse, but complementary methods and approaches

- Health promotion requires effective public participation

- Health professionals have a role in advocating for health

The Ottawa Charter, building on this discussion document and the Alma-Ata conference, was developed at the WHO's first International Conference on Health Promotion (WHO 1986). This identified three major strategies for health promotion, and five areas of action (see Table 17.2).

Beattie (1991) described approaches to health promotion as distributed along two dimensions: the first being the mode of intervention (authoritative or negotiated) and the second the focus of intervention (whether the individual or the collective) (see Fig. 17.2). Strategies at the top of his model (the more authoritarian) utilize medical authority to either redirect individual behaviours or to change policies in line with healthy choices; whereas those at the bottom rely on more collaborative or bottom-up strategies to improve the health of individuals or groups.

Strategies of health promotion

Health promotion is thus directed at a number of levels, from the individual and their lifestyles, to that of the community, and at the broadest level of international policy. An example of a campaign that combined individual and community approaches was

TABLE 17.2	The Ottawa Charter for health promotion	
Three strategies for health promotion		**Five areas of action**
Advocacy: for political, social and economic conditions favourable to health		• Build healthy public policy
		• Create supportive environments
Enabling: all people to have the control needed to achieve their fullest health potential		• Strengthen community actions
		• Develop personal skills
Mediating: coordinating action by governments, non-governmental actors, professionals and communities		• Re-orientate health services
Source: WHO (1986).		

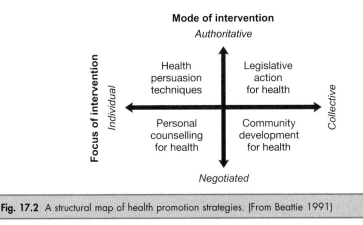

Fig. 17.2 A structural map of health promotion strategies. (From Beattie 1991)

'Heartbeat Wales', a primary prevention programme launched in 1985 that aimed to reduce the risk factors for heart disease in the Welsh population. This used advertising and market strategies to make healthy early choices the easier ones. Davison and colleagues (1991) analysed the cultural and social effects of this programme, noting first that it illustrated the 'prevention paradox'. This is the result of population strategies which entail getting the whole population to change their lifestyle when the benefit to most individuals is minimal – to prevent a small number of deaths requires that a large number of people change their behaviour. Given that this would not be a convincing message for most individuals, campaigns instead focus on simple messages such as 'eat more vegetables', or 'take more exercise'. However, Davison et al (1991) argue that lay epidemiology (the everyday beliefs people have about illness, its distribution and its causes) is rather more sophisticated than assumed by most health promotion campaigns. People notice that some 'low risk' individuals die of heart disease, whereas some 'high risk' individuals live to an old age. This illustrates another tension at the heart of public health practice, between the individual and collective levels of public health.

Despite a more holistic view at the level of theory and policy, it could be argued that a medical model and individualistic approach still dominates much practice in health promotion. Beattie (1991) notes that UK health agencies continue to use mass media campaigns such as those on drug use or HIV risk, despite little evidence that such educational interventions based on naïve views of behaviour change are effective.

SOCIOLOGICAL CRITIQUES OF PUBLIC HEALTH AND HEALTH PROMOTION

Sociology has contributed to our understanding of public health and health promotion, but has also provided a critique of them. Nettleton and Bunton (1995) identify three major strands in sociological analyses of health promotion practice:

- *structural critiques*, which focus on the ways in which the material conditions that give rise to ill health are marginalized in so much policy and practice

- *surveillance critiques*, which explore the role of health promotion practices in monitoring and regulating the population

- *consumption critiques*, which see lifestyle choices not as health 'risks' but as part of the ways in which we construct identities

BOX 17.2	Some key dates in the development of public health and health promotion
1848	1st Public Health Act
1854	John Snow causes the removal of the Broad Street pump handle
1872	2nd Public Health Act
1942	Beveridge Report identified five 'giant evils': want, disease, ignorance, squalor and illness
1946	NHS Act – removed clinics and dispensaries from local government control
1974	NHS Act – removed community health services from local authority control
1974	Lalonde Report
1978	1st International Conference on Primary Care, Alma Ata
1986	1st International Conference on Health Promotion produces the Ottawa Charter
1992	Rio Earth Summit generates Agenda 21
1999	DoH publishes *Saving Lives: Our healthier nation*
2000	Health Education Authority becomes Health Development Agency (HDA)
2005	DoH publishes *Choosing health: Making healthy choices easier*
2005	HDA functions are transferred to the National Institute for Health and Clinical Excellence
2006	Smoking banned in enclosed public places in Scotland
2007	Smoking bans introduced in Wales, England and Northern Ireland

These strands run through a number of debates in sociology about the cultural and social effects of public health and health promotion practice.

Victim-blaming

Early critiques of public health and health promotion practice focused on the ways in which these tended to 'blame the victim' for their own ill health. Robert Crawford (1977) argued that an ideology of victim-blaming had emerged as a result of rising healthcare costs in the context of both high public expectations of medicine, high expectations of 'entitlement' and a growing awareness of environmental health issues. Victim-blaming is, for Crawford, a political and ideological response in which the individual's lifestyle and behaviour is constructed as 'the problem' rather than the structural conditions that give rise to ill health, or constraints on ability to choose. Thus, campaigns encouraging mothers to cook healthier food for their children construct them as responsible for the health of their children whilst failing to address the higher costs of fresh fruit and vegetables, or the difficulties in accessing them from many of the more deprived areas of the UK.

Empowerment and the problem of choice

Thorogood (2002) discusses a problem at the heart of health promotion. Its aim is to promote healthy choices; yet it also valorizes empowerment, such that people make their own choices. Clearly there is a role for public policy in making the healthy choice the easy choice, but this also equates the healthy choice with the rational, obvious and moral one. What happens, asks Thorogood, to other legitimate choices? In the example of sexual health promotion, for instance, the healthy choice might be to use condoms to reduce the risk of sexually transmitted diseases – but discourses of health are rarely the primary ones individuals use in their everyday sexual lives, where pleasure, or the demonstration of trust may be more dominant.

Health promotion and governance

Petersen (1997) and Nettleton (1997) are among those who draw on the French historian Michel Foucault's work to explore the role of public health (specifically the 'new' public health) as one aspect of the 'governance' of contemporary societies. In this view, the surveillance needed to monitor risks for health and to manage them is an exercise that has made us all 'at risk' and in need of constant alertness to the project of health. The responsibility for managing those risks is shifted from the state to the individual, who has a duty to engage in 'processes of endless self-examination, self care and self-improvement' (Petersen 1997, page 194). Despite its emancipatory and egalitarian rhetoric, public health still has the primary goal of delineating the normal and abnormal; the healthy and unhealthy, and as such has a moral as well as technical role. Thus, it is part of the apparatus of the modern state that shapes our subjectivity, in that we learn to become risk-aware citizens whose obligation is to strive for better and better health.

293

Public health and the 'risk society'

The ways in which the technologies of health promotion and public health construct the population as 'at risk' have also been seen as an important element of what the German sociologist Ulrich Beck (1992) has called the 'risk society'. Beck argues that the contemporary age was characterized by societies being divided by their vulnerability to risks. The defining features of modern risks are that they are often invisible (such as carcinogens in food); omnipresent (affecting everyone) and derive not only from nature but from scientific progress itself. This has a number of implications for public health and health promotion. First, they have to address not only the risks of diseases and environments, but also complex issues arising from the effects of medicine itself. One example was the public debate over the Measles, Mumps and Rubella (MMR) vaccine in the UK. Media coverage of a link between MMR, bowel disease and autism led to a small decline in uptake of the vaccine, and a health promotion campaign designed to assure parents about its safety (Hobson-West 2003). Hobson-West examined the ways in which risk information was key to this controversy, in that public health promotion campaigns assumed that the public needed better and easier to understand information about risks; and that the proper way to present this was stressing individual choice and responsibility. This ignored, she argued, social and political aspects of the debate, such as the collective responsibility of immunization for 'herd immunity' and the issue of public trust in information sources.

Second, health promotion is responsible for the proliferation of risk in society, through generating ever more health issues for the public to address. We are constantly faced with messages about risks to monitor and minimize in the environment (the sun, radiation, hazardous waste), our lifestyles (smoking, insufficient exercise, food intake) and even medical interventions themselves (MMR, side-effects of medications). This proliferation contributes to what Giddens (1991) has identified as a defining feature of the modern age: that it is an age of anxiety, with excessive concern and uncertainty.

CHALLENGES IN POLICY AND PRACTICE

At the beginning of the 21st century, national policy on public health and health promotion illustrates some of the tensions around the philosophies of public health and debates around practice (summarized in Box 17.3). Policies have reflected political ideologies with, for instance, a 'Third Way' approach (discussed in Chapter 12) characterizing UK public health policy towards the end of the 20th century, as the Labour government attempted to move away from a purely individualistic approach towards a renewed focus on the social determinants of health. The 1999 publication *Saving Lives: Our Healthier Nation* had an explicit goal of addressing health inequalities and aimed 'to attack the breeding ground of poor health – poverty and social exclusion' (Department of Health 1999). Focusing on four main areas – cancer, coronary heart disease and stroke, accidents, and mental health – this policy introduced targets for action and encouraged greater partnerships between health and other sectors. However, more recently there has been a retreat from policies that address the structural cause of ill health and inequalities and a return to a more individualistic approach. In 2004, Derek Wanless reported on the state of the public health in England. He explicitly began his report with an individualistic framework, noting that 'Individuals are ultimately responsible for their own and their children's health' (Wanless 2004, page 4) and that progress on the public health would only be made if the public were to become 'fully engaged' in relation to their own health.

This illustrates a key challenge in public health policy – that of addressing the impacts of social inequality on health. Should health policy be directed 'upstream' at the causes of inequality itself (through, for instance, the taxation system) or at the outcomes, through directing more resources at those who suffer most from the effects of inequality?

In general, recent policies directed at health inequalities have used a 'targeting' approach, through directing resources specifically at the poorest areas of the country through such area-based initiatives as Health Action Zones, Sure Start (aiming to improve child development through integrated early education, family support and health services) and Neighbourhood Renewal. *Choosing Health: Making Healthier Choices Easier* (Department of Health 2005) has also stressed the individual level of responsibility, and sees the government's role as one of providing information and support to the public to motivate individuals to make the 'healthy' choices themselves.

A second challenge is implementing a less 'medical' model of public health and health promotion. One example perhaps is the introduction of the 2004 General Medical Service contract for GPs (general practitioners) in the UK. This aimed to incentivize GPs to do more public health and preventative work through setting targets on such clinical indicators as treating heart disease and patients with aspirin, reducing blood pressure, and

---

BOX 17.3 Some tensions in public health and health promotion theory and practice

- *Structural or individualist?* Should effort be directed primarily at the structural determinants of ill health, or 'downstream', at the level where interventions can have a measurable impact? If we want to reduce road traffic injuries, should we change transport systems to slow down cars or provide more road safety training for children?

- *The role of the State.* How far should the State interfere with the liberty of its citizens in order to protect the public health, or the health of individuals? Should it insist on vaccinations, ban hand guns, ban smoking in public places?

- *Science or activism?* Should public health professionals be value-free scientists, or political advocates?

achieving high rates of cervical screening. The target-driven approach, though, could be seen as increasing the medicalization of patients, encouraged to attend for more and more screening services and interventions.

Third, although international policy focused on inter-sectoral collaboration, addressing the broader determinants of health and including communities, this has proved difficult to implement at local, or even national levels. Healthy Cities projects are one example. These were set up to support local governments to develop healthy public policy in partnership with local communities and statutory sector agencies. However, evaluations of these projects have suggested that few manage to incorporate communities as active partners, and that the idealistic expectations of addressing social inequalities and radical social change were not met (Stern & Green 2005).

Public health and health promotion face, then, a number of challenges in improving population health and moving public policy in the direction of healthy policy. Some of these relate to debates in philosophy and values which underpin theory, and which impact on practice at the level of national policy and individual professional practice, including debate over the level of action, the role of the state and the role of medicine within public health (see Box 17.3).

References

Acheson D 1988 Public Health in England. Report of the committee of inquiry into the future development of the public health function. Department of Health, London

Armstrong D 1993 Public health spaces and the fabrication of identity. Sociology 27:393–410

Ashton J, Seymour H 1988 The new public health. Open University Press, Milton Keynes

Baum F 1998 The new public health: an Australian perspective. Oxford University Press, Oxford

Beaglehole R (ed) 2003 Global public health: a new era. Oxford University Press, Oxford

Beaglehole R, Bonita R, Horton R et al 2004 Public health in a new era: improving health through collective action. Lancet 363:2084–2086

Beck U 1992 Risk society: towards a new modernity. Sage, London

Becker MH 1974 The health belief model and personal health behaviour. Health Education Monographs 2:324–508

Beattie A 1991 Knowledge and control in health promotion: a test case for social policy and social theory. In: Gabe J, Calnan M, Bury M (eds) The sociology of the health service. Routledge, London

Crawford R 1977 You are dangerous to your health: the ideology and politics of victim blaming. International Journal of Health Services 7:663–680

Davison C, Davey Smith G, Frankel S 1991 Lay epidemiology and the prevention paradox. The implications of coronary candidacy for health education. Sociology of Health and Illness 13:1–19

Department of Health 1999 Saving lives: our healthier nation. CM 4386. TSO, London

Department of Health 2005 Choosing health: making healthy choices easier.

Giddens A 1991 Modernity and self-identity: self and society in the late modern age. Polity Press, Cambridge

Gilmore A, McKee M, Pomerleau J 2005 Tobacco: a public health emergency. In: McKee M, Pomerleau J (eds) Issues in public health. Open University Press, Maidenhead

Graham H 1987 Women's smoking and family health. Social Science and Medicine 25:47–56

Green J 1999 From accidents to risk: public health and preventable injury. Health, Risk and Society 1:25–39

Hobson-West P 2003 Understanding vaccination resistance: moving beyond risk. Health, Risk and Society 5:273–283

Lalonde M 1974 A new perspective on the health of Canadians. Ministry of National Health and Welfare, Ottawa

Macdonald G, Bunton R 1992 Health promotion: disciplinary developments. In: Bunton R, Macdonald G (eds) Health promotion: disciplines, diversity and developments. Routledge, London

National Centre for Social Research 2004 Health survey for England 2003. ONS, London

Nettleton S 1997 Governing the risky self: How to become healthy, wealthy and wise. In: Petersen A, Bunton R (eds) Foucault, health and medicine. Routledge, London

Nettleton S, Bunton R 1995 Sociological critiques of health promotion. In: Bunton R, Nettleton S, Burrows R (eds) The sociology of health promotion: critical analyses of consumption, lifestyle and risk. Routledge, London

Petersen A 1997 Risk, governance and the new public health. In: Petersen A, Bunton R (eds) Foucault, health and medicine. Routledge, London

Roberts I 2004 Injury and globalisation. Injury Prevention 10:65–66

Rothman KJ, Adami, H-O, Trichopoulos D 1998 Should the mission of epidemiology include the eradication of poverty? Lancet 352:810–813

Stern R, Green J 2005 Boundary workers and the management of frustration: a case study of two health city partnerships. Health Promotion International 20:269–276

Stott R 2006 Healthy response to climate change. British Medical Journal 332:1385–1387

Thorogood N 2002 What is the relevance of sociology for health promotion? In: Bunton R, Macdonald G (eds) Health promotion: disciplines, diversity and developments, 2nd edn. Routledge, London

Tones K, Green J 2004 Health promotion: planning and strategies. SAGE Publications, London

US Department of Health and Human Services 2004 The health consequences of smoking: a report of the surgeon general's. Centers for Disease Control, Atlanta

Vandenbroucke JP, Eelkman Rooda HM, Beukers H 1991 Who made John Snow a hero?' American Journal of Epidemiology 133:967–973

Wanless D 2004 Securing good health for the whole population. HM Treasury, London

WHO 1978 Primary health care: report of the international conference on primary health care. Alma-Ata USSR. 6–12th September, 1978. WHO, Geneva

WHO 1986 Ottawa Charter for Health Promotion, Presented at the First International Conference on Health Promotion, Ottawa, Canada, 21 November 1986

WHO 1984 Health promotion: a discussion document on the concepts and principles WHO, Copenhagen

CHAPTER

18 Measuring health outcomes

Ray Fitzpatrick

During the 20th century, health problems in the industrialized societies shifted steadily from the infectious diseases to chronic and degenerative diseases. Health services are now expected to have an impact on a diverse range of health problems that variously involve what can be called the 'five Ds': death, disease, disability, discomfort and dissatisfaction. The health services that have emerged to respond to such demands are of unprecedented size, diversity and complexity. Perhaps the greatest challenge now facing health services is to assess their impact on health problems. Now that public funds are an essential component of financial support for health care, governments of all political persuasions have begun to require evidence of the effectiveness of health services. At the same time, the health professions are also beginning to look more closely at the impact that their treatments and interventions might have. The common focus of such concerns is on assessing the outcomes of health care, that is, the impact on patients and populations of health services.

This chapter examines some of the different ways of conceptualizing and measuring health outcomes and some of the lessons to be gained from such evidence. In a discussion of the evaluation of health services, it is customary to distinguish between three different components of healthcare evaluation.

1. The structure of health care, which involves focusing on such matters as the numbers, distribution and qualifications of doctors, nurses and other health professionals.

2. The processes of health care, which are concerned with the therapeutic, diagnostic and other activities performed by health professionals for patients.

3. The outcomes of health care – these are the most important focus in evaluation and consider the ultimate results achieved for patients by health services.

MORTALITY

The first measure of outcome is important for a number of reasons. Most obviously, it is a central concern of clinicians and society to prevent deaths. From the perspective of measurement it is relatively simple to define compared with most other dimensions of health status. Moreover, particularly in industrialized societies, national recording systems have virtually complete information about deaths, something that cannot be said for most other measures of outcome.

Mortality rates can be used for a number of purposes. Thus, they indicate inequalities in health status between different parts of England and Wales. The highest standardized mortality ratios (SMRs) consistently occur in the northern Regional Health Authorities and the lowest in the south and west. The use of SMRs to examine inequalities between social and ethnic groups has been discussed in Chapter 8. Mortality rates can also be used to examine improvements over time. In England and Wales, life expectancy – a summary measure of the mortality rates prevailing at any time – increased for females from 42 years in 1841 to 80 years in 1997. Most of this improvement has occurred because of reductions in infant mortality; life expectancy at later ages has not improved so markedly: a woman aged 65 in 1841 could expect to live another 12 years; this figure had increased to 19 years by 2005. Nevertheless, mortality rates can be used to show significant progress in some areas in the recent past. Thus, among young men, there was a dramatic 44% reduction in lung cancer in the period 1975–87, a change almost entirely due to reductions in smoking and the tar content of cigarettes. Over the same period, mortality rates due to some other cancers, such as Hodgkin's disease, leukaemia and cancer of the testis, declined markedly as a result of medical interventions such as radiotherapy and chemotherapy. This is persuasive evidence that counterbalances the more pessimistic analyses of progress against cancer.

Infant mortality tends to be used as a particularly sensitive measure of the overall health of a country. Variations between countries in infant mortality are considered to be a reflection of social and economic conditions generally, as well as the quality of maternity and neonatal care.

◼ Avoidable mortality

One important approach to mortality statistics is to focus on deaths from certain conditions considered amenable to health-service intervention. Maternal and infant mortality can be used as indicators of the quality of obstetric and infant care. This approach has been extended to other causes of death where variations in death rates might indicate limitations of healthcare provision, particularly if deaths below particular ages are the focus of attention. For example, cervical cancer is regarded as, in principle, avoidable by a combination of screening and early treatment by surgery or radiotherapy. Similarly, preventive immunization or drug therapy for established cases is highly effective against tuberculosis, so that most mortality is in principle avoidable. Hypertensive disease can

BOX 18.1	Avoidable deaths and the NHS

1. Avoidable death rates vary in different areas of Britain

- Rates are influenced by social and environmental factors, e.g. deaths due to hypertensive/cardiovascular disease
- Figures for health authorities, when controlled for social and environmental factors, show variation (Charlton et al 1983)
- This variation is greater than could have occurred by chance

2. Are they due to the quality of health services?

- The positions of health authorities on 'league tables' of avoidable deaths have remained stable (Charlton et al 1986)
- Information on mortality is used as an indicator of quality of medical care, but have the social factors been properly allowed for in the analysis?

be detected by screening and ought to be amenable to dietary and smoking advice together with drug management (Box 18.1). This method can be used to compare the performances of different healthcare systems. A study of avoidable mortality rates in Europe over the period 1980 to 1997 showed that overall avoidable mortality rates improved approximately 2.5% per annum (Treurniet et al 2004). It was also possible to highlight important variations; for example, deaths from liver cirrhosis in the UK did not improve as rapidly as in other European countries, an indication of possible failures of health promotion in relation to alcohol consumption.

Hospital deaths

Deaths can nevertheless be an important alarm signal in health care and, as information systems become more effective and public concern over issues of quality increases, it can be expected that increasing attention will be given to hospital mortality data. A great deal of controversy followed the publication in the USA of the death rates for different hospitals of public sector (Medicare) patients. For example, mortality in a 30-day period following admission for pneumonia varied from 0 to 60% between different hospitals. It was argued that such evidence pointed to serious potential deficiencies in the quality of care of certain hospitals about which the public had a right to know. Similarly, death rates across all causes for admission in the NHS were found to vary across hospitals from 3.4% to 13.6% (Jarman et al 1999). However, technical objections can be raised regarding the quality of mortality data and incautious interpretations regarding their significance. In particular, account needs to be taken of the variation in the severity and complexity of illness of patients admitted to different hospitals. A study of patients admitted to NHS intensive care units found substantial and significant differences in death rates between units, with the worst mortality rate more than two-and-a-half times higher than the most favourable (Rowan et al 1993). However, when the study took account of severity of illness in the patients, variations in mortality were explained away for the majority of units, although 15% of units still had significantly higher death rates.

Of course, for many other kinds of hospital admissions, such as end-stage cancer, death will be the inevitable and accepted outcome and other criteria, such as the dignity of care, would be the most appropriate measure of quality. Again, as with avoidable mortality, there is a practical problem that deaths for particular hospital units are mercifully too infrequent an event to rely on for purposes of assessing outcomes and quality of care.

It is important to find explanations for why hospitals might have significantly different mortality rates after the severity of presenting illness has been taken into account. Studies of relatively simple-to-measure organizational factors such as whether a hospital has teaching or non-teaching status, is located in a rural or urban area and the number of hospital beds have not proved consistently important. For certain surgical procedures the greater the volume of the procedure performed, the lower the mortality rate, suggesting that experience and expertise acquired through practice improves the quality of outcomes. Other evidence shows that hospitals with more favourable mortality outcomes are more likely to use procedures (for example, thrombolytic agents, beta-blockers and aspirin for heart attacks) proven to be effective (Halm & Chassin 2001). Above all, evidence of poor outcomes for a hospital can provide real opprtunities for improvement. Wright and colleagues achieved a significant reduction in hospital deaths over a 3-year period, equivalent to 905 fewer deaths than expected, in an NHS hospital in the North of England, by conducting an audit and putting in place patient safety procedures and training (Wright et al 2006).

HEALTH STATUS AND QUALITY OF LIFE

For many health problems treated by health services, not only is death an uncommon and inappropriate measure of outcome but also, more importantly, the primary purpose of treatment is to improve the patient's functioning and well-being. Consider, for example, drug treatment for rheumatoid arthritis, epilepsy or migraine, hospice care of the terminally ill, or surgery for ulcerative colitis. In all such instances the focus is on the broad, pervasive effects that health problems have on the patient in terms of pain, disability, anxiety, depression, social isolation, embarrassment or difficulties in carrying on daily life. From the patient's perspective, health care is judged largely in terms of impact on these broader aspects of personal well-being. Patients themselves advocate that more research be conducted into the impact of treatments on these aspects of their lives. In recent years, outcome measures have emerged in an attempt to capture such aspects of patients' experiences. Frequently termed quality-of-life measures, they can often also be referred to as health-status instruments.

An early attempt to assess quality of life in patients in a systematic way was the Karnofsky Performance Index (Karnofsky & Burchenal 1949) (Table 18.1). The scale was designed particularly for use in the field of cancer and involves the clinician making a simple rating of the patient. It is still one of the more frequently used 'quality-of-life' scales and is very useful in drawing attention to those factors that matter to patients. It also helps health professionals predict which patients on a ward will require more attention and need more time and resources. Some of its disadvantages are considered here:

1. Is quality of life unidimensional? There is a fallacy behind the use of a unidimensional scale. Such a scale requires the assumption that a bed-bound person must have a quite poor score even if, for example, he or she is well adjusted to illness, receives full social support and sees life as fulfilling. Conversely, someone ambulant but otherwise depressed, isolated, with low self-esteem and anxious about health status would, nevertheless, receive a favourable score. In other words, instruments such as the Karnofsky Performance Index do not allow for the multidimensional nature of quality of life.

2. Is the scale reliable? It is not surprising, in view of the complex nature of quality of life, that the index is deficient in a basic requirement for such instruments in that it is not reliable; different raters disagree in applying the scale to patients.

TABLE 18.1	The Karnofsky performance index	
Description		**Score (%)**
Normal, no complaints		100
Able to carry on normal activities; minor signs or symptoms of disease		90
Normal activity with effort		80
Cares for self. Unable to carry on normal activity or to do active work		70
Requires occasional assistance but able to care for most of own needs		60
Requires considerable assistance and frequent medical care		50
Disabled; requires special care and assistance		40
Severely disabled; hospitalization indicated although death not imminent		30
Very sick; hospitalization necessary. Active supportive treatment necessary		20
Moribund		10
Dead		0

Reproduced with permission of Souvenir Press from Fallowfield (1990).

3. Is the scale valid? A serious deficiency is that clinicians sometimes disagree with patients' self-ratings on the scale. Indeed, it has more generally been found to be the case, across a wide range of healthcare settings, that health professionals make significantly different judgements of their patients' quality of life than patients themselves (Sprangers & Aaronson 1992). Such problems have underlined the need for instruments that patients can, whenever possible, complete themselves.

Health-status instruments

A large proportion of published clinical trials purporting to assess the impact of therapies on patients' quality of life rely on inaccurate evidence, such as the doctor's opinion or inappropriate laboratory measures. Where patients' perceptions of their health or quality of life are obtained in clinical trials, the questionnaires are often unvalidated or simplistic, and leave patients little scope for expressing their feelings. A review of quality of life measures in randomized controlled trials found a steady increase in the assessment of quality of life measures but, by 1997, still only 4.7% of trials overall included this dimension of outcome (Sanders et al 1998).

A number of instruments (variously termed 'health-status', or 'quality-of-life', instruments) have therefore emerged, designed to be used as questionnaires for self completion. One of the most widely used of such instruments is the Short-Form 36-Item (SF-36) Health Survey Questionnaire (McHorney et al 1994). The SF-36 contains 36 simple questions about the respondent's health. The items fall into one of eight scales addressing different aspects of subjective health: physical functioning, role limitations due to physical problems, role limitations due to emotional problems, social functioning, mental health, energy/vitality, pain and general health perception. The designers of the instrument have made considerable efforts to establish that the instrument is reliable (i.e. produces consistent responses if completed on different occasions not too far apart), and valid (for example, is able to distinguish individuals with different types and severity of health problem).

The SF-36 has now been used to examine the impact on individuals' subjective health of a number of different healthcare interventions.

A large number of health-status or quality-of-life measures are now available. Although different in style, content and general approach to measuring patients' problems, they generally tend to focus on those aspects of patients' daily lives that are most affected by ill health (Fitzpatrick et al 1992) (Box 18.2).

Instruments such as the SF-36 are ambitious in that they are intended to assess the impact on the patient's well-being and quality of life of a wide range of different health problems. It is often necessary to assess the patient's perspective with an instrument more specifically designed to be sensitive to one particular disease. One very typical and quite successful instrument of this kind is the Arthritis Impact Measurement Scale (AIMS), which, by means of simple questions, assesses the impact of rheumatic disease on patient well-being in areas such as mobility, dexterity, household activities, pain and depression. The instrument has been shown to be sensitive to improvements in patients within just 4 weeks of treatment with non-steroidal anti-inflammatory drugs (Anderson et al 1989). In a chronic disease such as rheumatoid arthritis, where improvements to the patient's condition can be quite subtle and undramatic, such instruments have a vital role to play in improving our understanding of outcomes, especially in view of evidence in rheumatology that they might be no less reliable and accurate than conventional laboratory and radiological measures and often provide the clinician with more meaningful information on the impact of treatment. Box 18.3 gives an example of how a questionnaire to assess patients' quality of life has been constructed in one particular field of medicine. The instrument described in the box now provides a validated assessment of quality of life in Parkinson's disease. Such measures provide essential information on outcomes not attainable from conventional clinical assessments for use in trials of the increasing number of medical and surgical treatments emerging for Parkinson's disease (Koller et al 2000).

Some observers argue that questionnaires such as those just described are still limited because they ask a standard set of fixed questions of everyone and do not leave much room for individuals' personal concerns or problems to be expressed if they happen not to be included as a questionnaire item (O'Boyle et al 1992). For this reason, several instruments have recently been developed in which respondents identify their own most important areas of life (family, religion, leisure activities or whatever) rather than respond to questionnaire items determined by the investigator. They can then rate how well they are doing in these personally nominated areas of life and also on subsequent occasions judge any changes for better or worse in these domains. Such approaches, commonly referred to as individualized measures, attempt to address the concern that quality of life is an essentially personal judgement.

BOX 18.2 Dimensions of quality of life usually assessed in health-status instruments

- Physical function, for example, mobility, ability to look after self
- Emotional well-being, for example, depression, anxiety, self-esteem
- Social function, for example, close attachments, social support, social integration
- Roles, for example, paid work, housework, child care
- Pain, for example, severity, frequency
- Other symptoms, for example, nausea, stiffness, fatigue

Reproduced with permission from Fitzpatrick et al (1992).

BOX 18.3   Constructing a quality-of-life instrument

- Objective: Parkinson's disease (PD) is a chronic degenerative disease mainly affecting individuals at older ages. There is no cure and treatment is designed to arrest the progression of symptoms and improve the quality of life. However, there is no specific measure of quality of life in PD
- Step one. Identify the problems: interview individuals with the problem. Allow them to say in their own words how PD affects them. Content analysis of interviews (tape-recorded) draws out a rich variety of themes
- Step two. Draw up questions: put together a long list (65+) of questions based on the results of Step one. Ask individuals with PD in the community to complete the questionnaire. Ask for their comments on items. Analyse results to find redundant or difficult items. Statistical analysis found that 39 questionnaire items could be used to assess eight important areas of life: mobility, activities of daily living, emotional well-being, stigma, social support, cognitions, communication, bodily discomfort
- Step three. Test the questionnaire: Again ask individuals with PD in the community to complete the (39-item) questionnaire. Ask some to repeat the task. Examine the results for internal consistency and test–retest reliability. Also ask patients in neurological clinics to complete the questionnaire to check that patterns of answers agree with other evidence of neurological problems for purposes of validity
- Result. A questionnaire that patients find easy to complete, that emphasizes issues that matter to them and that can be used to assess the course of illness and impact of interventions.

Reproduced with permission by Oxford University Press from Peto et al (1995) and Jenkinson et al (1995).

303

Adverse consequences of health care

Many medical treatments have harmful side-effects. This is the case in, for example, cancer therapies, which are designed to prolong life but which can have a variety of adverse effects at the same time. Cytotoxic chemotherapies can produce nausea, vomiting, hair loss and tiredness, as well as mood effects such as depression. In some cases, the costs to the patient from treatments outweigh benefits gained in terms of longevity. Quality-of-life measures allow us to give some quantitative expression to such adverse effects. Thus, Croog et al (1986) used a battery of quality-of-life measures to assess the impact of three alternative drugs for controlling hypertension. They measured general well-being, physical symptoms, sexual function, work performance, emotional state, cognitive function (e.g. memory), social participation and life satisfaction. Although achieving similar levels of blood pressure control, one drug stood out from the other two as having less harmful effects on quality of life. They found that some of the harmful side-effects of drugs produced broadly equivalent effects on quality of life to those found by individuals who have just lost their jobs. Broadly based measures of quality of life make it possible to detect and assess harmful effects that might occur in any of a wide range of aspects of patients' lives.

Attaching values to health

All healthcare systems have to make choices between different healthcare interventions; resources are not available to fund and provide all of the treatments that, in principle, are available. This requires extremely difficult choices to be made between interventions for very different health problems, e.g. between coronary bypass surgery, renal transplant, lipid screening and day hospitals for psychiatric patients. One of the many problems complicating such choices is that there is no single numerical scale in terms of which to measure the diverse states of health and illness treated by different healthcare programmes. Utility measurement is an approach that can be used to produce numerical values on a scale between 0 and 1 for all possible health states by assessing their relative value to individuals. In principle, it then becomes possible to assess in a standard way the improvements to health that can result from otherwise widely differing medical interventions.

A number of techniques have been developed to elicit how desirable individuals regard one health state compared with another. One such technique is the so-called standard gamble technique in which a subject is asked to choose between a particular state of ill health on the one hand and a gamble on the other hand. The gamble involves a hypo-thetical treatment that can cure the individual of the state of ill health, but with a partic-ular probability of death from the treatment. For states of ill health perceived by the subject to be very undesirable, one would expect the individual to prefer the gamble even with quite high probabilities of death. This probability is varied experimentally to reveal how ready the individual is to take the gamble rather than choose (hypothetically) to carry on living in the particular state of ill health being investigated. Data can be gath-ered from a sample of experimental subjects in such a way as to produce numerical values for a range of health states.

An alternative method (magnitude estimation) is to ask subjects to state how much worse they regard each of a number of ill-health states relative to one standard health state. One research group (Rosser & Kind 1978) asked subjects to rate the relative unde-sirability of 29 different states of illness produced by a matrix formed from combinations of two dimensions, varying degrees of distress and disability. The resulting relative values or 'utilities' of different health states are shown in Table 18.2. It is worth noting that some health states were rated as worse than 'dead' by judges. The research group found

TABLE 18.2 Valuation matrix of different health states[a]

Disability rating	Distress rating			
	No distress	Mild	Moderate	Severe
No disability	1.000	0.995	0.990	0.967
Slight social disability	0.990	0.986	0.973	0.932
Severe social disability and/or slight physical impairment	0.980	0.972	0.956	0.912
Physical ability severely limited (e.g. light housework only)	0.964	0.956	0.942	0.870
Unable to take paid employment or education, largely housebound	0.946	0.935	0.900	0.700
Confined to chair or wheelchair	0.875	0.845	0.680	0.000
Confined to bed	0.677	0.564	0.000	-1.486
Unconscious	-1.078	NA	NA	NA

Reproduced with permission by Oxford University Press from Drummond (1989).
[a] Healthy = 1.0, dead = 0.0. NA = not applicable.

that values attached to different health states were reliable in the sense that individuals' responses were consistent over time.

One of the challenging results of work about values in health is the discovery that individuals who have quite significant disability or poor health may consider their health more positively (for example rating themsleves as having a very high quality of life) than would healthy oberservers. This so-called 'disability paradox' raises quite major questions as to (1) how such differences arise and (2) whose values should be most important in decisions about health and health care (Albrecht 1999).

QUALITY-ADJUSTED LIFE-YEARS

Some health economists have argued that the values attached to different states of health and illness by methods such as those outlined above can be combined with survival data on years lived as a result of medical treatments to produce a generic output measure, the 'quality-adjusted life-year' (QALY) (Williams 1985). This standard, unitary means of expressing the benefits of medical treatments permits comparisons across treatments. Typically, information on QALYs has been combined with information about the costs of different treatment programmes (cost–utility analysis) and comparisons between programmes expressed in terms of costs per QALY gained, as in Table 18.3. It is argued that health authorities, faced with a scarcity of resources to meet all health problems, need to maximize their use of resources. The methodology of QALYs identifies treatments that maximize the use of resources by obtaining the greatest gain in terms of health for a unit of resource. Table 18.3 indicates that general practitioners giving advice to stop smoking is a dramatically more effective use of resources than, say, hospital haemodialysis. Such information appears to provide a more explicit and more rational basis for making decisions about the allocation of resources. However, the approach outlined above has generated intense debate (Box 18.4).

305

TABLE 18.3	'League table' of costs and QALYs for selected healthcare interventions (1983–4 prices)
Intervention	**Present value of extra cost per QALY gained (£)**
GP advice to stop smoking	170
Pacemaker implantation for heart block	700
Hip replacement	750
CABG for severe angina LMD	1040
GP control of total serum cholesterol	1700
CABG for severe angina with 2VD	2280
Kidney transplantation (cadaver)	3000
Breast cancer screening	3500
Heart transplantation	5000
CABG for mild angina 2VD	12600
Hospital haemodialysis	14000

Reproduced with permission by Oxford University Press from Drummond (1989).
CABG, coronary artery bypass graft; GP, general practitioner; LMD, left main disease; 2VD, two vessel disease.

BOX 18.4 Debate about QALYs

Arguments against
- There are no agreed methods – at least six methods have been developed (Froberg & Kane 1989)
- People's values differ and health means different things to different people
- Doctors rate states of ill health as less desirable than do patients (Rosser & Kind 1978)
- Even if the principle of 'league tables' is accepted, the methods of assessing costs and outcomes vary, therefore the results are problematic
- Can moral judgements be made scientific?
- QALYs condone cutting healthcare resources
- QALYs have unfair consequences, systematically disadvantaging some social groups, e.g. the elderly and terminally ill

Arguments in favour
- The current system of resource allocation is worse
- QALYs make decisions more open and accountable

PATIENT SATISFACTION

The patient's perspective

One source of evidence about the outcomes of health care that has, until recently, been all too frequently neglected is the patient's view. This neglect was partly due to the widespread assumption that the patient is insufficiently well informed to comment on his or her health care. Undoubtedly, there is also a tendency in many large bureaucratic organizations such as the National Health Service (NHS) to pursue internally generated routines and objectives without seeking external evidence of their reception by users. It should be clear that a primary objective of any healthcare system is to provide services in a manner that is acceptable to the patient. The Griffiths NHS Management Inquiry was highly critical of the failure of the NHS to act on this principle by systematically obtaining consumer feedback about the quality of services (DHSS 1983). Since that report, most health authorities have made much more effort to conduct such surveys.

There is also ample evidence from social scientific research to indicate how important the issue of patient satisfaction is. Patients who are dissatisfied with their health care are more likely not to follow the medical advice or regimen that they receive. In a sample of patients attending a neurological clinic for chronic headache, those who were more dissatisfied with the consultation (when interviewed afterwards) were significantly less likely to take the medication that had been prescribed for them (Fitzpatrick & Hopkins 1981). Similar results have been obtained between satisfaction and compliance in hypertension and paediatric clinics, and in general practice; dissatisfied patients are less likely to reattend for further care (Orton et al 1991) or might change their doctor (Rubin et al 1993).

A common distinction made in relation to health care is that between the technical and interpersonal aspects of care. Technical aspects of care refer to the technical competence with which treatment is provided. Interpersonal aspects focus on how doctors, nurses and other health professionals treat the patient – in other words, the degree of personal care and concern shown. Patient satisfaction is a particularly important indicator of interpersonal aspects of care. Thus, in a study of mothers attending a paediatric clinic with their children, the medical consultations were tape-recorded and analysed and mothers interviewed independently by researchers after the consultation to assess satisfaction (Korsch et al 1968). Satisfaction was higher when the doctor displayed a friendly manner to the mother. Satisfaction was also positively related to directly questioning mothers early in the consultation as to the main worries and concerns that had prompted the consultation. In a similarly designed study of general medical clinics in which analyses of tape-recorded consultations could be related to subsequent patient satisfaction, those patients who were given encouragement by the doctor to explain their medical problem in their own terms were significantly more satisfied than patients who reported their symptoms in response to more structured doctor-focused questioning (Stiles et al 1979). A study of patients attending primary care in England found that patients were significantly more satisfied after their consultations with the doctor if they felt that the doctor had showed sympathy, was interested in the patient's worries and discussed and agreed with the patient in partnership treatments for problems presented, behaviours all considered by the investigators to be examples of good 'patient-centred care' (Little et al 2001).

One of the more important of interpersonal skills in health care is giving information. Failures in this area are one of the most important sources of patient dissatisfaction. It can also be shown experimentally that efforts to improve the communication of information are appreciated by patients. Ley (1982) reported a study in which medical inpatients were allocated to one of three different patterns of communication. A 'placebo' group experienced the normal and routine pattern of communication from doctors. A 'control' group received in addition one visit from a junior doctor who discussed general matters not specifically related to the patient's admission. In the 'experimental' group the junior doctor, in the one visit to the patient, made a point of giving an explanation to the patient of the treatments and procedures he or she was receiving. All three groups subsequently completed questionnaires and the 'experimental' group produced significantly higher satisfaction scores.

Patient satisfaction studies also underline the importance of continuity and accessibility to patients. Women with breast cancer in remission were randomized between two alternative follow-up regimes, standard care requiring hospital-based check-ups at fixed intervals or primary-care-based follow-up by their own general practitioner. Although there were no differences in the detection of recurrences between the two groups, levels of satisfaction were significantly higher in the primary-care-managed group, women especially valuing speed and accessibility of primary care but also the advantages of seeing a doctor who knew them well and of consultations in which it was easier to discuss problems (Grunfeld et al 1999).

There are two distinct ways in which we can go about obtaining individuals' views in a survey on a subject like health care (Box 18.5). The choice will depend on circumstances. A general problem with all methods is that patients of different backgrounds tend to differ in readiness to express critical comments about health services. Younger patients, those with poorer health status and individuals with higher levels of education are more likely to express dissatisfaction.

Surveys of hospital care

To aid its deliberations, the Royal Commission on the NHS commissioned a survey of a sample of patients who had recently experienced either inpatient or outpatient treatment. The results of the national survey carried out by the Office of Population Censuses and Surveys are likely to be very similar to those that are obtained in local surveys of a particular hospital or district (OPCS 1978).

Table 18.4 shows that much of the dissatisfaction could be traced to problems of having to wait for outpatient appointments or hospital admission, and to the length of time

---

BOX 18.5 Obtaining views in a survey

There are two basic strategies to finding the views of patients. Either respondents are given a questionnaire to complete themselves or personal interviews are conducted to ask the questions. Advantages of the two approaches:

Self-completed questionnaire	Interview
Questions easy to standardize and process	More appropriate for sensitive or complex material
No interviewer bias	Easier to clarify ambiguous items
Low cost of data gathering	Rapport results in completion of questionnaire
Less need for trained staff	Scope to follow-up non-respondents

Reproduced with permission from Fitzpatrick (1991).

TABLE 18.4 Dissatisfaction with regard to aspects of the NHS

Outpatients	%	Inpatients	%
Information about progress	37	Woken too early	43
Time waiting for hospital transport	28	Information about progress	31
Waiting for first appointment	21	Food	21
Length of time at hospital	19	Waiting for admission	20
Adequacy of waiting room	18	Washing and bathing facilities	19
Length of wait to see doctor	16	Toilet facilities	15

Reproduced with permission of the Controller of HMSO and the Office for National Statistics from OPCS (1978).

---

waiting to see a doctor. Other complaints focused on amenities such as food and washing facilities in wards and the waiting room in outpatient clinics. A particularly large number in both patient groups were dissatisfied with information. A more recent survey of over 5000 patients attending 36 NHS hospitals found problems of communication still the main source of dissatisfaction, with 16% of patients receiving no explanation about their condition from the doctor and 60% receiving no advice about activities to do or not do after discharge (Bruster et al 1994).

It is surprising how similar are the results of surveys of patients' views of their hospital care across developed countries. Coulter & Cleary (2001) report the results of surveys using a standardized questionnaire with patients completed within a month of discharge from hospitals in UK, USA, Germany, Sweden and Switzerland. The problems that were most commonly reported by patients in all five countries were in the area of transition from hospital to community, such as advice about resumption of normal activities, about medication and danger signals to watch for at home. The area causing least problems as viewed by patients was physical comfort of the hospital. Importantly, when asked more general, global views of their hospital care, patients gave more positive ratings than might be predicted from their reports of specific problems, with the lowest level of dissatisfaction observed in Switzerland (3.7%) and the highest level of dissatisfaction (8.5%) in the UK.

Surveys of patient satisfaction have to be interpreted with caution because patients may experience a variety of specific problems arising during their care but still report themselves as satisfied. In a study of adult patients who had been admitted to any of five hospitals in Scotland included in the survey, the vast majority were very satisfied with their inpatient stay (Jenkinson et al 2002). Nevertheless over half of the patients who rated their hospital care as excellent still reported problems on 10% of specific aspects of their care. Some would conclude from such evidence that we should focus attention on the specific problems and experiences reported in surveys rather than whether patients are satisfied. The latter is too much influenced by feelings of gratitude and optimistic bias.

OUTCOMES AND THE EVALUATION OF SERVICES

Evaluation and the medical profession

One of the features that can distinguish a profession from other kinds of occupation is that it retains a very high level of control in assessing the value and quality of the product it provides to the public (see Chapter 15). Historically, the medical profession has exercised this control by means of a number of methods, such as monitoring the content and standards of the training provided for new or established members of the profession or by penalizing individual doctors who fail to uphold required professional standards. In Britain, the General Medical Council (GMC) was established – after lengthy negotiations between the State and the newly emerging medical profession in the middle of the nineteenth century – as one of the main institutions to ensure satisfactory performance by doctors. However, health care has now become so complex and costly that traditional methods of upholding professional standards are no longer sufficient. Moreover, society has changed profoundly since the nineteenth century. The State is now intimately involved in health care through funding medical services with public money. It seeks evidence that such funds are well spent. In the USA, in addition to the federal government's concern about public healthcare spending, industry has become concerned about the value of medical services because so much is paid for from employers' insurance contributions. In other words, powerful forces such as government and business are seeking clearer evidence of the value of health care. In addition, consumers have also become more knowledgeable, more demanding and more sceptical in their dealings with health professionals.

The medical profession has not only faced external pressures to evaluate its activities. From within, epidemiologists such as Cochrane (1972) have argued that insufficient attention has been given to the scientific appraisal of the impact on health of medical interventions. The response of the medical profession to such pressures has been to take more seriously its responsibility to examine and monitor the quality and value of its services, in particular by practising medical audit. Medical audit has been defined as 'looking at what we are doing with the aim of making improvements in patient care and use of resources' (Difford 1990). It is conventional to distinguish between audit of process, in which the focus is the evaluation of medical activities (normally against agreed standards), and audit of outcome in which the question concerns the impact of activities upon illness. The latter is, as this chapter establishes, more difficult, so that most audit has been concerned with examining process, by methods such as reviewing samples of case notes, analysing hospital statistical data or comparing local use of procedures such as X-rays against published expert advice.

▦ Evaluation and the future of health care

At least three different views can be taken of the impact that measurement of outcomes can have on health care. For many observers, the evaluation of outcomes will be a fundamental turning point in the history of medicine, allowing for explicit, rational, scientific answers to all the problems arising from current uncertainties as to the value of medical treatments. As is examined in Chapter 19, outcomes research must address the enormous variations in the rates at which many medical and surgical treatments are performed, even among populations with similar levels of medical need. The hope is that all parties – the doctor, the patient and the purchaser – will have access to clearer information as to the likely results of investigations and treatments, and will, therefore, be able to make more informed decisions about health care.

A second position about future developments in this area is to adopt a more cautious stance and to argue that, at present, the advocates of outcomes measurement are expressing something of an article of faith. Despite enormous advances in computers and information systems, we are a very long way from the kinds of integrated systems that can monitor the longer-term impact of medical interventions in populations, and the kinds of practical and valid measures of outcome that can be used on a large scale are only just now beginning to be developed and examined. To understand the outcomes of most procedures, long-term studies integrating hospital and community data, to an extent that is not yet feasible outside of very special research contexts, will be required.

There is also a third, longer-term view of these developments. Analysts of both British and American health care (Ham 1981) have suggested that two distinct interest groups have tried to shape the future of health care. One group – the 'professional monopolizers' – have sought to defend the traditional privileges and practices of the medical profession, particularly the clinical autonomy of the doctor. A second group – 'the corporate rationalizers'– emphasize the many irrationalities and inefficiencies that bedevil healthcare systems when traditional professional autonomy is left unchecked by planning and evaluation. According to such analyses there has for a very long time been a stalemate in health policy between these two conflicting philosophies, and the present debate over outcomes is unlikely to result in decisive shifts. According to this view, for the foreseeable future health services will defy precise measurement of their value because of the inherent uncertainties and complexities of medical practice. Whatever the future direction of medical care, the assessment of outcomes will remain a central concern of health services.

References

Albrecht G Devlieger P 1999 The disability paradox: high quality of life against all the odds. Social Science and Medicine 48:977–988

Anderson J, Firschein H, Meenan R 1989 Sensitivity of a health status measure to short term clinical changes in arthritis. Arthritis and Rheumatism 32:844–850

Bruster S et al 1994 National survey of hospital patients. British Medical Journal 309:1542–1546

Charlton J et al 1983 Geographical variation in mortality from conditions amenable to medical interventions in England and Wales. Lancet i:691–696

Charlton J, Lakhani A, Aristidou M 1986 How have 'avoidable death' indices for England and Wales changed? 1974–78 compared with 1979–83. Community Medicine 8:304–314

Cochrane A 1972 Effectiveness and efficiency. Nuffield Provincial Hospitals Trust, London

Coulter A, Cleary P 2001 Patients' experiences with hospital care in five countries. Health Affairs 20:244–252

Croog S et al 1986 The effects of antihypertensive therapy on the quality of life. New England Journal of Medicine 314:1657–1664

Department of Health and Social Security (DHSS) 1983 NHS management inquiry. HMSO, London

Difford F 1990 Defining essential data for audit in general practice. British Medical Journal 300:92–94

Drummond M 1989 Output measurement for resource allocation decisions in health care. Oxford Review of Economics and Politics 5:59–74

Fallowfield L 1990 The quality of life: the missing measurement in health care. Souvenir Press, London

Fitzpatrick R 1991 Surveys of patient satisfaction: I – Important general considerations. British Medical Journal 302:887–889

Fitzpatrick R, Hopkins A 1981 Patients' satisfaction with communication in neurological outpatient clinics. Journal of Psychosomatic Research 25:329–334

Fitzpatrick R et al 1992 Quality of life measures in health care. I: Applications and issues in assessment. British Medical Journal 305:1074–1077

Froberg D, Kane R 1989 Methodology for measuring health-state preferences – III: Population and context effects. Journal of Clinical Epidemiology 42:585–592

Grunfeld E et al 1999 Comparison of breast cancer patient satisfaction with follow-up in primary care versus specialist care: results from a randomised controlled trial. British Journal of General Practice 49:705–710

Halm E, Chassin M 2001 Why do hospital death rates vary? New England Journal of Medicine 345:692–694

Ham C 1981 Policy making in the National Health Service. Macmillan, London

Jarman B et al 1999 Explaining differences in English hospital death rates using routinely collected data. British Medical Journal 318:1515–1520

Jenkinson C et al 1995 Self reported functioning and well-being in patients with Parkinson's disease. Age and Ageing 24:505–509

Jenkinson C, Coulter A, Bruster S et al 2002 Patients' experiences and satsifaction with health care: results of a questionnaire study of specific aspects of care. Quality and Safety in Health Care 11:335–339

Karnofsky D, Burchenal J 1949 The clinical evaluation of chemotherapeutic agents in cancer In: MacLeod C (ed) Evaluation of chemotherapeutic agents. Symposium at New York Academy of Medicine. Columbia University Press, New York, p 191–205

Koller W et al 2000 Randomised trial of tolcapone versus pergolide as add-on to levodopa therapy in Parkinson's disease patients with motor fluctuations. Movement Disorders 16:858–866

Korsch B, Goszzi E, Francis V 1968 Gaps in doctor patient communications: 1. Doctor patient interaction and patient satisfaction. Paediatrics 32:855–871

Ley P 1982 Satisfaction, compliance and communication. British Journal of Clinical Psychology 21:241–254

Little P et al 2001 Observational study of effect of patient centredness and positive approach on outcomes of general practice consultations. British Medical Journal 323:908–911

McHorney C, Ware J, Lu J 1994 The MOS 36-Item Short Form Health Survey (SF-36): III Tests of data quality, scaling assumptions and reliability across diverse patient groups. Medical Care 32:40–66

O'Boyle C et al 1992 Individual quality of life in patients undergoing hip replacement. Lancet 339: 1088–1091

Office of Population Censuses and Surveys (OPCS) 1978 Royal commission on the National Health Service: patients' attitudes to the hospital service. HMSO, London

Orton M et al 1991 Factors affecting women's response to an invitation to attend for a second breast cancer screening examination. British Journal of General Practice 41:320–323

Peto V et al 1995 The development and validation of a short measure of functioning and well-being for individuals with Parkinson's disease. Quality of Life Research 4:241–248

Rosser R, Kind P 1978 A scale of valuations of states of illness: is there a social consensus? International Journal of Epidemiology 7:347–358

Rowan K et al 1993 Intensive care society's APACHF II study in Britain and Ireland – II: outcome comparisons of intensive care units after adjustment for case mix by the American APACHE II method. British Medical Journal 307:977–981

311

Rubin H et al 1993 Patients' ratings of outpatient visits in different practice settings. Journal of the American Medical Association 270:835–840

Sanders C et al 1998 Reporting on quality of life in randomised controlled trials. British Medical Journal 317:1191–1194

Sprangers M, Aaronson N 1992 The role of health care providers and significant others in evaluating the quality of life of patients with chronic disease: a review. Journal of Clinical Epidemiology 45:743–760

Stiles W et al 1979 Interaction exchange structure and patient satisfaction with medical interviews. Medical Care 17:667–679

Treurniet H, Boshuizen H, Harteloh P 2004 Avoidable mortality in Europe (1980–1997): a comparison of trends. Journal of Epidemiology and Community Health 58:290–295

Williams A 1985 Economics of coronary bypass grafting. British Medical Journal 291:326–329

Wright J et al 2006 Learning from death: a hospital mortality reduction programme. Journal of Royal Society of Medicine 99: 303–308

Organizing and funding health care

Ray Fitzpatrick

Over the course of the 20th century, health care developed from a collection of small-scale and low-cost services to a complex, labour-intensive and diverse industry. In modern industrialized societies a large and generally growing proportion of resources is now devoted to health care. For example, in the United States 15% of all national resources are devoted to health care and it is confidently predicted that this proportion will increase, not least as the population ages. As the size and scope of this industry have expanded, so too have individuals' rights and expectations with regard to health. Governments have thus become increasingly committed to making health services available to their citizens. The very scale of modern health care has prompted governments of all political persuasions to raise fundamental questions. How effective are health services? How efficient are they in delivering health care? Ultimately, the common theme of such questions concerns the value of modern health care. The answers are often sought by looking for lessons from alternative systems of health care. The most striking feature of modern health care is the diversity of funding and organization in different countries. This chapter describes the different types of healthcare system that have emerged in industrialized societies and the ways they shape the practice of medicine, and then examines the strengths and weaknesses of different systems.

TYPES OF HEALTHCARE SYSTEM

A basic requirement for any product or service such as health care is that some method is needed to permit consumers to obtain the product from the producer. The simplest method to understand is the market, wherein the consumer purchases the product directly from the producer at a price agreed between the two parties at the time of the transaction. This is the basic principle behind many transactions in modern industrial societies, and indeed, until quite recently, was the dominant means of providing and obtaining health services. However, health services have tended to evolve away from basic market transactions in two respects. First, potential consumers of health services have increasingly preferred to take out insurance to cover possible costs of health care, rather than face unpredictable and often expensive costs incurred at the time of illness. Second, an additional party has mediated between the producer and consumer of health care to provide resources necessary for the provision of health care. This 'third party', very often the government, but also employers, trade unions, sickness funds, insurance societies and charities, has tended to become increasingly influential in the way services are provided. The more that third parties provide funds directly to the producers (hospitals, doctors and the pharmaceutical industry) to allow them to provide care to those entitled to services, either because of citizenship or an adequate record of insurance contributions, the further the system has evolved away from market mechanisms.

All healthcare systems can be understood in terms of the different ways in which transactions occur between these three key parties. In particular, systems differ in the extent to which market versus third-party mechanisms, particularly public provision, dominate transactions and, more specifically, in the ways that individuals obtain insurance against healthcare costs. A simple typology distinguishes four major alternative systems of health care that can be found in western industrialized societies (Field 1973) (Box 19.1).

The socialized systems of health care have probably experienced the most dramatic changes in recent years. In theory, these systems provided comprehensive care to all citizens without user charges. Services were planned centrally to maximize efficient and fair use of resources. It became increasingly clear, however, that behind this ideal model of health care there were major deficiencies, as the healthcare system of countries such as Russia received only 2% of gross national product, resulting in major shortages of basic drugs and other facilities (Field 1995). Moreover, unofficial bribing was often necessary

---

BOX 19.1 Alternative systems of health care

1. **The pluralistic health system**
   - A wide variety of coexisting schemes (insurance, fee-for-service) provide funds
   - Healthcare facilities owned by wide variety of institutions (private, State, federal)

2. **The health insurance system**
   - Resources gathered by third party as compulsory insurance from individuals and employers

3. **The health service system**
   - Most facilities owned by the State
   - Doctors independent but receive most of their income from the State

4. **The socialized health system**
   - All facilities owned by the State
   - Most healthcare personnel are salaried State employees

for patients to obtain adequate care, and major inequalities existed in access to health care between political elites and other groups. As the former socialist societies have moved toward markets and privatization, their healthcare services have also changed, the preferred model now being based on health insurance contributions from employees and their employers, which insurance agencies pay as fees to clinics and hospitals (Curtis et al 1995).

An even greater diversity of forms of health care may be found in non-western societies. A full classification would need to include the traditional systems of healing that have developed in India and China over many hundreds of years. In both these countries traditional medicine has provided sophisticated diagnostic and therapeutic methods that have developed completely independently of western biomedical science. However, the rapid social and economic changes that these countries are currently experiencing are having dramatic impacts on their healthcare systems. For example, during its Socialist period, China evolved a comprehensive system of primary care to cover its largely rural population. 'Bare-foot doctors' with minimal medical training and facilities provided a simple but comprehensive primary care service, referring to secondary medical centres the problems that they could not address. The system was funded collectively by the rural commune. However, in the 1980s agriculture was privatized and this collective form of rural medical care virtually disappeared to be replaced by fee-for-service, with the result that illness creates major financial suffering to poorer families (Liu et al 1995). Meanwhile, the growing urban populations of China increasingly receive health care through insurance plans provided by the employer, with marked differences in coverage between plans. Social and economic growth has thus been accompanied by growing inequalities between regions and social groups in China (Hsiao 1995).

■ Payment mechanisms

In addition to the wide variety of organizational arrangements that have emerged in different western countries, there are also major differences in the methods of paying doctors and these can also exert considerable influence on the nature of medical care. We can distinguish three major types of method, although in most healthcare systems a mixture of the methods can coexist and, often, individual doctors are paid by more than one method.

Fee-for-service involves the patient paying the doctor a fee for each separate item or element of care for which the doctor wishes to charge. In its simplest and historically earliest form, this involves direct patient payments at the time of use. This is still one of the most important methods of paying for health bills in the USA, involving 28% of all personal health expenditure. Insurance systems have emerged in most western countries that reduce or eliminate the need for direct patient payments. However, very often the medical profession has insisted on retaining fee-for-service as their method of payment, with the fees being reclaimed from federal and provincial government (Canada), from the patient's private insurer (USA), or from sickness funds (Germany).

Capitation reimburses the doctor by paying a fixed, usually annual, sum for each patient under his or her care. It is most naturally a method employed in primary care where the doctor has a continuous list or 'panel' of patients for whom he or she is responsible. Britain and Holland are two of the main examples.

Salary is the last method and involves an employer paying the doctor an annual income in return for his or her services. It is the method for paying hospital doctors in Britain, Sweden and Germany.

Unfortunately, there is no perfect method of paying doctors. Each method is known to have certain potentially harmful effects on the provision of health care. The most serious and most clearly documented problems are those associated with fee-for-service. This system encourages doctors to perform those procedures specifically rewarded by fees, which in most systems tend to be technical investigations and more interventionist treatments. To put it bluntly, many fee-for-service systems do not recognize talking to the patient as a distinct item of service! Fee-for-service requires more mechanisms than other methods of payment to control potentially wasteful treatments or investigations. Another problem that tends to occur in countries where doctors are paid by fee-for-service is that doctors tend to be poorly distributed geographically, as economic incentives encourage concentrations in more affluent areas.

Capitation provides more financial incentives that encourage doctors into 'under-doctored' areas. Among its main limitations are that it does not provide financial rewards for good quality care (as income is unrelated to quality or amount of activity) and might encourage doctors to refer-on difficult medical problems.

Salaried payment is also not without problems. In principle, it requires the doctor to be more concerned about pleasing his or her superiors or employers, who determine rewards and promotions, and less concerned with pleasing the patient. Generally, the medical profession has been quite conservative, preferring to keep to the particular system of payment historically established in each country. However, an overall trend can be detected for more doctors to be paid on a salaried basis, typically as employees of an organization.

Health expenditure in different countries

Western countries vary not only in how they organize and fund health services, but also – most dramatically – in the amount of funds devoted to health care. Comparisons of levels of expenditure are not easy because of problems of what is included and excluded in the category of health care in different countries, and also because of unstable exchange rates for countries' currencies. Nevertheless, the most recent figures produced on a systematic standardized basis show differences in levels of expenditure between countries that have remained fairly stable over time (Table 19.1). It is clear that there are considerable differences between countries that might all be regarded as similarly advanced industrial

TABLE 19.1	The per capita expenditure on health, the percentage of wealth (GNP) spent on health and the various mortality rates for selected countries for 2002–3					
Country	Per capita expenditure on health (US $)	Health expenditure as proportion of GNP (%)	GNP[a] per capita (US $)	Life expectancy (years), male	Life expectancy (years), female	Infant mortality (per 1000 live births)
USA	5274	14.6	37870	75	80	7
Denmark	2835	8.8	33570	75	80	4
Germany	2631	10.9	25290	76	81	4
Sweden	2489	9.2	28910	78	82.	3
France	2348	9.7	24730	76	83	4
Holland	2298	8.8	26230	76	81	5
Canada	2222	9.6	24470	76	83	5
UK	2031	7.7	28320	75	80	5

Adapted from The World Bank (2005).
[a] GNP estimates differ slightly from those used to calculate proportions in column two.

societies, whether expressed as absolute amounts of expenditure or as proportions of the gross national product (GNP), used as the most reliable measure of countries' overall wealth. Table 19.1 shows that, for example, the USA spent more than 2.5 times as much per capita as the UK. It is also clear that some countries at very similar levels of wealth in terms of GNP (for example Sweden and UK) spend quite different amounts of their wealth on health care.

A number of different explanations have been offered to account for the differences between countries in their levels of expenditure. One factor that can play a role is the level of health professionals' earnings, especially those of doctors, which are undoubtedly high in countries such as the USA. A very different explanation would point to the important role of the general practitioner in systems like the NHS in acting as a filter or gatekeeper and limiting access to more expensive hospital facilities. Another factor that clearly distinguishes systems like the USA and the UK is that the former is an open system in which no actor – the doctor, the patient, the hospital, the insurance company or the government – has the full capacity and incentives to control the volume of medical activities and the costs that ensue. Typically in the USA, doctors or hospitals bill patients' insurance companies, who ultimately recover their costs from patients' employers, who hope in turn to pass on these costs to the general public in prices to the consumer. The healthcare system in the USA has historically been a highly inflationary one because of this capacity of actors to pass on their costs, and this process stands in direct contrast to the UK, where a closed financial system operates in that the total amount of finance available to the NHS is set and controlled centrally by the Treasury and, to a large extent, cannot be expanded further.

However, the most general explanation offered to explain differences in countries' levels of healthcare expenditure is that the greater a country's wealth, the greater will be not only the amount but also the proportion of the wealth devoted to health care. Support for this view comes from analyses of data (such as in Table 19.1) for a number of different countries that produce highly significant correlations between countries' GNP and the proportion of GNP allocated to health care (Maxwell 1981). Such analyses can also be used to predict the level of health care that might be expected for a particular country, given its GNP. It has been suggested that, for example, the USA consistently spends more than expected and the UK less than might be expected from its GNP. However, others have argued that such analyses are inappropriate and use misleading exchange rates to calculate standardized expenditures (Parkin et al 1989).

VARIATIONS IN MEDICAL CARE

It is not surprising, in view of these differences in funding, to discover that the extent of medical intervention also varies between countries. Thus the rate of surgery in the USA and Canada is at least twice that in the UK, once differences in population size and structure have been taken into consideration. A study of hysterectomy (McPherson 1990) showed the age-standardized rate per 100 000 women as 700 in the USA, 600 in Canada, 450 in Australia, 250 in the UK and 110 in Norway. Similar international variations could be shown for tonsillectomy, cholecystectomy and prostatectomy. These international differences are not confined to surgery. Aaron & Schwartz (1984) showed a wide range of differences between the USA and the UK. In the USA, twice as many X-ray examinations were carried out per person; there was six times greater computer tomographic scanning capacity; three times more kidney dialysis treatment was provided; and between five and ten times more hospital intensive-care beds were available.

Variations within countries

Much of the international variation in rates of medical treatments can be accounted for in terms of general differences in economic prosperity of different countries. There is also a tendency for fee-for-service systems of paying the doctor to be associated with higher use of technical procedures such as investigations, and greater resort to active treatments, such as surgery, because such forms of care tend to be more financially rewarding (Abel-Smith 1976). However, it has become increasingly apparent that there are variations in surgical and medical procedures within countries that are as great as those between countries. It is less easy to explain such variation in terms of gross economic incentives. A recent study by Weinstein and colleagues (2006) showed a staggering 20-fold variation in rates for certain forms of spinal surgery in Medicare patients across the United States. Two New England cities, which were socially and demographically similar – Boston and New Haven – were examined in more detail. Although Boston had 2.3 times higher rates for carotid endarterectomy, the rates for cholecystectomy and hysterectomy were two-thirds, and for coronary bypass surgery only half, of those in New Haven (Wennberg et al 1987). Similar variations have been found in different regions of the NHS. For example, rates for hysterectomy per 100 000 women have been found to vary between 181 in Mersey and 287 in North-East Thames, whereas rates for tonsillectomy varied from 144 in Trent to 251 in North-East Thames (McPherson et al 1981).

Explanations for medical variations

Studies showing variation in the performance of treatments between areas within a country raise fundamental issues. It is extremely unlikely that variation in morbidity in the populations served could explain very much, if any, of the wide variations found in such studies. Moreover, it is unlikely that differences in consumer demand could explain large amounts of the differences in treatment rates prevailing in populations of similar social composition. One factor that is clearly implicated is supply. It can be no coincidence that the two-fold differences in surgical rates in the USA compared with the UK are mirrored by there being twice the number of surgeons per capita in the USA. However, where studies have attempted systematically to examine the effects of supply (McPherson et al 1981) it has been found possible to explain only a small amount of the variation in rates of treatment this way. It is clear that, for many procedures, the main problem is inherent uncertainty about the appropriate indications for treatment and the precise value of treatment in terms of outcomes.

It is known that clinicians can vary enormously in the diagnostic and history-taking procedures used in making decisions about elective surgery (Bloor 1976). However, to produce large and consistent differences in rates between areas, such individual differences in clinical opinion and approach must also be influenced by local or regional preferences or customs, otherwise the effects on variations in treatment rates produced by individual differences in clinical style would be cancelled out. Therefore, at the heart of any explanation of variations in treatment rates are professional uncertainty, lack of agreement about the indications for intervention and the value of intervention. Local and international variation is known to be greater for procedures such as tonsillectomy, prostatectomy and hysterectomy, over which professional uncertainty is greater than for procedures such as cholecystectomy, where some degree of consensus has emerged (Wennberg et al 1982).

CRITERIA FOR EVALUATING HEALTH SYSTEMS

▩ Healthcare expenditure and health status

The main reason why so much uncertainty surrounds many medical and surgical procedures is that they have not been evaluated properly. It is very difficult to distinguish specific effects of a medical therapy from other possible causes of change in the course of illness, such as placebo effects and spontaneous changes in the underlying disorder. For this reason it is often argued that only a randomized controlled trial (RCT), where patients are randomly allocated between the treatment group and a control group and differences in subsequent health status compared between the two groups, is adequate to distinguish real treatment effects. Very few medical interventions have been evaluated by means of such demanding methods (Cochrane 1971). In the example of the study of spinal surgery by Weinstein and colleagues (2006) cited above, an important factor explaining the enormous varations with which surgery is used in different parts of the USA is the lack of any clear scientific evidence from randomized controlled trials to show the best ways of managing severe back pain. Some would argue that, especially when RCTs might pose ethical problems because of the need to withhold treatment, medical treatments can still be reasonably evaluated by less exact methods such as, for example, longitudinal observational studies in which the impact of therapies on groups of patients is recorded and compared with untreated comparison groups. However, such studies are still all too rare (McPherson 1990).

Greater uncertainty surrounds the relationship between overall levels of healthcare expenditure and benefits in terms of health status. Table 19.1 compares the expenditure figures for health care in a range of western countries with a number of the most recently available health-status measures. Life expectancy is a global measure that summarizes the mortality rates prevailing at all ages. It is apparent from Table 19.1 that the USA, despite spending much more on health care than other countries, does not enjoy more favourable life expectancy than countries such as Holland and Canada, with quite low per capita healthcare expenditure. The infant mortality rate is a quite widely used indicator not only of infant health status but also of whole populations. Again, it is clear that the USA does not enjoy infant mortality rates commensurate with its high healthcare expenditure.

Other analyses of the relationship between countries' levels of healthcare expenditure and mortality rates have similarly failed to find evidence of the negative correlation that might reasonably be expected (Cochrane et al 1978, Maxwell 1981). Indeed, the one variable that tends to predict mortality rates from such comparisons of national data is the gross national product (GNP) – the overall level of wealth of the country (Cochrane et al 1978). This would, of course, be consistent with the arguments of McKeown that, historically, social and economic factors have exerted far greater influence upon health than have medical measures (see Chapter 1). In view of the evidence that mortality rates are largely influenced by social, economic and environmental factors rather than medical care, it might well be argued that mortality rates are not appropriate measures of health status with which to compare countries' healthcare systems. Rather, it might be argued, the main impact of health services is intended to be upon morbidity. In particular, the objectives of health services are to reduce the impact of illness in terms of pain, discomfort, disability and other aspects of health status. However, as indicated in Chapter 18, instruments for measuring these outcomes of health services have only recently been developed and there are numerous logistic and methodological problems that would make the comparative assessment of different healthcare systems extremely difficult. At present, therefore, the only available data with which to evaluate the effectiveness, in terms of impact upon health, of different healthcare systems is mortality.

Efficiency

There are a number of different ways in which one might evaluate the quality of different health services. Box 19.2 lists the widely cited criteria of Maxwell (1984). From the above discussion it is clear that there are basic difficulties in examining the effectiveness of healthcare systems, particularly problems of measuring outcomes. The scope for using the other five criteria is examined briefly below.

Efficiency is a term that is frequently applied to health care but seldom used with much clarity. The efficiency of an engine is the relationship between the actual and the theoretically possible amount of energy used to achieve a desired output. The closer the machine gets to the lowest level of energy use considered possible, the greater its efficiency. In human systems one normally compares the costs of two or more alternative ways of achieving the same output or result, with the less costly alternative being regarded as more efficient. The scope for increasing efficiency in health services is potentially enormous. For example, in a wide range of problems, outpatient or day-case care can be substituted for longer inpatient management; or the nurse or general practitioner can replace more costly hospital care. Efficiency is examined by health economists using techniques such as cost–benefit analysis, in which all the costs of two or more alternative therapies or ways of organizing care are compared. This requires taking into account the costs of alternative treatments, such as any additional burden imposed on the family or other carers, as well as formal healthcare costs.

Constant efforts are made in all healthcare systems to achieve 'efficiency savings'. However, in practice, this often means reducing levels of spending available, which should not be confused with real improvements in efficiency because saving money can often be associated with deteriorating efficiency.

Efforts have been made to measure efficiency more directly, but the exercise has proved particularly difficult. One solution has been the development of 'performance indicators' (such as average length of hospital stay, throughput of patients per annum and turnover interval between cases occupying a bed), which can be measured for different units, hospitals and districts. However, such measures can be quite misleading. A unit might appear to be performing more efficiently if patients' mean length of hospital stay is lower than other units. However, a full cost–benefit analysis might show that this short length of hospital stay involved transferring higher costs to the community by premature discharge, together with unresolved complications of treatment that actually led to many

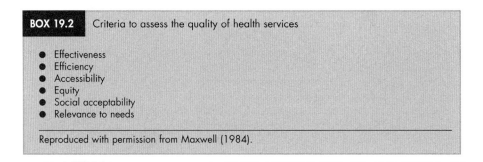

BOX 19.2   Criteria to assess the quality of health services

- Effectiveness
- Efficiency
- Accessibility
- Equity
- Social acceptability
- Relevance to needs

Reproduced with permission from Maxwell (1984).

patients being readmitted. It is also possible that varying lengths of stay in different units are due to different levels of severity of disease in the patients admitted.

It is even more difficult to compare healthcare systems in terms of efficiency. In general, the length of stay in hospitals in the USA is considerably shorter than in Britain. Economic pressures have been the main factor driving down lengths of stay in the USA. Unfortunately, lengths of stay tend to be a matter of local practice and tradition, and optimum length of stay has rarely been subjected to the kind of scientific examination adopted by Deyo et al (1986), who were able to show from a randomized controlled trial that shorter lengths of bed rest were as effective in the management of back pain as longer stays.

Another aspect of efficiency would include consideration of 'bureaucracy' or administration costs of health care because such costs do not apparently make a direct contribution to patient care. The NHS fares particularly well compared with most other systems. For example, it has been estimated that the USA spends as much as 22% of its health expenditure on administration costs, compared with about 6% required by the NHS (Himmelstein & Woolhandler 1986). High administration costs arise from a combination of fee-for-service and the need to itemize and bill every procedure. It is of note that, as the NHS began to experiment with 'internal markets', both health authorities and hospitals required a great deal more information of this kind and administration costs rose sharply.

Accessibility

This criterion is concerned with how readily available health services are. The healthcare system with the most visible problem is the more market oriented one of the USA, in which some 15–20% of the population have inadequate healthcare insurance. No other western healthcare system permits this degree of financial inaccessibility. Given that, for those who are insured in the USA, out-of-pocket expenses at the time of seeking care are higher than in European systems, it is remarkable that consultation rates are no different between systems. A different kind of problem of access is the need to wait for admission for treatment. This would appear to be very much more of a problem for the publicly funded and provided services of Britain and Sweden and is one major reason why in both these countries proposals have been implemented to increase the incentives for hospitals to reduce waiting times by a more competitive structure of revenue.

Equity

Equity with regard to health involves addressing some very complex issues, especially when trying to compare the performance of different healthcare systems. Thus a distinction can be made between equality of access (the extent to which different social groups have access to health services) and equality of health status (the extent to which different social groups enjoy similar levels of health). As other chapters in this book have shown, social differences in health status can be caused by a wide range of social, economic and environmental factors and the scope for intervention by health services, no matter how broadly defined, can be modest. Some would therefore argue that it is more reasonable to confine attention to comparing the efforts of different healthcare systems to achieve equality of access, although even with this more modest criterion there could be substantial social and cultural factors influencing use of health services. Other problems complicating quantitative comparisons of inequalities are that the social groupings (such as classes) are not consistent between countries and that social and cultural factors can influence individuals' perceptions of their health status (see Chapter 3).

321

With regard to social differences in health status, it is clear that all European and North American societies continue to experience differences in mortality between social groups, and the view that social democratic welfare states or Socialist societies have eradicated such differences is misguided (Illsley 1990). Thus a comparative study of Denmark, Finland, Norway, Sweden, Hungary and England and Wales showed that in all countries mortality among men with the highest level of education was 40–60% lower than men of the lowest educational level (Lahelma & Valkonen 1990). In general, some of the lowest inequalities in health status appear to be found in Sweden, a country that has probably the strongest and most active commitment to welfare policies. Nevertheless, even in Sweden there are occupational and regional inequalities in mortality arising from work hazards, dietary- and alcohol-related diseases and other unexplained environmental factors (Diderichsen 1990).

All healthcare systems have taken some steps to reduce or eradicate differences of access by income. At one extreme, a substantial proportion of the population in the USA does not have full access to health care because of inadequate insurance. Such individuals have to resort to a 'second-class' system of publicly funded health care, which has experienced particularly tight financial restrictions in the last 10 years. At the other extreme, financial barriers to access are largely removed from most European systems, and further steps have tended to be taken centrally to reduce regional inequalities of access. Particularly successful was the impact on the NHS of the Resource Allocation Working Party (RAWP), which resulted in England and Wales having the least regional inequalities in the geographical distribution of doctors when compared to France, Germany and Holland (Townsend & Davidson 1982).

Social acceptability

The general trend is for users of health services to express positive satisfaction overall with their healthcare system. For example, in a survey of over 25 000 patients across 17 different countries, the vast majority were satisfied with their primary care services, despite the enormous variations in organization and delivery across systems (Wensing et al 2004). However behind such positive overall views, patients seem commonly to experience problems that appear to have a great deal in common across systems. In a study of patients' views of being an inpatient in Germany, Sweden, Switzerland, UK and USA similar problems were reported (Coulter & Cleary 2001). Patients in all systems did not feel that staff communicated well with them. Their care did not seem well coordinated. They often did not feel they were treated with respect; for example, staff talking about them in their presence as if they were not there. In all systems patients did not feel as fully involved in decisions about their care as they wished. By contrast in all five countries, satisfaction with the physical comfort of inpatient stay was quite high. Overall it is striking how similar are patients' expectations of health care and how similar are the strengths and weaknesses of modern health care's capacity fully to meet such expectations.

Relevance to health needs

Relevance is the last important criterion emphasized in Maxwell's list for evaluating health services. At the extreme it is possible to conceive of a healthcare system that takes little or no account of the health needs of the population it served. Thus it has often been a key problem in third world countries that the healthcare system has developed largely to conform to the standards of western high-technology medicine and, although relevant to the needs of urban social and political elites, it has failed to address the often more basic health needs of the rural majority populations. Such stark failures of relevance are less easy to identify in western healthcare systems and involve major initial difficulties in defining the health needs of populations.

Nevertheless, one very promising line of research has begun to open up the more focused and manageable issue of appropriateness. To what extent are the treatments provided in a healthcare system appropriate to the patients who receive them? The methodology for addressing this question is complex and can take different forms, but one approach essentially involves asking representative samples of relevant clinicians to rate the appropriate indications for a particular medical or surgical intervention (for example, which test results, past medical history and other patient characteristics would be appropriate indications for someone to undergo coronary artery bypass graft (CABG)). These agreed indications are then used to analyse the characteristics of samples of patients who have actually undergone the particular procedure. This methodology has been largely used in the USA and has produced quite startling results. Retrospective analyses of case records showed that for patients who received carotid endarterectomy, about one-third were rated as appropriate, one-third equivocal and one-third inappropriate. Similarly, one-quarter of coronary angiographies and one-quarter of endoscopies were rated as equivocal or inappropriate (Brook 1990). These studies lend support to the view that a substantial proportion of the treatment provided in the USA might be of questionable value in terms of outcomes and could occur as much out of a more general optimistic bias and faith in technology in American culture or, more cynically, because of strong financial rewards built into fee-for-service medicine.

This methodology has now been applied cross-nationally. Two panels of physicians and surgeons, one from the USA and one from the UK, were asked to rate a large number of indications in the form of elements of case histories, in terms of appropriateness for coronary angiography and also for CABG (Brook et al 1988). The American panel rated a much larger number of case-history indications as being appropriate for either procedure. The sets of indications of the two panels were then applied to real case histories. First, they were applied to two samples of American patients who had undergone coronary angiography. The American panel's ratings resulted in 17% and 27% being rated as inappropriate, whereas the British panel's ratings identified 42% and 60% as inappropriate. The ratings of indications were then applied to another sample – American patients who had undergone CABG. By the American criteria 11% of operations were inappropriate; by the British criteria this figure was 15%. There are, therefore, quite powerful differences of views about the scope for benefit from medical treatment in medicine, despite the fact that medical science and medical training are very similar in the two countries.

The World Health Organization reported a very ambitious programme to assess the performance of all healthcare systems comparatively and quantitatively (WHO 2000). The framework used to compare healthcare systems involved assessment against three criteria: (1) impact on health; (2) responsiveness; and (3) financial fairness. The first criterion is more self-evident and assesses impact of healthcare systems on health status. The other two criteria go beyond what has usually been assessed by bodies such as WHO. Responsiveness focuses upon how well healthcare systems have respect for users of the service and demonstrate a client orientation as reflected in measures such as patients' reports about being given appropriate information about their health problems (see Chapter 18). Financial fairness is considered to occur when all households contribute a similar proportion of income to health care regardless of health status or level of use of the health service (Murray & Frenk 2001).

The report that emerged from the WHO combined statistical evidence for all countries' healthcare systems in relation to the three criteria into a single rank-ordering of countries

(WHO 2000). It caused considerable controversy, partly because the countries ranked as having the most successful healthcare systems (France, Italy and Spain; ranked 1st, 2nd and 3rd respectively) were unexpected. Just as controversial, the USA, which spends far the greatest proportion of its wealth on health, ranked only 37th. More importantly, the report received considerable methodological criticism. It was felt that insufficiently robust data existed to measure many of the properties of healthcare systems in a standardized way (Almeida et al 2001). Moreover, basic definitions were criticized. It was argued that the view of fairness that all households contribute the same proportion of spending on health failed to take account of countries' intentions to be fair by funding health care through some degree of progressive taxation (i.e. higher rates of taxes borne by those with higher incomes). The WHO definition of fairness did not acknowledge that different households had different levels of need. The approach was also criticized for exaggerating the role of health care in determining health (Navarro 2000). The response to such criticisms is to argue that governments and populations need comparative information on their healthcare systems to assess strengths and weaknesses and that only by the development of more valid methods can an evidence base for how to organize healthcare systems be developed (Murray & Frenk 2001).

MARKETS VERSUS REGULATION IN HEALTH CARE

In many respects the many complex difficulties faced by healthcare systems can be subsumed into two broad types of problem. First, healthcare systems need to obtain adequate funds to pay for the healthcare needs of the populations they serve and mechanisms are required to ensure that such funds do not outstrip the capacity of the funder to pay. Second, mechanisms are required to improve the effectiveness and efficiency of health services, particularly in the light of evidence of ineffectiveness and inefficiency of the kind briefly reviewed in this chapter. No healthcare system appears to have addressed either problem satisfactorily and there is a constant and increasingly international search for solutions to both problems. Again, to simplify the discussion, it is possible to detect two alternative strategies that have been pursued by governments, sickness funds, health providers and other agencies concerned with the provision of health care in attempts to address the twin problems just identified. One strategy has focused on competition. It has sought to intensify the scope of market forces in the field of health care. The hope has been that competition between providers of health care would force them to reduce their costs as well as maximize their efficiency and effectiveness in accordance with the logic of market competition in other spheres of commerce. The second and contrasting strategy has been to introduce regulation into the operations of the healthcare system. Faced with evidence or inefficiencies such as wide and unaccountable variations in clinical practice and use of resources, this solution has attempted to use methods of centralized planning and managerial control of health budgets. The competitive strategy is best characterized by the American system and the regulation/planning strategy is more typical of European systems.

The competitive strategy was pursued in the USA throughout the 1980s. Government finance for planning of health services was withdrawn and instead support was given to encourage competition, especially to promote the development of Health Maintenance Organizations (HMOs). HMOs were established in which a group of health providers offered a complete package of healthcare services to consumers at an annually agreed price. It was hoped that HMOs would compete with each other in terms of the attractiveness of the package of services offered and their price. Finally, competition was encouraged by increasing the proportion of health bills paid out-of-pocket by the patient in the hope that this would increase consumer sensitivity to costs. To date, there has been little evidence that procompetitive strategies have succeeded in the main objective of driving down the highly inflationary costs of American health care.

The planning and regulatory strategies of European health services are too diverse to encompass in a brief chapter. To varying degrees in each country, regulation has included efforts to set overall limits to expenditure on health care, particularly in the hospital sector, by setting doctors' fees, regulating the introduction of high-technology medicine. This strategy has been largely successful in containing costs, but analysts are less happy with the evidence of continued inefficiencies and unexplained variations in most European systems, and countries such as Sweden and Britain continue to be concerned with the unresponsiveness of their healthcare systems to the consumer and the persistence of waiting lists as unresolved problems.

Partly because of their perceived lack of consumer responsiveness but more particularly to control costs, many European systems were, in the 1990s, subjected to major changes intended to induce greater market competitiveness. In the very different systems of the UK, Holland and Sweden, the distinction between purchasers and providers of care was sharpened and providers (particularly hospitals) were given greater incentives to compete for patients on whose behalf the health authorities in the UK and Sweden and the sickness funds in Holland purchased care (Ham & Brommels 1994). However, the benefits of competition predicted by neoclassical economic theory have not produced greater efficiency and effectiveness in the field of health care, whether in Europe or in the USA (Glaser 1993). Some of the problems exacerbated by greater competition, such as the perceived oversupply of hospitals in large cities, have needed traditional European mechanisms of planning and regulation to address them (Ham & Brommels 1994).

■ Convergence of healthcare systems?

Some observers (Enthoven 1990, Ham et al 1990) have argued that pure strategies of either market competition or central planning and regulation have failed to address the key problems of health services and have suggested that there is now evidence in many healthcare systems of a convergence towards a mixed approach combining elements of both strategies. Again, it is impossible to encompass all the varieties of strategy emerging in each country, but some commonly occurring themes can be detected. One theme is that of 'peer review', in which clinical decisions that could result in large use of resources, such as admission to hospital and decisions about surgery, are subject to external review by colleagues. This has gone much further in the USA, where peer review is current and intended to have a direct influence on the use of resources, than in Europe, where it has, to date, been largely retrospective and used more for educational purposes, as in medical audit.

The second theme is the development of information systems to monitor and measure the activities and outcomes of health care. The intention is to use increasingly sophisticated information technology to inform all the parties to health care – the doctor, the patient and the purchaser in particular – about the efficiency and effectiveness of healthcare activities (Ellwood 1988).

A third common theme emerging in healthcare systems to varying degrees is the desire to separate out the purchaser of health care (such as the health authority or sick fund) from the provider (such as hospitals) and to increase the degree of choice that the purchaser has between different providers. In systems such as those in the UK, Holland and Sweden, the intention is to induce competition within a publicly funded system. The hope is that a system that incorporates all three elements (peer review, increased attention to audit of outcomes and scope for funders to choose between providers who compete in terms of quality and price) will produce a solution to the many dilemmas of modern medical care.

The need to ration

One of the most controversial problems facing healthcare systems of all types is the need to decide mechanisms of allocating limited healthcare resources in relation to competing demands. 'Rationing' is an emotive short-hand term used in this context and suggests a process of explicit and deliberate decisions about resource allocation. In reality, many healthcare systems have implicitly rationed without formally deciding to do so, because, for example, low-income individuals are not able to purchase health care or because delays or queues discourage numbers of patients from obtaining care.

However, as medical technology continues to develop and new treatments and health-care costs escalate, governments across Europe and North America have had to devise more morally explicit principles whereby healthcare resources are allocated. A number of alternative principles could be used (Box 19.3). Unfortunately, these principles can conflict with each other (Harrison & Hunter 1994). For example, patients for whom current treatments are ineffective would be denied health care if the criterion of effectiveness were applied strictly, whereas they would receive services under principles of need or equity. All of the principles are difficult to operationalize. There are, for example, no agreed ways of defining or determining need. Any healthcare system is therefore likely to have to make trade-offs or compromises between principles rather than rigorously adhere to one.

The National Institute for Health and Clinical Excellence (NICE) was set up to provide authoritative guidance to the NHS on interventions. It is expected that the health service take full account of NICE guidelines in determining what is publicly provided. It has been criticized for taking too much notice of economic evidence about cost effectiveness and decisions not to recommend particular drugs for public funding can be highly

---

BOX 19.3 Alternative principles for allocating healthcare resources between conflicting demands

1. Effectiveness
- Resources are allocated to those treatments that have the greatest effect on outcomes in terms of health.

2. Cost-effectiveness
- Resources are allocated according to the principle of effectiveness, but also take account of costs in relation to effectiveness (i.e. favouring treatment with the best cost–benefit ratio).

3. Need
- Resources are allocated to those patients or patient groups with the greatest need.

4. Equity
- Resources are allocated on a principle of a basis of fairness or equity between individuals and patient groups.

5. Chance or 'fair goes'
- Resources are allocated by some form of random process so that everyone has a similar chance of care, or 'first come first served' principles.

Reproduced with permission by the Institute for Public Policy Research from Harrison & Hunter (1994).

controversial. Nevertheless it is striking that many other healthcare systems have now created similar systems to use best evidence to identify interventions that should be provided from public funds.

Health authorities are also increasingly consulting the public about how health services should be prioritized by means of postal surveys or public meetings. However, the results of such consultation exercises have served only to complicate decisions, partly because public responses are heavily influenced by the wording of the questions and partly because the principles on which the public makes its choices differ from those considered important by doctors or managers. The public appears more impressed by the acute and high technology services and to value less preventive interventions such as health education or services for mental illness (Brown 1995).

There are therefore no simple solutions to the problem of providing health services that meet every desirable objective for health. This chapter has illustrated the diversity of forms that advanced healthcare systems have adopted in the search for optimal solutions.

References

Aaron H, Schwartz W 1984 The painful prescription. The Brookings Institution, Washington DC

Abel-Smith B 1976 Value for money in health services. Heinemann, London

Almeida C et al 2001 Methodological concerns and recommendations on policy consequences of the World Health Report 2000. Lancet 351:692–697

Bloor M 1976 Bishop Berkeley and the adenotonsillectomy enigma. Sociology 10:44–61

Brook R 1990 Relationship between appropriateness and outcome. In: Hopkins A, Costain D (eds) Measuring the outcomes of medical care. Royal College of Physicians, London

Brook R et al 1988 Diagnosis and treatment of coronary disease: comparison of doctors' attitudes in the USA and the UK. Lancet i:750–753

Brown S 1995 Assessing public opinion on investment in health services. International Journal of Health Services 6:15–24

Cochrane A 1971 Effectiveness and efficiency. Nuffield Provincial Hospitals Trust, London

Cochrane A, St Leger A, Moore F 1978 Health service input and mortality output in developed countries. Journal of Epidemiology and Community Health 32:200–205

Coulter A, Cleary P (2001) Patients' experiences with hospital care in five countries. Health Affairs 20:244–52

Curtis S, Petukhova N, Taket A 1995 Health care reforms in Russia: the example of St Petersburg. Social Science and Medicine 40:755–766

Deyo R, Diehl A, Rosenthal M 1986 How many days of bed-rest for acute low back pain? A randomised clinical trial. New England Journal of Medicine 315:1064–1070

Diderichsen F 1990 Health and social inequalities in Sweden. Social Science and Medicine 31:359–367

Ellwood P 1988 Outcomes management: a technology of patient experience. New England Journal of Medicine 318:1549–1556

Enthoven A 1990 What can Europeans learn from Americans? In: Health care systems in transition. Organization for Economic Cooperation and Development (OECD), Paris

Field M 1973 The concept of the 'health system' at the macrosociological level. Sociology, Science and Medicine 7:763–785

Field M 1995 The health crisis in the former Soviet Union: a report from the 'post-war zone'. Sociology, Science and Medicine 41:1469–1478

Glaser W 1993 The competition vogue and its outcomes. Lancet 341:805–812

Ham C, Brommels M 1994 Health care reforms in the Netherlands, Sweden, and the United Kingdom. Health Affairs 13:106–119

Ham C, Robinson R, Benzeval M 1990 Health check: health care reforms in an international context. Kings Fund Institute, London

Harrison S, Hunter D 1994 Rationing health care. Institute for Public Policy Research, London

Himmelstein D, Woolhandler S 1986 Cost without benefit: administrative waste in US health care. New England Journal of Medicine 314:441–445

Hsiao W 1995 The Chinese health care system: lessons for other nations. Sociology, Science and Medicine 41:1047–1056

Illsley R 1990 Comparative review of sources, methodology and knowledge. Sociology, Science and Medicine 31:229–236

Lahelma E, Valkonen T 1990 Health and social inequalities in Finland and elsewhere. Sociology, Science and Medicine 31:257–266

Liu Y et al 1995 Transformation of China's rural health care system. Sociology, Science and Medicine 41:1085–1094

Maxwell R 1981 Health and wealth. Lexington Books, Lexington, MA

Maxwell R 1984 Quality assessment in health. British Medical Journal 288:1470–1472

McPherson K 1990 International differences in medical care practices. In: Health care systems in transition. Organization for Economic Cooperation and Development (OECD), Paris

McPherson K et al 1981 Regional variations in the use of common surgical procedures. Sociology, Science and Medicine 15A:273–288

Murray C, Frenk J 2001 World health report 2000: a step towards evidence-based health policy. Lancet 357:1698–1700

Navarro V 2000 Assessment of the world health report 2000. Lancet 356:1598–1601

Parkin D, McGuire A, Yule B 1989 What do international comparisons of health care expenditures really show? Community Medicine 11:116–123

Townsend P, Davidson N 1982 Inequalities in health: the Black report. Penguin, Harmondsworth

Weinstein JN et al 2006 United States' trends and regional variations in lumbar spine surgery: 1992–2003. Spine 31:2707–2714

Wennberg J, Barnes B, Zubkoff M 1982 Professional uncertainty and the problem of supplier-induced demand. Sociology, Science and Medicine 16:811–824

Wennberg J, Freeman J, Gulp W 1987 Are hospital services rationed in New Haven or overutilised in Boston? Lancet i:118

Wensing M et al 2004 Impact of national health care systems on patient evaluations of general practice in Europe. Health Policy 68:353–357

World Bank 2005 World development indicators 2005. The World Bank, Washington DC

World Health Organization (WHO) 2000 World health report 2000. WHO, Geneva

Index

329

331

335